"There is abundant evidence that people with even long-standing diabetes can improve their health dramatically—and practically reverse their condition. Gabriel Cousens shows you how to tackle this disease through lifestyle intervention, explaining how a low-fat, vegan diet could save your life. *There Is a Cure for Diabetes* is an extraordinary tool that will guide you in your journey to fight diabetes and regain your health."
       —Neal Barnard, MD, Physicians Committee for Responsible Medicine

"With this book, Gabriel Cousens takes his place among the world's leading physician-healers. A synthesis of his thirty-five years of clinical experience, *There Is a Cure for Diabetes* presents a practical, comprehensive, and highly effective holistic approach for treating and curing one of our most common diseases. It is the greatest contribution to the treatment of diabetes I've encountered in the forty years since I began my medical training."
       —Dr. Rob Ivker, DO, ABHM, co-founder and past president of the American Board of Holistic Medicine and author of *Sinus Survival*

"As a doctor who has treated diabetes for nearly thirty years, I can tell you with certainty that the standard medical protocols and management of this illness are not only inappropriate, they're absurd. In sharp contrast, Gabriel Cousens has developed a protocol for successfully restoring the health and well-being of diabetics, sparing them the pain and agony of unnecessary and inevitable amputations, obesity, blindness, and premature death. If followed, his advice provides diabetics freedom from their illness and enriches the quality of their lives."
       —Daniel Nuchovich, MD, director of Jupiter Gardens Medical Center and Jupiter Institute of the Healing Arts

"Gabriel Cousens has clearly established himself as the world's leading medical authority on diabetes. His Tree of Life program is proven to completely reverse Type-2 diabetes and markedly improve the condition of those suffering from Type-1 diabetes."
       —David Wolfe, author of *Superfoods* and *Eating for Beauty*

"The beauty of Gabriel's work is that he's not just putting forward an interesting theory—the people he's cured of diabetes are living proof that it works. The truths in [*There is a Cure for Diabetes*] go behind diabetes—they're a sensible lifestyle choice for all human beings."

—*The Mother* magazine

"Packed with information and references to studies and other scientific papers that can make your head spin. [Cousens's] years of tireless scientific research for the living foods community is a precious gift for those of us seeking a much healthier lifestyle. All in all, *There Is A Cure For Diabetes* is an excellent book for a raw foodist library."

—**Raw Food Right Now!**

"*There is a Cure for Diabetes* is a comprehensive guide—not to living with diabetes but for learning how to live without it. It is about embracing a culture of life rather than a culture of death. In reading this book, do not expect an approach of moderate changes to your lifestyle—adding this, or subtracting that—this is about total physical and spiritual transformation."

—**Spiritualitea.com**

There Is a
Cure

The 21-Day+ Holistic
Recovery Program

for Diabetes

REVISED EDITION

Gabriel Cousens, MD

Forewords by
Sandra Rose Michael, PhD,
and DNM Brian R. Clement, PhD, NMD, LNC

North Atlantic Books
Berkeley, California

Published by
North Atlantic Books
P.O. Box 12327
Berkeley, California 94712

Cover design by Suzanne Albertson and Jared Krikorian
Book design by Suzanne Albertson

Printed in the United States of America

There Is a Cure for Diabetes: The 21-Day+ Holistic Recovery Program, Revised Edition is sponsored by the Society for the Study of Native Arts and Sciences, a nonprofit educational corporation whose goals are to develop an educational and cross-cultural perspective linking various scientific, social, and artistic fields; to nurture a holistic view of arts, sciences, humanities, and healing; and to publish and distribute literature on the relationship of mind, body, and nature.

MEDICAL DISCLAIMER: The following information is intended for general information purposes only. Individuals should always see their health care provider before administering any suggestions made in this book. Any application of the material set forth in the following pages is at the reader's discretion and is his or her sole responsibility. If you are on insulin, you must consult your physician because you could go into insulin shock on this program without proper insulin regulation.

North Atlantic Books' publications are available through most bookstores. For further information, call 800-733-3000 or visit our website at www.northatlanticbooks.com.

Library of Congress Cataloging-in-Publication Data

Cousens, Gabriel, 1943–
    There is a cure for diabetes: the 21-day+ holistic recovery program / Gabriel Cousens; foreword by Brian R. Clement.—Rev. ed.
        p. cm.
    Summary: "This substantially revised edition offers an innovative approach to the prevention and healing of what Dr. Gabriel Cousens, a leading medical authority in the world of live-food nutrition, calls chronic diabetes degenerative syndrome (CDDS), his new definition of diabetes"—Provided by publisher.
    Includes index.
    ISBN 978-1-58394-544-5
1. Diabetes—Diet therapy. 2. Vegetable juices. 3 Low-calorie diet. 4. Glycemic index. I. Title.
RC662.C68 2013
616.4'620654—dc23   2012022832

1 2 3 4 5 6 7 Malloy 18 17 16 15 14 13

Printed on recycled paper

ACKNOWLEDGMENTS

There Is a Cure for Diabetes has been an interesting collective effort over 40 years, of input mostly from clients, who have been my main teachers, and of inspiration from the pioneers of the live-foods movement, each illuminating another aspect of the live-food approach to healing diabetes naturally. These people include **Viktoras Kulvinskas, MS**, who specifically offered his insights in the importance of enzyme therapy for diabetes; **Dr. Brian Clement** of Hippocrates Health Institute; and **Reverend George Malkmus** of Hallelujah Acres. All expressed their experience in confirming the viability of a live-foods approach to diabetes reversal.

Dr. Edmond Bordeaux Szekeley, over a period of 30 years (1940–70), healed all manner of diseases, including diabetes, with a live-food diet. **Max Gerson, MD**, made some of the earliest and best-publicized public healings with live foods, including healing Dr. Albert Schweitzer of diabetes. I also want to acknowledge **Paavo Airola, ND, PhD**, who shared his insights on healing diabetes as a key nutritional mentor for eight years. I appreciate the pioneering work of **Neal Barnard, MD**, and the practice of **John McDougall, MD**, which clinically support the general efficacy of a plant-source diet for diabetes reversal.

To my two inspiring and guiding enlightened spiritual teachers, **Swami Prakashananda** and **Swami Muktananda Paramahansa** from India, who both had diabetes and showed how it could be managed with a simple vegan diet. With gratitude to my assistant, **Joshua Sedam**, for the second edition, which is almost entirely a new book. Joshua Sedam's work allowed this new edition to be accomplished more quickly and thoroughly than I could have done on my own. Special thanks to my master student and Essene priestess **Marcela Benson, MA** (www.holisticnutritionstudio.com), a graduate of my Spiritual Nutrition Masters Program, who has helped bring those teachings to the Spanish speaking world of South and Central America as well as Spain and who has updated the diabetes food preparation training and the recipes and teaching of the Phase 1.0 diet. This effort was done with profound love for all the people who want to learn how to heal diabetes and seek the wisdom of conscious evolution. Marcela Benson dedicates her work in loving memory of her father **Ernesto Tobal** who never had the good fortune to find this information and to all the mothers and fathers who will read this book and heal themselves embracing the path of health for their children and the world. Thank you to master student Stella Morris for helping Marcela revise and finalize the order and content of these recipes.

To my wonderful partner, **Shanti Golds Cousens**, whose love and support for this book is greatly appreciated, and who leads the Tri-Yoga aspect and helps with client support of the Dr. Cousens's Diabetes Recovery Program—A Holistic Approach in the United States. Thank you to nurse **Ariel Krzys**, who helped compile much of the newer client data, and who, along with **India Aubrey**, has been key in client support for the Dr. Cousens's Diabetes Recovery Program—A Holistic Approach and one-year follow-up support program.

I also want to thank the collaborators in the film *Simply Raw: Reversing Diabetes in 30 Days*; **Keith Lyons**, who provided essential support through the birth of the film; **Michael Bedar**, who helped this process; and **Alex Ortner**, who has helped get *Simply Raw* out to the world.

To the service of God, who inspired me to write the second edition of this new breakthrough book and to carry on the teachings of Genesis 1:29 as the spiritual and nutritional blueprint for the healing of diabetes:

> See, I give you every seed-bearing plant that is upon all the earth, and every tree that has seed-bearing fruit; they shall be yours for food.

And the inspiration of God through Moses Rabineau in Devarim (Deuteronomy) 30:19–20:

> I call heaven and earth to witness this day against you, that I have set before thee life and death, blessing and cursing: therefore choose life, that both thou and thy seed may live: that thou mayest love the Lord thy God, and that you mayest obey God's voice and cleave to the Divine: for the Divine Presence is thy life and length of days.

CONTENTS

Contents

CHAPTER 3

A Preliminary Theory of Diabetes 107

CHAPTER 4

Dr. Cousens's Diabetes Recovery Program— A Holistic Approach 183

CHAPTER 5

Dr. Cousens's Diabetes Recovery Program— A Holistic Approach: New Results from the Last 120 Diabetic Participants 283

CHAPTER 6

Happy Continuation: Living in the Culture of Life 405

CHAPTER 7

Culture of Life Cuisine 429

FOREWORD

Sandra Rose Michael, PhD, DNM
Minister of Health, Republic of New Lemuria

It is a joy and honor to endorse this groundbreaking work of Dr. Gabriel Cousens. His book creates a model for transforming international and national health in a fundamental but critical way, increasing general quality of life and longevity as well as treating diabetes in particular. In 2005, I was invited to participate in the first International Care Congress, sponsored in Istanbul by the World Health Organization and attended by heads of more than 60 nations; the focus was on the issues of population aging. The statistics presented proved that globally the old, overmedicalized disease model is not working, and according to the Istanbul Declaration on Global Aging and Care, "the best insurance for quality of life in older age is health, and promoting health throughout the life course is the surest way to sustain and guarantee healthy aging." Preventing and curing diabetes, a global pandemic now affecting 27 percent of people over the age of 65 in the United States, along with its concomitant accelerated aging symptoms, including severe atherosclerotic disease, cardiovascular disease, degenerative neuropathies, degenerative kidney disease, and a doubled rate of Alzheimer's disease (also known as Type-3 diabetes), are powerful ways to sustain and guarantee health and longevity.

The brilliant work of Dr. Cousens's second edition of *There Is a Cure for Diabetes* goes far beyond the original book published in 2008. It is essentially a new book. In this book, he introduces the concept of chronic diabetes degenerative syndrome (CDDS), thus revealing a new and clinically useful way of understanding the chronic degenerative aging process labeled "diabetes." In this chronic degenerative process, there is a continuum from imbalanced blood sugars going above 100 to glucose spiking, prediabetes, and finally full-blown diabetes. This clear description of the progressive degenerative process, which Dr. Cousens has clinically and meticulously documented in his own practice, gives us a powerful understanding of how to reverse it.

It is helpful to appreciate that diabetes is accelerated aging that literally can take 10–19 years off of one's life and, for many, reduce the quality of life for decades on end. By labeling this progressive, degenerative syndrome and describing it, Dr. Cousens gives us a way to identify and reverse it—even the allegedly impossible Type-1.

Obviously if we can understand the process and have a way to reverse it, it significantly impacts our ability to optimize the transition from a degenerative painful aging process to a healthy, relatively pain-free longevity process. He defines Type-2 diabetes as an accelerated, chronic, degenerative aging process that is primarily a genetic and epigenetic toxic downgrade, resulting in a leptin, insulin, and/or metabolic dysregulation (including protein, lipid, and carbohydrate imbalances) and driven by a chronic inflammatory process. This breakthrough definition gives us a way to clinically intervene and prevent this disease not only on an individual basis but also on a national and worldwide basis. The key to stopping this inflammatory process, as Dr. Cousens points out, is to understand the toxic diet that gives rise to it. This is primarily a diet high in sugar (complex and simple carbohydrates), high in cooked animal fat and trans fats, and low in fiber. The major offenders are white flour, white sugar, high fructose corn syrup, and a variety of heavily sugared junk foods and soft drinks. These are compounded by a lifestyle of obesity, lack of exercise, stress, general toxic exposure (including pesticides, herbicides, chemical poisons, and heavy metals), and accelerated by mineral, antioxidant, and vitamin deficiencies. Additionally, ongoing radiation exposure (such as from Fukushima, depleted uranium, body scanners, and smart meters) and electro-smog cause DNA and thyroid damage, further augmenting this global pandemic of diabetes. A signal that more serious degeneration is going on is the onset of insulin and/or leptin resistance. This chronic aging process is complicated by toxic degenerative epigenetic memory programs. These toxic metabolic memories, Dr. Cousens points out, must and can be turned off to stop an ongoing cardiovascular, renal, neurological, cerebral, and retinal degeneration. This appears to be the secret to his success in not only healing and preventing diabetes but reversing some of its most treacherous symptoms.

The breakthrough in Dr. Cousens's study of 120 people is that he has developed a simple, potent dietary approach using a diet calorically composed of 25–45 percent complex carbohydrates of live leafy greens, sprouts, and vegetables; 25–45 percent raw plant fat; and 10–25 percent plant-source protein. It appears from his discussion that the 100 percent live-food, plant-source-only diet is the key ingredient in making this dietary approach so successful at healing diabetes. What is remarkable about this rather simple, dedicated approach is the results. Extraordinarily, 61 percent of non-insulin-dependent diabetics are off all medication and healed in just 3 weeks. Twenty-four percent of the insulin-dependent Type-2 diabetics (similar to Type-1s in that their bodies cannot produce sufficient insulin) are off all insulin with fasting blood sugars less than 100 in 3 weeks. Even more extraordinary is 21 percent of Type-1 diabetics, which every medical school would consider impossible to heal, are able to come off all insulin and maintain a fasting blood sugar under 100 in the short time of 21 days. *Dr. Cousens has clearly cracked the diabetes code.* In this book, he gives us a sophisticated and rather new theory of how to heal both Type-1 and Type-2 diabetes based on his successful clinical results. This may even be the foundation for reversing Type-3 diabetes, or Alzheimer's, and other diseases associated with aging.

The significance for me, as a person committed to uplifting public health and bringing educational awareness to the longevity process and age reversal on an international level (who has successfully utilized primarily raw, plant based protocols for nearly 40 years), is that Dr. Cousens has given us a successful model of how to reverse pathologically accelerated aging, or CDDS, which applies successfully to not only diabetes but the whole aging mechanism. The key is translating Dr. Cousens's diabetes-focused work into national programs globally for not only preventing and treating diabetes but also optimizing the longevity process for everyone. Although his book does not specifically talk about aging beyond the dietary aspects, Dr. Cousens does lecture around the world on how to protect not only diabetics but all who are aging. Although there is much overall work on aging that goes far beyond diet, which Dr. Cousens is the first to point out in his lectures, the dietary approach to protecting against and even reversing diabetes is a fundamental approach that can be brought into national policies throughout the world.

This is exactly what Dr. Cousens is now doing with his understanding of diabetes. He has already set up nutritional, nonprofit, diabetes-prevention and health-education training centers in the United States, Nigeria, Ghana, Ethiopia, and Mexico, with other countries patiently waiting to work with him. This book is a wealth of information and a foundation, based on his clinical experience, for preventing and treating diabetes worldwide. In this context, this book is not only theoretically outstanding and clinically extraordinary but provides humanity with the tools to prevent and heal the scourge of diabetes which has afflicted approximately 366 million people, with one person dying from this affliction every 7 seconds and millions suffering from the chronic debilitating aspects of this disease. This book is a powerful contribution to the rapid restoration and continued evolution of health on the planet.

FOREWORD

Brian R. Clement, PhD, NMD, LNC
Director, Hippocrates Health Institute

There Is a Cure for Diabetes is a well-written, concise compilation of sound research, common-sense suggestions, and clinical experience that demonstrates a proven way to prevent and eradicate diabetes. This book is undoubtedly one of the most—if not the most—significant books ever written to address this disease. Gabriel Cousens, MD, is a caring professional who delivers a heartfelt, inspiring message and a practical plan that, based on my own experience over the past 40 years, results in the swift and permanent elimination of Type-2 diabetes for those who choose to take responsibility for their lifestyle. The plan may also produce potentially significant reductions in insulin dosages for people with Type-1 diabetes. Type-2 diabetes is directly linked to lifestyle choices; it does not deserve the status of having billions of dollars spent on it for research and drug development, marketing, and institutions that protect corporate and government interests and their industry profits. Diabetes and the promotion of a drug-dependent "cure" by multinational pharmaceutical companies and the medical community are the real global epidemics that are destroying the possibility of a healthy, drug-free life for millions worldwide. Maintaining health is much simpler than is purported in the journals of medicine and mainstream media, and Dr. Cousens is a leader in showing us how. *There Is a Cure for Diabetes* is essential reading for anyone who desires lifelong health and a saving grace for current and future generations who wish to be free from diabetes.

INTRODUCTION

Healing Diabetes Is a Shift in Consciousness

Society is always taken by surprise by any new example of common sense.

Ralph Waldo Emerson

No physician can ever say that any disease is incurable. To say so blasphemes God, blasphemes Nature, and depreciates the great architect of Creation. The disease does not exist, regardless of how terrible it may be, for which God has not provided the corresponding cure.

Paracelsus

It's supposed to be a professional secret, but I'll tell you anyway. We doctors do nothing. We only help and encourage the doctor within.

Albert Schweitzer, MD

This second edition is written with more than 120 Type-1 and Type-2 diabetics through our program versus 11 for the first edition. These 120+ diabetics have provided me with a much deeper insight into what I now call a "chronic degenerative diabetes syndrome" (CDDS). My clinical experience with these 120 people is that Type-2 diabetes is a curable disease. Although allopathic teachings label Type-1 and Type-2 diabetes as incurable, my current clinical experience with the last 120 clients is that in 21 days, 61 percent of those with Type-2 non-insulin-dependent diabetes mellitus (NIDDM) and 24 percent of those with Type-2 insulin-dependent diabetes mellitus (IDDM) are healed—meaning a fasting blood sugar (FBS) of less than 100 and no medications. Approximately 31.4 percent of Type-1 diabetics were off all insulin in three weeks and approximately 21 percent of Type-1 diabetics were off all insulin with a FBS less than 100. From my 40 years of clinical experience as a holistic medical doctor, and that of live-food therapeutic centers since the 1920s when Max Gerson, MD, healed Albert Schweitzer of diabetes with live foods, the fact that diabetes is a curable disease is common knowledge in the live-food community. Diabetes is not a fixed sentence; it is not our natural condition and has only become a problem of pandemic proportions since the 1940s. The word pandemic comes from the Greek *pan-*, meaning "all," plus *demos*, meaning "people or population," thus, *pandemos*, or "all the people." A pandemic is an epidemic that becomes very widespread and affects a whole region, a continent, or the world. This book gives a new insight and theory into looking deeply at the underlying causes of diabetes, which I now label CDDS, on both the pandemic-global and the personal level. It affirms to readers that there is a consistent scientific process to achieve rapid reversal from the misery of a diabetic physiology to a joyous and healthy physiology.

Although many people have a genetic susceptibility to Type-2 diabetes, the true causes (which activate the genetic potential physiology of diabetes) lie in a personal and world lifestyle and diet that pulls the trigger on the diabetes gun. This diabetogenic personal and world lifestyle and diet includes the following, on the level of individual responsibility: a diet high in refined simple and complex carbohydrates; high amounts of cooked animal protein and saturated fats with their trans-fatty acids produced from cooking (and especially frying oils at high temperatures and hydrogenation), as well as vegetable-based trans-fatty acids; low-fiber food; caffeinated beverages; smoking; a lifestyle devoid of love and exercise; high stress; and watching television programming. Diabetogenic contributing factors on a planetary level include living in a degraded environment in which the air, earth, and water are, according to the Environmental Protection Agency, filled with 70,000 different toxic chemicals, heavy metals, agrochemicals, and other toxic substances—65,000 of which are potentially hazardous to our health.

The Environmental Defense Council reports that more than four billion pounds of toxic chemicals are released into the environment each year, including 72 million pounds of known carcinogens. In addition, we live in a mental and emotional environment filled with messages of stress and death from the media, including news of constant wars and terrorism infecting the planet. These degenerate conditions and lifestyles and a high-carbohydrate, junk-food diet that create diabetes emanate from these modern human-created realities, which, taken together, we are calling the Culture of Death.

The cure, on the most profound level, is to move away from a global and personal lifestyle of the Culture of Death, to embrace the lifestyle of the Culture of Life. On a personal level this means choosing to live in a way that promotes life and well-being for oneself as well as the planet. It means creating a diet and lifestyle in which there is naturally minimal or no incidence of diabetes. Individually, this means a diet that is organic; moderately low glycemic; moderate-low plant-source-only carbohydrate (25–45 percent, primarily from leafy greens, green vegetables, and sprouts); at least 80 percent live food; high in mineral content; 25–45 percent plant-source-only, raw fat (no animal protein or fat and no trans fats from animal or plant sources); 10–25 percent protein; low-insulin index; well hydrated; individualized; and of modest food intake. For it to be successful, it needs to be a cuisine that is sustainable for the duration of one's life and prepared and eaten with love. Collectively, it means creating a world culture where all people have access to healthy, organic food and water, decent shelter, and a living environment free of chemicals and pollutants. Healing diabetes in this personal and global context is an act of love for oneself and the living planet. This love is an expression of the Culture of Life.

The teaching of this book is that humanity is created to be vibrant, alive, and healthy. As it says in Deuteronomy 30:19 from 3,400 years ago: "Today, I have set before you life and death and a blessing and a curse. You must choose life in order that you and your children shall live." Things have not changed. Humanity still has that choice. This book is about empowering individuals, health professionals, as well as national and global policy makers to make that choice. Even in the most adverse circumstances, it still is possible for motivated individuals and nations to heal on the Dr. Cousens's Diabetes Recovery Program—A Holistic Approach as an act of love and consciousness.

The inspiration for this book began with a movie on diabetes and live foods (*Simply Raw: Reversing Diabetes in 30 Days*) that was made at the Tree of Life Rejuvenation Center U.S. in Patagonia, Arizona. The original idea was to do a film on the effect of being raw for 30 days. I strongly suggested that it would be more interesting to the general public to witness on film the effect of live foods on diabetic, McDonald's Culture-of-Death individuals. Based on my clinical experience in healing diabetes naturally with motivated people, I was confident that these principles and approach would work with this more typical group of diabetic people. It seemed like an interesting exploration of how it would work for a group of people totally unfamiliar with live-food cuisine and way of life. The results were amazing. Of the six who started the program, only one dropped out. By the fourth day, four were off their insulin or oral hypoglycemic medications, and one Type-1 diabetic was down from 70 units of insulin per day and moving toward the 5 units he reached by the end of the month. The other of the two Type-1 diabetics, whose FBS chart appears later in the book and who was diagnosed with Type-1 diabetes by doctors in a hospital setting, dropped from 20 units of insulin and a blood sugar as high as 300 to a normal fasting blood sugar of 73 after two weeks on the program and has remained in the mid-80s to 90s for the past eight years. As of the release of this book's second edition, eight years later in 2012, he remains cured of Type-1 diabetes. Another participant, who had severe neuropathy in his lower limbs, numbness in his scrotum and feet, was suffering from mental deterioration and confusion, and was preparing to have a foot amputated, recovered completely from the neuropathy and became mentally clearer. The tissue of his foot also healed and his blood sugar dropped to normal range in the first two weeks. The disappearance of painful neuropathy on this program is a common occurrence. Two of the women who had been living with a blood sugar of 300-plus while on medications dropped to blood sugars of 109 and 111 by the end of the month without medications. Most of the other participants' blood chemistries also became normal after one month. Mental states became clear and joyous in all participants.

On realizing the powerful effect of 30 days of live food with specific diabetic supplements and herbs on participants' physical and mental states, and on their diabetes in particular, it became clear that I had developed a program that could be applicable and successful for all types of diabetics, as this group was representative of the Western populace. Dr. Cousens's Diabetes Recovery Program—A Holistic Approach is more powerful than even the 30-day raw approach seen in the film. With the 120 clients who have entered the program, the record of healing is progressively better than with the first 11, and I am shocked at the increase in of Type-1 diabetes healing. Literally two-thirds of the last two groups of Type-1 diabetics came off all insulin and had an FBS less than 100, and 31.4 percent of the Type-1 diabetics are off all insulin with FBS heading toward 100. I have now developed a working theory to explain these dramatic results, and I am no longer considering them a fluke.

The overall program includes a minimum seven-day green juice fast (for Type-2 diabetics) in the first week, which greatly accelerates the reversing of the diabetic degenerative physiological process, and low-glycemic green avocado smoothies for Type-1 diabetics. Based on research by Dr. Stephen Spindler, it is my theory that the calorie restriction activated by the fast turns on the antiaging and theoretically the antidiabetic genes. This is then followed by dietary intake of a 25–45 percent moderate-low complex carbohydrate live-food, plant-source-only diet. The participant is invited to enjoy a delicious, healthy, healing, plant-source-only, organic cuisine that limits all carbohydrates to leafy greens, high-fiber vegetables, and sprouts and has no limitations on plant-source fats and protein. There are no processed, junk, or GMO foods or white sugar or white flour. This is the powerful secret of the success of this program. In the second week, a four-day course shows people how to let go of their belief that diabetes is incurable. It also shows people how to let go of all the psychological programming and habits that create the diabetes lifestyle. In the third week, people learn how to prepare moderately low-glycemic foods and a healthy healing cuisine. There then is a one-year follow-up that supports people in staying on the program. This includes nurse support calls and a once-a-month live videoconference with Dr. Cousens at DrCousens.com.

This book covers the global diabetes pandemic, the causes of diabetes, the follow-up support program, and provides an in-depth discussion of the synergistic reasons of why this program is so successful, as well as a dramatic new theory and program for understanding and reversing CDDS, which is the driving force behind Type-2 diabetes. CDDS includes the dynamics of glucose spiking with normal FBS as well the prediabetes syndrome. The healing approach in this book works for all levels of CDDS.

There Is a Cure for Diabetes contains over 900 references. Most are primary sources of information, which include hundreds of other researchers' scientific publications, spanning many decades, supporting a nutritional approach to diabetes reversal and healthy living in general. Some of the statistics on diabetes and research findings vary. For example, the Centers for Disease Control estimate 27 million diabetics and 57 million prediabetics in the United States. But the rate of diabetes in the world is changing so rapidly that it seems any statistics are low estimates. I have chosen to include the variances, rather than to average them. The variations show the state of the knowledge and information and should not be interpreted as contradictions.

Make no mistake: Liberating ourselves from the cultural, nutritional, and personal habits that contribute to the manifestation of diabetes not only helps us to heal ourselves and realize better health but is an act of love and consciousness that contributes to a multilevel positive transformation of society. This is not only an approach that leads to the prevention and healing of CDDS and diabetes; it outlines the fundamentals of a healthy diet as both rejuvenating and leading to a generally healthier, happier, and more ecological life for yourself and the whole living planet. I have already started such Culture of Life humanitarian diabetes prevention and treatment programs in Mexico, Ghana, Nigeria, Cameroon, Ethiopia, and New Guinea, and for Mexican farm workers in the United States and Native Americans; I am now moving toward a preliminary program in Ethiopia. Once one understands the dynamics of individual healing, it is fundamental to expand it to a community and natural approach.

Only one question is left to the reader: Do you love yourself and the planet enough to want to heal yourself of diabetes and help the world switch from the Culture of Death, which is the ultimate cause of diabetes, to the Culture of Life, which brings love, peace, abundance, and health to yourself and the planet?

With heartfelt blessings to your health, joy, and spirit,

Gabriel Cousens, MD

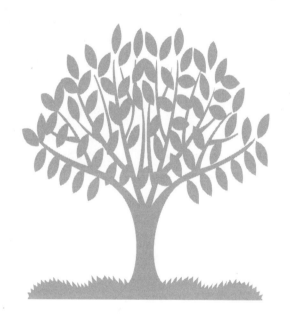

CHAPTER 1

Diabetes Pandemic: World,
Nations and Cultures, Cities

The World

Worldwide, diabetes has reached pandemic proportions. Data published in December 2006 in the International Diabetes Federation's (IDF) *Diabetes Atlas* show that the disease now affects a staggering 246 million people worldwide, with 46 percent of all those affected in the 40-to-59 age group. In 2013 it may be closer to 366 million, with 100 million diabetics in India alone. Previous figures underestimated the scope of the problem, while even the most pessimistic predictions fell short of the current figure. The new data predict that the total number of people living with diabetes will skyrocket to 380 million within 20 years if nothing is done.[1] Diabetes, mostly Type-2, now affects 5.9 percent of the world's adult population, with almost 80 percent of the total in developing countries. The regions with the highest rates are the Eastern Mediterranean and Middle East (where 9.2 percent of the adult population is affected) and North America (with 8.4 percent affected). The highest numbers, however, are found in the Western Pacific, where some 67 million people have diabetes, followed by Europe with 53 million. According to the CDC, as of January 2011, 8.3 percent of the U.S. population have diabetes; 11.3 percent of adults 20 years and older and 27 percent of adults 65 years and older have diabetes. (Twenty-seven percent of those with diabetes do not know they have the disease.) Thirty-five percent of adults 20 to 64 years old and 50 percent of those 65 and older have prediabetes. That is a total of 26 million Americans with diabetes and 79 million with prediabetes.

The World Health Organization (WHO) warns that deaths due to diabetes will increase globally by as much as 80 percent in some regions over the next 10 years.[2] Professor Pierre Lefèbvre, former president of the IDF, explains: "It is estimated that over 3.8 million deaths can be attributed to diabetes each year. That is 8,700 deaths every day; or six deaths every minute." He adds that "the dramatic rise in diabetes prevalence that can be found mainly in low and middle income countries is of particular concern." According to the WHO in 2007, by 2025, the largest increases in diabetes prevalence will take place in developing countries, where the number of people with diabetes will increase by 150 percent.[3] With no action to defuse this increase, it is estimated that total direct health care expenditures on diabetes worldwide will be up to 396 billion international dollars (ID) in 2025. This means that the proportion of the world's health care budget spent on diabetes care in 2025 will be between 7 percent and 13 percent—most likely closer to 13 percent.[4]

According to a WHO report,[5] deaths from diabetes will increase by 80 percent in the Americas, by 50 percent in the Western Pacific and the Eastern Mediterranean regions, and by more than 40 percent in

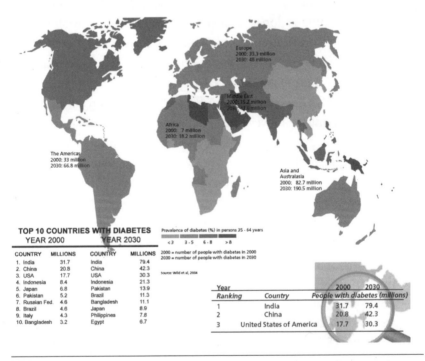

FIGURE 1. Diabetes prevalence by region, current and projected. (The graph shows 2000 data for the top 10 countries and projected data for 2030.)

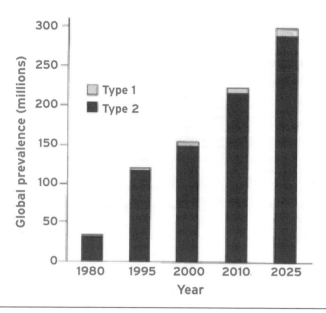

FIGURE 2. Estimated global prevalence of Type-1 and Type-2 diabetes

Africa over the next 10 years. It may seem strange that the developing world, which is often associated with hunger and inadequate nutrition for children, is now experiencing an epidemic of Type-2 diabetes, a disease usually associated with a wealthy and unhealthy lifestyle. This can be explained by the high degree of urbanization in some countries such as India that has brought adaptation to the lifestyles from industrialized countries, resulting in diseases such as diabetes related to this new lifestyle.[6] Epidemiologically, diabetes mellitus has been linked to the Western lifestyle and is uncommon in cultures consuming a more historical and indigenous diet.[7,8] As populations switch from their native diets to the "foods of commerce," their rate of diabetes increases, eventually reaching the same proportions seen in Western societies.[9]

As we look at this pandemic, we need to be clear that it is worldwide. In short, we can call it a metabolic time bomb: Of the estimated now 57 million people diagnosed with prediabetes in the United States alone,[10] about 10 percent will develop full-blown diabetes each year, shortening life-spans by 10 to 19 years and accounting for about 210,000 deaths

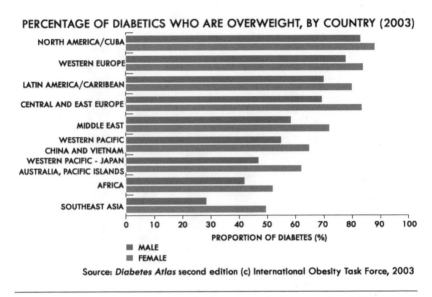

PERCENTAGE OF DIABETICS WHO ARE OVERWEIGHT, BY COUNTRY (2003)

Source: *Diabetes Atlas* second edition (c) International Obesity Task Force, 2003

FIGURE 3. Percentage of diabetics who are overweight, by country, 2003

per year from diabetes. An infant born in 2000 in the United States has a better than one-in-three chance of developing diabetes. For those in certain ethnic groups such as Native American, Puerto Rican, Mexican, and Chinese, that projection may even be increased to one in two. African Americans and Latinos have about twice the risk of developing Type-2 diabetes. Type-2 diabetics are about three-to-four times more likely to develop clinical depression than nondiabetics.

With my program there is explicit hope for Type-2 diabetes being completely reversed in a relatively short time. The good news is that with the Dr. Cousens's Diabetes Recovery Program—A Holistic Approach, Type-2 diabetes is not necessarily a death sentence; rather, it is a benign disease if it is appropriately addressed.

The message is apparent. Uncontrolled diabetes is a forced death march for those who are not willing to make the effort to heal themselves and a disaster in progress for the cultures and economies of nations worldwide. This book outlines a clear and safe approach to addressing the individual and global issue of diabetes, and in that context is a way forward for policy makers and all people who want to reverse this preventable trend. Type-2 diabetes is a pandemic wake-up call to the world to change its diet and lifestyle relying on junk food and high-sugar and high-saturated animal fat, trans-fatty-acid, and pesticide- and herbicide-laden food. First, we must understand the full extent of the problem among nations and cultures. An obvious result of this discordant diet and lifestyle is obesity. We need to be clear: Obesity does not cause diabetes but is also a symptom of the diet and lifestyle that create diabetes. It is an indicator that is easy to associate with diabetes and helps us track the diabetic trend: close to 90 percent of Type-2 diabetics are overweight.

Nations and Cultures

At the time of this revised publication, the three countries with the most diabetics are India (50.3 million), China (43.2 million), and the United States (27 million), followed by Russia (9.6 million) and Germany (6 million). Below is a 2006 chart of sugar consumption in the "top three." Notice a pattern?

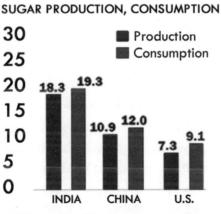

FIGURE 4. Sugar production and consumption in India, China, and the United States, 2005-6

Asia

India has the largest diabetic population in the world, with an estimated 50.3 million Type-2 diabetics. The WHO predicts that deaths from diabetes in India will increase by 35 percent over the next 10 years. In China, the number of people with Type-2 diabetes is likely to reach 50 million in the next 25 years. There is a noticeable trend toward diabetes in Asian countries.

We do not have to look far to understand why. About 14 percent of Asian children are obese. That's about twice the normal obesity rate of their parents. In Japan, the prevalence of Type-2 diabetes among junior high schoolchildren has almost doubled, from 7.3 per 100,000 in 1976–80 to 13.9 per 100,000 in 1991–95. Type-2 diabetes now outnumbers Type-1 diabetes in Japanese children.[11] In China, the number of obese people has tripled since 1992 to 90 million as Western fast-food cuisine has become more popular and people are becoming more materially prosperous.

This is pointing to a problem that is obviously very serious through-out the world, including Asia, where people in nations such as Korea, China, and Japan are up to 60 percent more genetically susceptible to diabetes than Caucasians, even though currently their national rates may be lower because they have not fully assimilated the more diabe-togenic Western cultural diet.

The Americas

Based on 1994 extrapolations from prevalence studies, there are now about 37 million people with diabetes in the Americas (approximately 26 million in the United States and 13 million in Latin America and the Caribbean). This accounts for one-quarter of the world's total population suffering from diabetes. According to projections, the most dramatic increase is predicted to be in Central America, with an increase close to 100 percent. (Estimates vary—we are providing what we consider reasonable estimates from the literature.) In the Caribbean islands, prevalence is expected to increase by 74 percent, compared to 40 percent for South America and 25 percent for the United States and Canada.[12]

Recent changes in mortality profiles in the Americas (between 1980 and 1990) indicate that diabetes is the seventh leading cause of death and the third most common chronic condition leading to high mortality. Hispanics are the fastest-growing minority group in the United States, with one out of two Hispanic women developing diabetes. Data from the Third National Health and Nutrition Examination Survey (NHANES III) showed that minority persons with diabetes in the United States, particularly Mexican Americans, were more likely to have poorer glycemic control than African Americans and non-Hispanic whites.[13]

> Organic and nutritious foods make a meaningful impact on children's health that lasts throughout life.
> **Jorge Valenzuela, Save the Children**

There is a growing awareness in Spanish-speaking communities of the importance of healthy nutrition and of the disaster of Type-2 diabetes. I am working with John David Arnold, PhD, international director of the League of United Latin American Countries (LULAC), and with Jorge Valenzuela, head of Save the Children and Mexico executive director on these issues.

> Diabetes is the unnecessary scourge of humanity that, unless prevented, will continue to evolve in future generations until it wipes us off the face of the planet.
> **John David Arnold, PhD,**
> **international director of LULAC**

D. Z. Jackson, in the pages of the January 11, 2006, edition of the *Boston Globe*, aptly commented on the tidal wave of diabetes cases in the United States: "Type 2 diabetes is sweeping so rapidly through America we need not waste time giving children bicycles. Just roll them a wheelchair."[14]

In the United States, estimates by the Centers for Disease Control and Prevention (CDC) are 20.8 million diabetics diagnosed and about 20 million who are considered prediabetic. In 2004, about 1.4 million adults in the United States between ages 18 and 79 were diagnosed with diabetes. From 1997 through 2004, the number of new cases of diagnosed diabetes increased by 54 percent.[15] This means there was an increase from 4.8 to 7.3 percent of the population. Diabetes was a very rare illness in 1880, with only 2.8 persons out of every 100,000 having diabetes. The formal prevalence of diabetes in the Native American population in 2002 was 15.3 percent, which is an increase of 33.2 percent from 1994. This is more than 50 percent greater than the general U.S. population. The informal estimate among all tribes according to diabetes activist Dennis Banks, American Indian Movement leader, is close to 90 percent. From 1990 to 1998, the number of newly diagnosed diabetics among people younger than 34 increased by 71 percent in the U.S. Native American populations. Diabetes-related deaths have jumped 45 percent since 1987, while death rates from heart disease, stroke, and cancer have actually decreased. Diabetes deaths are independent of those general trends.

In response to a study published in the January 1, 2003, issue of the *Journal of the American Medical Association* (*JAMA*), which used Behavioral Risk Factor Surveillance System (BRFSS) data to show a recent increase in diagnosed diabetes as well as a significant association between overweight and obesity and diabetes, CDC director Dr. Julie L. Gerberding stated, "These increases are disturbing and are likely even underestimated. What's more important, we're seeing a number of serious health effects resulting from overweight and obesity." Dr. Gerberding added, "If we continue on this same path, the results will be devastating to both the health of the nation and to our healthcare system."[16]

Why we are overweight is associated with overnutrition. Americans at the beginning of the twenty-first century are now consuming more food and several hundred more calories per person per day than did their counterparts in the late 1950s (when per capita calorie consumption was at the lowest level in the last century), or even in the 1970s. The U.S. food supply in 2000 provided 3,800 calories per person per

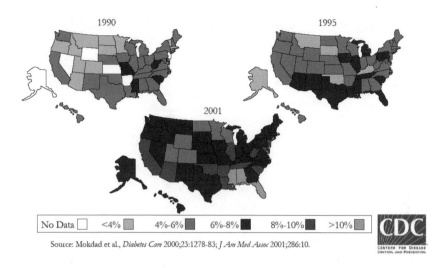

FIGURE 5. Diabetes trends among adults in the United States, 1990, 1995, 2001

day, 500 calories above the 1970 level, and 800 calories above the record low in 1957 and 1958. Of those 3,800 calories, the USDA's Economic Research Service (ERS) estimates, roughly 1,100 calories are lost to spoilage, plate waste, and cooking and other losses, putting dietary intake of calories in 2000 at just under 2,700 calories per person per day. ERS data suggest that average daily calorie intake increased by 24.5 percent, or about 530 calories, between 1970 and 2000. Of that increase, grains (mainly refined grain products) contributed 9.5 percentage points; added fats and oils, 9.0 percentage points; added sugars, 4.7 percentage points; fruits and vegetables together (which are our Culture of Life antidiabetogenic foods), only 1.5 percentage points.[17]

Diabetes as a Cause of Death

According to the CDC, diabetes was the sixth leading cause of death listed on U.S. death certificates in 2002. (Other reports suggest it is fifth or seventh—regardless, we need to pay attention.) This ranking is based on the 73,249 death certificates in which diabetes was listed as the underlying cause of death. According to death certificate reports, diabetes contributed to a total of 224,092 deaths.

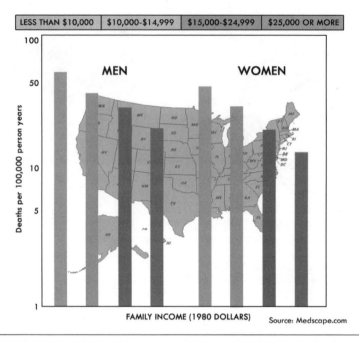

FIGURE 6. Diabetes death rates among adults, age 45 and older, by family income and gender

Still, diabetes is likely to be underreported as a cause of death. Studies have found that only 35–40 percent of decedents with diabetes had it listed anywhere on the death certificate and only 10–15 percent had it listed as the underlying cause of death. Overall, the risk for death among people with diabetes is about twice that of people without diabetes of similar age.

Diabetes mortality and family income show a strong relationship, according to data from the National Longitudinal Mortality Study for 1979 to 1989. For people 45 and older, the age-adjusted death rate in the United States from diabetes decreased as family income increased. The relationship between family income and death from diabetes was similar for men and women; for both sexes, mortality from diabetes decreased at each higher level of family income. The diabetes death rate among women in families with incomes below $10,000 was three times the death rate of those with incomes of $25,000 or more; among men, the death rate among the lowest income group was 2.6 times that of the highest income group.[18]

Diabetes is strongly associated with economic factors that differ from industrialized nations to developing nations. In developed countries, "low-income" means poor access to healthy foods, the most affordable diet being a higher and cheaper caloric carbohydrate diet that actually creates a diabetic physiology—nutrient-poor foods high in calories from processed sugar and hydrogenated oils. These cheap calories come at a high health price for the lower class, as seen in Figure 7.

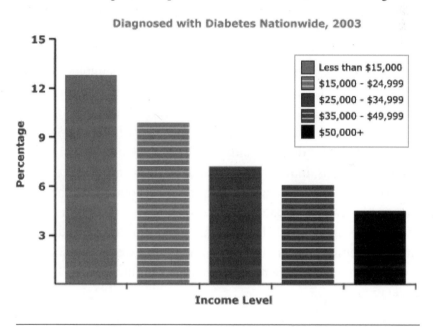

FIGURE 7. Percentage diagnosed with diabetes nationwide, 2003, by income level (Source: U.S. Centers for Disease Control and Prevention)

In England, as in the United States, the poor are 2.5 times more likely to develop Type-2 diabetes than the general population and 3.5 times more likely to develop serious complications. In these societies obesity is nearly 50 percent higher among poor women, and they are 50 percent more likely to be smoking. In Northeastern England, diabetes is 45 percent higher in women and 28 percent higher in men than the national average. People from black and minority ethnic groups are up to six times higher.

Africa

In Africa, the current figure of 13.6 million people with diabetes is expected to almost double in the next 25 years, reaching just under 27 million, according to Professor Jean-Claude Mbanya, vice-president of the IDF: "Of concern is also the early onset of diabetes, particularly in sub-Saharan Africa, where more and more people in their thirties and early forties are developing Type-2 diabetes. They run a high risk of diabetes complications such as heart disease and foot ulcers at an early age."[19]

Until recently, there was a lack of data on the epidemiology of diabetes mellitus in Africa. Over the past decade, information on the prevalence of Type-2 diabetes has increased, albeit still limited, but there is still a lack of adequate data on Type-1 diabetes in sub-Saharan Africa. For Type-2 diabetes, although the prevalence is low in some rural populations, moderate and even high rates have been reported from other countries. In low diabetes prevalence populations, the moderate to high rates of impaired glucose tolerance is a possible indicator of the early stage of a diabetes epidemic.[20] I am currently introducing a simple screening program in Nigeria and Ghana, which hopefully will give some more accurate results. According to the African Diabetes Federation,

> The prevalence of Type-2 diabetes is low in both rural and urban Bantu communities, but is ten times more prevalent in Muslim and Hindu communities in Tanzania and South Africa, and in the Chinese community in Mauritius. Type-1 diabetes, while still rare, is becoming increasingly prevalent. [Diabetes prevalence is higher in urban, migrant and African-origin populations living abroad.] Diabetes is already a major public health problem in Africa and its impact is bound to increase significantly if nothing is done to curb the rising rate of impaired glucose tolerance (IGT), which now exceeds 16 percent in some countries.[21]

The Middle East

In Israel, mostly among the large non-European immigrant population, the diabetes rate is already 7 percent of the population, with some 400,000 people diagnosed with diabetes. Another 600,000 suffer from some form of prediabetes or the metabolic syndrome (Syndrome X), which is strongly associated with insulin resistance among Jewish immigrant populations such as Yemenites, Kurds, and Ethiopians who, in their indigenous environment, had extremely low rates of diabetes. Upon arrival in Israel, they took on the more European junk-food culture, stopped exercising, and began experiencing skyrocketing incidence of diabetes. Yemenites are the ethnic group with the highest incidence of the disease.

In one study of Arab men and women from the Galilee in Israel, Dr. Mohammed Abdul-Ghani, a family physician and diabetes expert in the town of Nahf, discovered that 26 percent of his patients were diabetic and didn't know it, while 42 percent had impaired glucose tolerance and were at risk. Only 31 percent had no diabetic symptoms. This isn't just about Israeli Arabs; in Saudi Arabia, at least 25 percent of the population has diabetes, and in Bahrain, about 32 percent have diabetes. It is possible there is something in the Arab genetics that predisposes them to the chronic degenerative diabetes syndrome (CDDS) as the result of a diet high in sugar and lamb.

In the Arab countries, high levels of overweight and obesity exist particularly among women, in countries as diverse as Egypt and the Gulf states, including Saudi Arabia. Obesity rates are 25–30 percent in Saudi Arabia and Kuwait, with the United Arab Emirates and Bahrain not far behind. In Iran, obesity rates vary from rural to urban populations, rising to 30 percent among women in Tehran. In northern Africa, the prevalence of obesity among women is high. Half of all women are overweight (body mass index, or BMI, greater than 25), with rates of 50.9 percent in Tunisia and 51.3 percent in Morocco, and obesity rates (BMI > 30) in women of 23 percent in Tunisia and 18 percent in Morocco, representing approximately a threefold increase over 20 years.[22]

Europe

The WHO estimates 53 million diabetes cases in Europe as of 2007 and projects 64 million by 2025. In England, there are 1.4 million diabetics, and the number of people in the UK with diabetes is predicted to reach 3 million by 2010.

Diabetes has been known to the world for thousands of years. Hippocrates noted it. The Sanskrit term for diabetes mellitus, *madhumeda*, appeared in Ayurvedic texts thousands of years ago. Madhumeda translates as "honey urine" because the ancient practitioners first diagnosed the disease by testing the patient's urine to see if it, like honey, attracted ants.[23] It was portrayed in ancient Egyptian wall paintings showing somebody having what we call a muscle-wasting disease and urinating copiously. One of the earliest known records of diabetes spoke of frequent urination, or "polyuria," as a symptom on papyrus written by Hesy-Ra, a Third Dynasty Egyptian physician.[24] During the first century CE, Arateus described diabetes as "the melting down of flesh and limbs into urine," and Galen of Pergamum, a Greek physician, felt diabetes was a form of kidney failure.[25] Then it was rare; today, it is pandemic. What we are seeing today is a commentary on the state of mind and consequent lifestyle of our world culture. The behavior and lifestyle habits that create Type-2 diabetes are Crimes Against Wisdom. It is this lifestyle and diet of refined white sugar, saturated animal fat, and junk food that causes a metabolic disorder of carbohydrate, lipid, and protein metabolism.

Yes, diabetes has a very clear genetic component, especially for Type-2 diabetes. Type-1 diabetes also has a genetic component, but the genetic component is a significantly less important factor. Both of these may be associated with gestational diabetes (diabetes during pregnancy). Type-2 is also associated with vitamin and mineral deficiencies. The key deficient minerals are magnesium, chromium, vanadium, manganese, and potassium. It is associated with lack of exercise and obesity. It has become a pandemic because people are not living in a way that brings them into balance with themselves or the living. They are living the lifestyle of the Culture of Death and not the Culture of Life. This is why we call it a *Crime Against Wisdom*, an ancient Ayurvedic phrase that describes the situation.

Cultures

Type-2 diabetes seems to have the highest rates in indigenous cultures where they have minimal genetic defense. When indigenous cultures come in contact with processed, adulterated, high white-sugar and white-flour foods, and move from an active to a more passive lifestyle with its concomitant obesity, they are at serious risk for diabetes.

The association between poor diet and obesity is strong. From a dietary perspective, obesity is primarily connected to a diet high in sugar and complex carbohydrates. Americans have become conspicuous consumers of sugar and sweet-tasting foods and beverages. Per capita consumption of caloric sweeteners, mainly sucrose (table sugar made from cane and beets) and corn sweeteners (notably high-fructose corn syrup), increased 43 pounds, or 39 percent, between 1950–59 and 2000. In the year 2000, each American consumed an average 152 pounds of caloric sweeteners. That amounted to more than two-fifths of a pound, or 52 teaspoons per person per day.[26] This is something unheard of in human history. Dr. Thomas Cleave did a historical survey after World War II of indigenous cultures to which white sugar and white flour had been introduced. He found that in every culture in which there was an outbreak of Type-2 diabetes, the disease occurred approximately 20 years after white sugar and white flour were introduced. That's a very clear statement. Although it is commonly thought that diabetes is a blood sugar imbalance, it is actually a chronic degenerative disorder that affects protein metabolism, fat metabolism, and carbohydrate metabolism. This metabolic imbalance is interwoven with diet and lifestyle characterized by obesity and lack of exercise primarily combined with high processed sugar and high carbohydrates in general and secondarily with high animal fat and protein and low-fiber foods. A much greater percentage of the uneducated and lower classes develop diabetes, and more specifically, a great many Native

Americans, African Americans, Asians, and Hispanics suffer from it.

We only have to go back a little bit in history to see that this pandemic is relatively new. We have been on the planet for perhaps 3.2 million years. The Pima Indians had only one single documented case of diabetes by 1920. Their cousins, the Tarahumaras, who have stuck with a natural diet, have only 6 percent incidence of diabetes. Meanwhile, their genetic relatives the Pimas have up to 51 percent incidence, and in 2011, the unofficial estimate is as high as 90 percent incidence. In 1970, the Pimas' ability to fish was compromised by some river dams, and they turned more to Western culture junk foods. The rate skyrocketed when genetics and a diabetogenic Western diet merged. The rate of diabetes is dramatically affected by the genetics for diabetes in a particular culture, and many scientists believe genetics may explain the obesity problem among Native Americans. The first U.S. researcher to learn about the Mexican Pimas was Leslie O. Schulz, professor of health sciences at the University of Wisconsin-Milwaukee. With the cooperation of the tribe, she has established a clinic and research site to test several hypotheses about this contrast in diabetes rates. Since 1991, she has made some 15 trips to Maycoba, as well as many visits to the Gila River reservation.

Her "thrifty gene" theory is as follows:[27] Before food preservation and transportation methods were developed in the United States, indigenous populations in North America relied exclusively on locally produced food, in the same way indigenous Mexican populations such as the Pimas do today. When the harvest was poor, people ate less. Long periods of drought and famine were especially common in desert regions, such as the area the Pimas inhabit.

"The theory is that Native Americans have what is called the 'thrifty gene,'" Schulz explains. "They're genetically geared to conserving and being thrifty in terms of their calories, so that they don't waste it in case a famine comes along. They're going to be the ones to survive."

The continual availability of food in the United States today appears to have contributed to the Pimas' problems with obesity, Schulz says. The thrifty gene, which allowed Indians to survive long periods of famine in Mexico, works against them on the Gila River reservation. "All of a sudden, there's this constant food supply, like we have now, 24 hours a day. We never have the famine, so that's why they become so much more overweight. Then, being overweight, they develop the Type-2 diabetes that goes with that."

Total Prevalence of Diabetes by Race/Ethnicity[28]

Non-Hispanic Whites: 13.1 million, or 8.7 percent, of all non-Hispanic whites age 20 years or older have diabetes.

Non-Hispanic Blacks: 3.2 million, or 13.3 percent, of all non-Hispanic blacks age 20 years or older have diabetes. After adjusting for population age differences, non-Hispanic blacks are 1.8 times as likely to have diabetes as non-Hispanic whites.

Hispanic/Latino Americans: After adjusting for population age differences, Mexican Americans, the largest Hispanic/Latino subgroup, are 1.7 times as likely to have diabetes as non-Hispanic whites. If the prevalence of diabetes among Mexican Americans is applied to the total Hispanic/Latino population, according to the CDC, in 2006, about 13.5 percent of Hispanic/Latino Americans age 20 years or older would have diabetes. Sufficient data are not available to derive estimates of the total prevalence of diabetes (both diagnosed and undiagnosed diabetes) for other Hispanic/Latino groups. However, residents of Puerto Rico are 1.8 times as likely to have diagnosed diabetes as U.S. non-Hispanic whites.

American Indians and Alaska Natives: 99,500, or 12.8 percent, of American Indians and Alaska natives age 20 years or older who received care from Indian Health Service (IHS) in 2003 had diagnosed diabetes. Some 118,000 (15.1 percent) American Indians and Alaska natives age 20 years or older have diabetes (both diagnosed and undiagnosed). Taking into account population age differences, American Indians and Alaska natives are 2.2 times as likely to have diabetes as non-Hispanic whites.

Asian Americans and Pacific Islanders: The total prevalence of diabetes (both diagnosed and undiagnosed) is not available for Asian

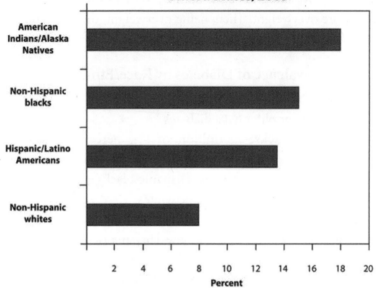

Estimated age-adjusted total prevalence of diabetes in people aged 20 years or older, by race/ethnicity— United States, 2005

Source: *For American Indians/Alaska Natives, the estimate of total prevalence was calculated using the estimate of diagnosed diabetes from the 2003 outpatient database of the Indian Health Service and the estimate of undiagnosed diabetes from the 1999-2002 National Health and Nutrition Examination Survey. For the other groups, 1999-2002 NHANES estimates of total prevalence (both diagnosed and undiagnosed) were projected to year 2006.*

* Graph and information obtained from CDC (Center for Disease Control and Prevention) website at http://www.cdc.gov/diabetes/pubs/estimates05.html#prev4 on December 1, 2006.

FIGURE 8. Estimated age-adjusted total prevalence of diabetes in people age 20 years or older by race/ethnicity, United States, 2005

Americans or Pacific Islanders. However, in Hawaii, Asians, native Hawaiians, and other Pacific Islanders age 20 years or older are more than twice as likely to have diagnosed diabetes as Caucasians after adjusting for population age differences and are more susceptible than Caucasians to being overweight. Similarly, in California, Asians are 1.5 times as likely to have diagnosed diabetes as non-Hispanic whites. Other groups in these populations also have increased risk for diabetes.

Cities

New York City is an amplified microcosm of this information. There are 800,000 people with diagnosed diabetes in New York City—one in eight people. It is the only major disease in the city that is growing. The percentage of diabetics in New York City is about a third higher than the rest of the nation and cases have been increasing about twice as fast as nationally. In the past 10 years, New York City has seen a 140 percent increase in diabetes. The proportion of diabetics is higher than that of Los Angeles, Chicago, or Boston. In New York, the diabetic rate is highest where there are ethnic groups with high genetic tendencies.

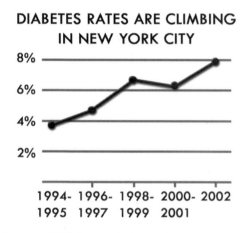

DIABETES RATES ARE CLIMBING IN NEW YORK CITY

Sources: NYC Dept. of Health & Mental Hygiene; US Centers for Disease Control and Prevention; World Health Organization

FIGURE 9. Diabetes rates in New York City (Source: NYC Department of Health and Mental Hygiene)

It is worst in East Harlem, where the health department survey shows that 16–20 percent, or up to one in five, adults had diabetes around the turn of the century. The only place that is higher is among the Pima Indians in Arizona, where approximately 50–90 percent suffer from diabetes. In East Harlem, diabetes-related amputations are also higher than in any other part of the city. And of course that is also the location of the highest percentage of people who are overweight—people who have bad food habits, exercise very little, and have significant poverty.

According to the CDC, one in three children born in the United States is expected to become diabetic in their lifetimes. New York is not the only place where diabetes is epidemic. As quoted in *The Daily Texan* in 2005, "In President George W. Bush's home state of Texas, state health services commissioner Dr. Eduardo Sanchez said, 'Half of Texas children born after the year 2000 will develop diabetes.'"

Age as a Factor

Diabetes also increases with age. It could almost be considered a marker of accelerated aging.

In 2005 one in five New Yorkers 65 years and older had diabetes, but by 2010, 25 percent of all people in the United States over the age of 60 have developed Type-2 diabetes. New York is not even the most overweight. In New York, 20 percent are overweight, while 20–30 percent are overweight in the rest of the country. But it is in New York, as in England, that Type-2 diabetes is very much connected with race, genetics, and money. It seems to have an inverse relationship to income. Poverty seems to be associated with less access to fresh fruits and vegetables, exercise, and health care and more empty carbohydrate calories. New York's poverty rate is approximately 20 percent, which is higher than the nation's 12.7 percent.

African Americans, Latinos, Mexican Americans, and Puerto Ricans have a diabetes rate close to twice that of white people. In England, we see the same kinds of racial ratios. Asian Americans and Pacific Islanders also appear more susceptible, and they seem to develop diabetes at lower comparative weights. There is no question that genetics plays a role, but our lifestyle is the determining factor. Our collective world lifestyle is one big Crime Against Wisdom.

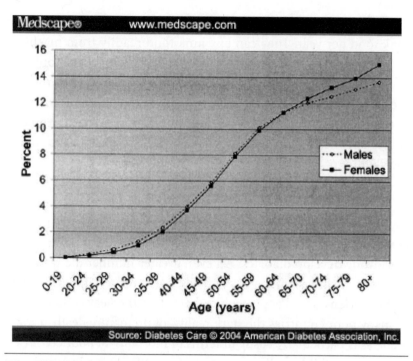

FIGURE 10. Diabetes rates in men and women, up to age 80 or older (Source: American Diabetes Association, Inc., *Diabetes Care*, 2004)

In New York City—home to a pretty educated group—a 2002 health department survey found that 89 percent of diabetics didn't know their HgbA1c levels.[29] The HgbA1c is called the glycosylated hemoglobin test; this important test measures the level of sugar that binds nonenzymatically to hemoglobin and thus helps monitor the degree of diabetes. Any HgbA1c result above 5.7 is considered diabetic. In New York City, half the grade schoolers are overweight, and roughly one in four are obese (more than 20 pounds overweight). While the state was trying to promote more exercise, the city actually passed a school budget with less exercise. According to the CDC, nationwide daily participation in gym class has dropped to 28 percent in 2003, from 42 percent in 1991. The federal government of the United States had actually made proposals to cut the exercise time even less. Diabetes reflects the imbalance of the culture.

American kids are watching 20,000 hours of commercials for junk food per year. They can buy junk food readily from machines in their schools. We act as if this is not really happening, but data of the diabetes pandemic show the hard-core reality. The dramatic increase in Type-2 diabetes among children is an ominous symptom of the Culture of Death lifestyle. How much more suffering and disability do we need to wake up from this deadly lifestyle and diet of the Culture of Death?

Costs to Society

By 2025, the largest increases in diabetes prevalence will take place in developing countries. Each year an additional seven million people worldwide develop diabetes. An even greater number die from cardiovascular disease made worse by diabetes-related lipid disorders and hypertension.[30] People with diabetes face the near certainty, and in many poor countries the stark reality, of premature death. Type-1 diabetes is particularly costly in terms of mortality in poor countries, where many children die because access to life-saving insulin is not subsidized by governments (who, in some countries, even place high taxes on purchased insulin). Often, insulin is not available at any price. Recent studies in Zambia, Mali, and Mozambique highlight a stark reality: A person requiring insulin for survival in Zambia will live an average of 11 years. A person in Mali can expect to live for 30 months. In Mozambique, a person requiring insulin will be dead within 12 months.[31] In Tanzania, mortality of patients with insulin-dependent diabetes was found to be 40 percent after a mean of five years.[32] The main causes of death in those dying in hospitals were ketoacidosis (50 percent) and infection (32 percent), mirroring the patterns observed in Europe and the United States in the preinsulin era.[33] Using WHO figures on years of life lost per person dying of diabetes, this translates into more than 25 million years of total life lost each year to the disease and into reduced quality of life caused by the preventable complications of diabetes.[34]

Economic Impact

The estimated economic impact of diabetes is considerable and is becoming most noticeably felt in the poorest countries, where people with diabetes and their families bear almost the entire cost of whatever medical care they can afford. In Latin America, families pay 40–60 percent of diabetes care costs out of their own pockets, and in India, the poorest people with diabetes spend an average of 25 percent of their income on private care. Most of this money is used to stay alive by avoiding fatally high blood sugar levels.

Because diabetes is increasing faster in the world's developing economies than in its developed ones, it is the developing world that will bear the brunt of the future cost burden. More than 80 percent of expenditures for medical care for diabetes are made in the world's economically richest countries. Less than 20 percent of expenditures are made in the middle- and low-income countries, where 80 percent of people with diabetes will soon live. The United States is home to about 8 percent of the world's population living with diabetes and spends more than 50 percent of all global expenditure for diabetes care.

In the United States in 1997, the total medical expenditures incurred by people with diabetes was $77.7 billion, or $10,071 per capita annually for medical products and services, compared with $2,669 for people without diabetes.[35] Related ailments are costly, as well: $30,400 for a heart attack or amputation, $40,200 for a stroke, and $37,000 for end-stage kidney disease. The CDC estimated that the annual cost of diabetes in the United States by 2002 was in the range of $264 billion.[36] The following are key cost elements:

- $132 billion total (direct and indirect)
- $92 billion direct medical costs
- $40 billion indirect costs (disability, work loss, premature mortality)

Government budgets worldwide will face the immense strain of diabetes care on disability payments, pensions, social and medical service, and revenue loss.

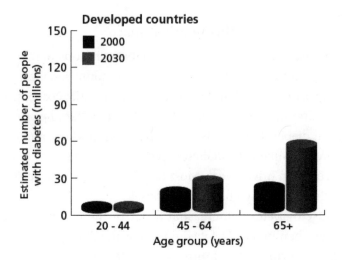

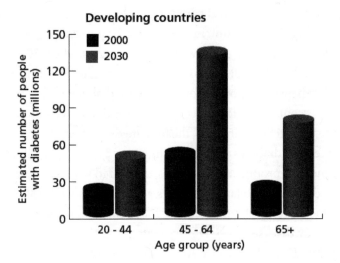

Diabetes affects all people in society, not just those who live with the disease. WHO estimates that mortality from diabetes, heart disease, and stroke costs about 250 billion international dollars (ID) in China, ID225 billion in the Russian Federation, and ID210 billion in India in 2005. Much of the heart disease and stroke in these estimates was linked to diabetes. WHO estimates that diabetes, heart disease, and stroke together will approximately cost as follows:

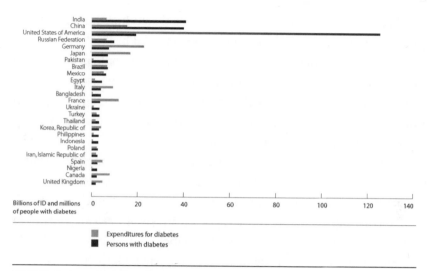

FIGURE 11. Annual health expenditure for diabetes (international dollars) compared to people with diabetes in the 25 countries with the largest numbers of people with diabetes in 2007

- $555.7 billion in lost national income in China over the next 10 years
- $303.2 billion in the Russian Federation
- $333.6 billion in India
- $49.2 billion in Brazil
- $2.5 billion even in a very poor country like Tanzania

These estimates are based on lost productivity, resulting primarily from premature death. Accounting for disability might double or triple these figures.

Diabetes also has a negative impact upon a person's general health condition and work performance. In 2003, the CDC found that 33.6 percent of U.S. adults with diabetes reported at least one day of poor mental health for each 30 days; 53.9 percent reported at least one day of poor physical health; and 62.8 percent reported at least one day of either poor mental or physical health. Also, 32.6 percent of adults with diabetes were unable to perform their usual activities at least one day per month due to either poor mental or physical health.

If we actually followed the diet of prevention we could probably save hundreds of billions in direct and indirect costs, but are we going to do that—that is the question. Why not do the obvious? Roughly $40 billion in federal subsidies are going to pay corn growers so that corn syrup is able to replace cane sugar. Corn syrup has been singled out by many health experts as one of the chief culprits of rising obesity, because corn syrup does not deter the appetite. Since the advent of corn syrup, consumption of all sweeteners has soared, as have people's weights.

According to a 2004 study reported in the *American Journal of Clinical Nutrition*, the rise of Type-2 diabetes since 1980 has closely paralleled the increased use of sweeteners, particularly high-fructose corn syrup. Data collected from the study of 51,603 nurses in the United States found that women who drank one serving of nondiet soda or fruit punch daily, which was sweetened with either sugar or high-fructose corn syrup, were an average of 10.3 pounds heavier than women who drank less than one per month. The study was conducted over four years. In addition, the sugar consumers had an 82 percent increased risk of developing Type-2 diabetes. "The message is: Anyone who cares about their health or the health of their family would not consume these beverages," said Walter C. Willett of the Harvard School of Public Health, who helped conduct the study. "Parents who care about their children's health should not keep [processed-sugar beverages] at home."[37] Dr. Willett's statement makes the point clearly: The profits made from the Culture of Death lifestyle are in direct conflict with our ability to care for our children and ourselves. The ability to love and care for our children and ourselves is a healthy characteristic of the Culture of Life. Do we choose life or do we choose death?

Research also indicates that high-fructose corn syrup interferes with the heart's use of key minerals like magnesium, copper, and chromium, in addition to being implicated in elevated blood cholesterol levels and the creation of blood clots. These factors contribute to cardiovascular disease—the leading cause of death among diabetics. High-fructose

IN 1997, AMERICANS CONSUMED THREE-FOURTHS MORE CALORIC SWEETNER PER CAPITA THAN IN 1909

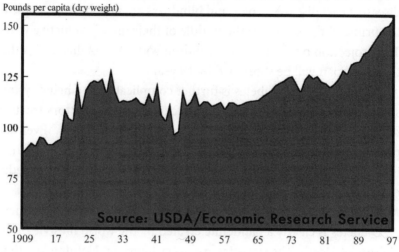

FIGURE 12. Sugar consumption among Americans, 1909-97

corn syrup has also been found to inhibit the action of white blood cells so that they are unable to defend the body against harmful foreign invaders.[38]

There are no real accidents here. This is very straightforward and is a clear and ongoing tragedy. The American Diabetes Association estimates that diabetes cost about $132 billion in 2005. To put this cost in perspective: all the cancers together in United States cost about $171 billion a year. We have a major epidemic, and we are only making the problem worse.

There are many secondary causes to this pandemic. Some doctors are a little concerned, as increasing numbers of children are given antipsychotic drugs for anxiety and conditions like autism. This is because these drugs can promote weight gain and therefore elevate the risk of diabetes. The antipsychotic Zyprexa, for example, has been implicated in causing weight gain and diabetes. With increased weight, there is increased diabetes. Little research has been done on the long-term impact of Type-2 diabetes on children, over their life-span. The chronic complications that follow tend to happen approximately 15 years after the onset. This means that life-limiting complications such as kidney disease, heart disease, stroke, and blindness are now hitting people in the prime of their lives, in the middle of their most productive years. The projection by the CDC for children with Type-2 diabetes is that their life-span will be shortened by 19 years.

The treatment of diabetes is further complicated by a belief system stated by the *New York Times* and backed by most doctors treating diabetes: "Diabetes has no cure. It is progressive and fatal." Even the preliminary results of our research are showing this to be a myth. It is a myth because we did not previously have widespread knowledge of how to reverse it naturally, although as early as 1920, Max Gerson, MD, healed Albert Schweitzer, MD, of diabetes with a live-food diet.

Diabetes is clearly a pandemic created by the world lifestyle of the Culture of Death. The statistics are overwhelming. Nothing less than the health of whole societies is at stake. What is needed is to help the world transition into the Culture of Life, which must be done on a personal basis. Before we talk about how we can easily reverse our current pandemic to a world without diabetes, we need to scientifically investigate personal lifestyle habits that create diabetes and, from this science-based approach, develop a program that can help us choose prudent lifestyle habits that will create a nondiabetic, healthy physiology.

Notes

1. International Diabetes Federation. "Diabetes epidemic out of control." December 4, 2006. http://www.idf.org/home/index.cfm?node=1563.

2. World Health Organization. "Preventing chronic diseases: A vital investment." 2005. http://www.who.int/chp/chronic_disease_report/en/index.html.

3. World Health Organization. "Preventing chronic diseases."

4. International Diabetes Foundation. "Diabetes deaths to increase dramatically over next ten years." October 5, 2005. http://www.idf.org/node/1295.

5. World Health Organization. "Preventing chronic diseases."

6. World Diabetes Foundation. "Diabetes facts." http://www .worlddiabetesfoundation.org/composite-35.htm.

7. Burkitt, D, and Trowell, H. *Western Diseases: Their Emergence and Prevention*. Cambridge: Harvard University Press, 1981.

8. Vahouny, G, and Kritchevsky, D. *Dietary Fiber in Health and Disease*. New York: Plenum Press, 1982.

9. Murray, M T. "Diabetes mellitus." *Natural Medicine Journal*, April 1998, 5.

10. In a cross-section of U.S. adults ages 40 to 74, tested from 1988 to 1994, 33.8 percent had impaired fasting glucose (IFG), 15.4 percent had impaired glucose tolerance (IGT), and 40.1 percent had prediabetes (IGT or IFG or both). Applying these percentages to the 2000 U.S. population, about 35 million adults ages 40 to 74 would have IFG, 16 million would have IGT, and 41 million would have prediabetes.

11. Kitagawa, T, Owada, M, Urakami, T, and Yamauchi, K. "Increased incidence of non-insulin dependent diabetes mellitus among Japanese schoolchildren correlates with an increased intake of animal protein and fat." *Clin Pediatr (Phila.)*, 1998, 37: 111–15.

12. Pan American Health Organization. *Health in the Americas*. Washington, DC, 1998.

13. Stem, M P, and Mitchell, B D. "Diabetes in Hispanic Americans." In *Diabetes in America*, 2nd ed, 631–59. Washington, DC: National Institutes of Health, 1995.

14. Jackson, D Z. "Diabetes and the trash food industry." *Boston Globe*, January 11, 2006.

15. CDC, National Center for Health Statistics, Division of Health Interview Statistics. Data from the National Health Interview Survey, 2004–5. http://www.cdc.gov/nchs/data/series/sr_10/sr10_232.pdf.

16. http://www.cdc.gov/brfss/training/interviewer/01_section/09_diabetes.htm.

17. USDA. *USDA Agriculture Fact Book 2001–2002*. Washington, DC: GPO, 2002.

18. Hodgson, T A. National Center for Health Statistics, Centers for Disease Control and Prevention. Unpublished estimates. 1997. See also Herman, W H, Teutsch, S M, and Geiss, L S. "Diabetes mellitus." In *Closing the Gap: The Burden of Unnecessary Illness*, ed. Amler, R W, and Dull, H B. New York: Oxford University Press, 1987.

19. International Diabetes Federation. "Online press release, April 2005." http://www.idf.org/sites/default/files/attachments/IDF-Africa-Action -Plan-FINAL.pdf.

20. Motala, A A, Omar, M A, and Pirie, F J. "Diabetes in Africa.

Epidemiology of type 1 and type 2 diabetes in Africa." *J Cardiovasc Risk*, April 2003, 10(2): 77–83.

21. International Diabetes Federation, African Region. http://www.idf.org /sites/default/files/attachments/IDF-Africa-Action-Plan-FINAL.pdf.

22. Mokhtar, N, Elati, J, Chabir, R, Bour, A, Elkari, K, Schlossman, N P, Caballero, B, and Aguenaou, H. "Diet culture and obesity in northern Africa." *J Nutrition,* 2001, 131:887S–892S.

23. *Alternative Medicine*, February 2007, p. 64.

24. Cherewatenko, V. *The Diabetes Cure.* New York: Harper Resource, 2000, p. 13.

25. Ibid.

26. USDA. *USDA Agriculture Fact Book 2001–2002.*

27. University of Wisconsin-Milwaukee Graduate School. "Solving a diabetes mystery: Leslie Schulz is providing new insight into the high rate among Pima Indians in Arizona." http://www.uwm.edu/Dept/Grad _Sch/Publications/ResearchProfile/Archive/Vol21No1/schulz.html.

28. American Diabetes Association. "Total prevalence of diabetes and prediabetes." http://www.diabetes.org/diabetes-basics/diabetes-statistics.

29. Steinbrook, R. "Facing the diabetes epidemic: Mandatory reporting of glycosylated hemoglobin values in New York City." *New Eng J Med*, February 9, 2006, 354(6): 545–48. http://content.nejm.org/cgi/content/ full/354/6/545?ck=nck.

30. International Diabetes Federation. "Did you know?" http://www .mannkindcorp.com/Collateral/Documents/English-US /Diabetes%20Fact%20Sheet.pdf.

31. International Diabetes Federation. "The human, social, and economic impact of diabetes." http://www.positiveidcorp.com/files/Fixing_the _Black_Hole_in_Diabetes_Management.pdf.

32. McLarty, D G, Kinabo, L, and Swai, A B M. "Diabetes in tropical Africa: A prospective study, 1981–87. II. Course and prognosis." *BMJ*, 1990, 300: 1107–110.

33. Joslin, E P. *The Treatment of Diabetes Mellitus*. 4th ed. Philadelphia: Lea and Febiger, 1928, p. 384.

34. International Diabetes Federation. "The human, social, and economic impact of diabetes."

35. Centers for Disease Control and Prevention. *National Diabetes Fact Sheet*. Washington, DC: U.S. Department of Health and Human Services and the Centers for Disease Control and Prevention, 1998.

36. These estimates of the economic cost are supported by the findings in a study by the Lewin Group, Inc., for the American Diabetes Association and are 2002 estimates of both the direct (cost of medical care and services) and indirect costs (costs of short-term and permanent disability and of premature death) attributable to diabetes.

37. Stein, R. "A regular soda a day boosts weight gain: Non-diet drinks also increase risk of diabetes, study shows." *Washington Post*, August 25, 2004. http://www.washingtonpost.com/wp-dyn/articles /A29434-2004Aug24.html.

38. McVitamins. "High-fructose corn syrup." http://www.mcvitamins.com /high-fructose-corn-syrup.htm.

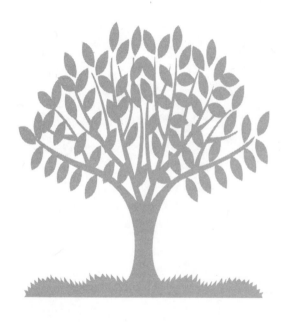

Diabetic Lifestyle Habits
and Risk Factors

When we break the natural laws, they break us. In this chapter, you are going to read about some things that you may hold dear as part of what you see as your lifestyle identity. It is very important that you acknowledge the healthy part of yourself that does not want diabetes, or the diet and lifestyle that created it, to be your life experience anymore. Letting go of diabetogenic lifestyle habits is part of the healing process; it includes any attachment one may have had to the diabetic identity that one may be carrying. "My precious burdens," Walt Whitman said, "My precious burdens I carry them wherever I go."

What we will investigate now are our precious burdens, and in Chapter 4, I will discuss life practices that will help us let go of these and to create a Culture of Life lifestyle that activates the best things possible for us as individuals. If you are having any doubt as you read this book cover to cover, see the client results in Chapter 4. What you will see is the reality that you want for yourself, for your family, and for society. Hold in your mind the potential that you can be one of the healthiest, most vibrant people you know. I am going to guide you to achieving just that. With this in mind, let's look at these diabetes-creating lifestyle patterns that need to be transformed to help reverse and prevent Type-2 diabetes and/or the chronic diabetes degenerative syndrome (CDDS).

Risk factors associated with the Culture of Death are listed as follows. We'll look at them one by one in this chapter, along with other issues of diabetes such as accelerated aging, genetics, diabetes in children, insulin resistance, gestational diabetes, Alzheimer's associated diabetes, and cancer associations. The personal lifestyle habits, choices, and predisposing diseases that are diabetogenic include:

- Inactivity, especially television watching
- Overweight and obesity—including the causal behaviors of

eating a processed-cooked-pasteurized-irradiated food diet,
having a high-glycemic and high-insulin index diet, eating a
low-fiber diet, eating meat, and ingesting food-borne envi-
ronmental toxicity (including that found in fish)
- Dairy and meat consumption
- High-stress lifestyle and hypertension
- Candida
- Depression
- Metabolic syndrome (Syndrome X)
- Toxicity of heavy metals and drinking water
- Vaccinations
- Caffeinated beverages
- Smoking

Inactivity

According to the U.S. Centers for Disease Control (CDC), 37.7 percent
of diabetics report being physically inactive. Inactivity promotes Type-2
diabetes and even increases insulin needs in Type-1 by not access-
ing the benefit of special proteins that transport glucose into the cells.
Essentially, exercise works like taking an insulin shot because it reduces
blood glucose levels. Working your muscles more often and making
them work harder improves their ability to use insulin and absorb glucose. This puts less stress on your insulin-making pancreatic beta cells.

A new theory on how exercise serves to work like insulin stems from
information that there are special proteins called GLUT-4 transporters
that usher glucose into the muscle cells. Exercise causes GLUT-4 transporters to rise to the surface of the cellular membrane, where they can
shuttle circulating glucose into the cell, increasing insulin sensitivity
and decreasing insulin needs. Findings from the Nurses' Health Study
and Health Professionals Follow-Up Study suggest that walking briskly
for a half hour every day reduces the risk of developing Type-2 diabetes
by 30 percent. The benefits of exercise, with suggestions and data, will
be presented at greater length in Chapter 3.

Television Programming

Let's look at television watching specifically. A study by the American Diabetes Association followed 41,811 men ages 40 to 75 over a 10-year period. A direct association was observed between television watching and risk of developing diabetes. The men who reported sitting in front of a television more than 19 hours per week were more than 150 percent more likely to become diabetic than those who watched less than three hours a week. "Bubble gum for the eyes," Steve Allen called it. Television watching is another form of inactivity, and as was just pointed out, increasing evidence suggests that exercise is protective against the development of Type-2 diabetes mellitus.

Every two hours per week you spend watching television instead of pursuing something more active increases the chances of developing diabetes by 14 percent.[1]

Overweight and Obesity

It is important to understand overweight and obesity, taken together or separately, as a reflection of the Culture of Death diet and lifestyle, as an underlying cause of insulin resistance and diabetes, and as a Culture of Death lifestyle association that may be associated with television watching as well. Data from the CDC shows that among diabetics, 82.1 percent are overweight or obese, and 48.1 percent are obese based on self-reported height and weight. Overweight or obesity is a precondition for many of the preventable causes of death now experienced in the developed world. A special report in the *New England Journal of Medicine* found that obesity is now such a significant factor that "it is larger than the negative effect of all accidental deaths combined (e.g., accidents, homicide, and suicide), and there is reason to believe that it will rapidly approach and could exceed the negative effect that ischemic heart disease or cancer has on life expectancy."[2] They continue: "From our analysis of the effect of obesity on longevity, we conclude that the steady rise in life expectancy during the past two centuries may soon come to an end."

Let's look at some of the theoretical underlying causes of overweight and obesity.

Processed, Cooked, Pasteurized, and Irradiated Food

There is no necessity to sell out our health and shorten our lives so that someone else can profit from marketing longer-shelf-life, so-called "convenience foods." To continue to eat these foods is to reaffirm membership in the Culture of Death.

When you cook food, according to the Max Planck Institute, you coagulate 50 percent of the food's protein. Other research shows that 60–70 percent of vitamins and minerals and up to 95–100 percent of phytonutrients are destroyed when food is cooked. Processing, cooking, pasteurization, and irradiation are all food-handling methods that destroy the antidiabetogenic qualities of our foods given to us in their natural state. Because of these processes that destroy the nutritional value of the food by at least 50 percent, we end up needing to eat more food to get the nutritional value that we would have gotten with the uncooked food in its whole state. This additional eating leads to overweight. This has significant implications for why we use a nutrient-dense live-foods diet, as discussed in Chapter 4. In addition, the junk-food diet fills us with empty calories, leaving us more hungry and further craving food.

For example, to make this point crystal clear, shopping in the center aisles of the supermarket (where the processed foods are) can create diabetes. Adam Drewnowski, an obesity researcher at the University of Washington, wanted to figure out why it is that the most reliable predictor of obesity in America is a person's low economic status. Drewnowski gave himself a hypothetical dollar to spend, using it to purchase as many calories as he could. He discovered that he could buy the most calories per dollar in the middle aisles of the supermarket, among the towering canyons of processed food and soft drinks. Drewnowski found that a dollar could buy 1,200 calories of cookies or potato chips but only 250 calories of carrots; that his dollar bought 875 calories of soda but only 170 calories of orange juice.[3] This is a possible insight into why people of low economic means have the highest rates of diabetes in Western cultures.

Going deeper into the psychospiritual level, as we contrast the Culture of Death with the Culture of Life, it is my teaching that "there is never enough food for the hungry soul." The Culture of Death creates a hungry, empty soul experience, which we try to fill with food as a substitute for love and connection. The Culture of Life fills our souls with love.

Glycemic Index and Insulin Index

A high-glycemic diet is one that includes any white sugar, any white flour, white rice, honey, maple syrup, alcohol, wheat, any junk food, fruit juices, and most fruit (except berries, cherries, lemons, limes, and grapefruit, which are relatively low on the glycemic index). A high-glycemic diet also includes cooked beets and carrots, rutabaga, summer squash, cooked yams, pumpkin, parsnips, and white potatoes, as well as apricots, figs, grapes, raisins, melons, mangos, bananas, papaya, pears, peaches, plums, pineapple, sapote, cherimoya, rambutan, durian, dates, and dried fruits. All fruit juices, carrot juice, and beet juice are also high-glycemic foods. High insulin index foods, which are low on the glycemic index but still moderately diabetogenic, include meat, fish, chicken, and dairy.

I recommend against eating fruit for three to six months until the fasting blood sugar (FBS) stabilizes at 100 or below, and then only low-glycemic fruit such as berries, cherries, citrus, cranberries, and an occasional green apple.

Low Fiber

Fiber is the part of the plant that cannot be digested or absorbed by the body. It is a carbohydrate that is obtained from vegetables, fruits, nuts, and seeds. Fiber is either water soluble or water insoluble. Water-soluble fiber is especially good for people with diabetes because it delays the pace at which food passes through the stomach. This allows a slower rate of absorption of glucose into the bloodstream, which reduces the glycemic roller coaster. It also improves insulin sensitivity, combating insulin resistance and helping insulin do its job of ushering glucose into the cells.

According to Dr. Julian Whitaker, MD,

One of the earlier studies demonstrating the power of dietary fiber in the treatment of diabetes was conducted by Perla M. Miranda, RD, MS, and David L. Horwitz, MD, PhD, FACp, and published in the *Annals of Internal Medicine* in 1978. Each of eight subjects who had insulin-dependent diabetes consumed either 20 grams of dietary fiber per day in the form of high-fiber bread or a mere 3 grams of fiber. All other factors of the diet were kept constant, as was the patients' insulin dosage. On the low-fiber intake, the average blood glucose level of the patients was 169.4 mg/dl. During the period of higher fiber intake, the mean blood sugar level was 120.8 mg/dl.[4]

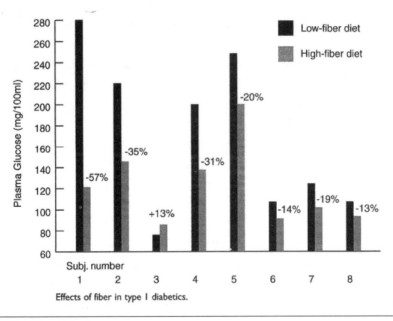

FIGURE 1. Effects of fiber in Type-1 diabetics (Source: Julian Whitaker, *Reversing Diabetes*, p. 116)

High Animal Fat: Meat Eating

A quarter pound of beef raises insulin levels in diabetics as much as a quarter pound of straight sugar.

Diabetes Care **7, 1984, p. 465**

Cheese and beef elevate insulin levels higher than "dreaded" high-carbohydrate foods like pasta.

American Journal of Clinical Nutrition **50, 1997, p. 1264**

A single burger's worth of beef, or three slices of cheddar cheese, boost insulin levels more than almost two cups of cooked pasta.

American Journal of Clinical Nutrition **50, 1997, p. 1264**

We have been hinting that a successful reversal of diabetes takes us back to high-enzyme live food and unprocessed food, which is part of the Culture of Life. This is a diet similar to what the human organism has been eating for perhaps 3.2 million years. A shift happened about 10,000 years ago, when farming and herding came into the forefront of the tribal cultures and we began to switch to a grain-based and herding civilization. Herding meant the introduction (for the first time in human history) of high amounts of flesh food and grain into the diet regularly. Before that, the human species did not eat a lot of meat. According to Robert Leakey, one of the leading medical anthropologists in the world, the human diet was primarily a plant-source "chimpanzee" diet with an occasional mouse or rat. Through simple logic, one can see that a brown bear is clearly more carnivorous than a human by looking at its claws and teeth, and yet a brown bear eats a diet of 95–97 percent raw plant food. The longest-living Hunza people of northern Pakistan live on a diet that contains less than 1 percent meat. Consider that between 1840 and 1974, the quantity of meat eaten per person in the United States increased five times over. During roughly the same time, the United States went from being the healthiest nation in world in 1900, out of 100 surveyed, to "dead" last in 1990.[5]

The diet that historically and currently has been best for health and prevention of Type-2 diabetes, as well as my newly defined CDDS, is one that is medium-to-low complex carbohydrate, non-animal-fat or protein, moderate plant fat, moderate protein, low-insulin producing, and high in fiber. In World War II, Professor H. P. Himsworth noted that when food shortages removed the white flour, white sugar, and excessive meat protein and fats from the typical British diet, the death rate from diabetes fell 50 percent.

Studies have shown that Seventh-Day Adventist men who ate meat six or more days a week had 3.8 times greater risk of having diabetes mentioned on the death certificate as compared with those Seventh-Day Adventists who were lacto-ovo vegetarians.[6] However, the unexpected finding was that 20 years prior, at the outset of the study, those who were nondiabetic were more apt to get diabetes if they were customarily in the habit of consuming meat.

In *The China Study*, T. Colin Campbell, PhD, relates a study that measured diets and diabetes in a population of Japanese American men in Washington State. These men, sons of Japanese immigrants to the

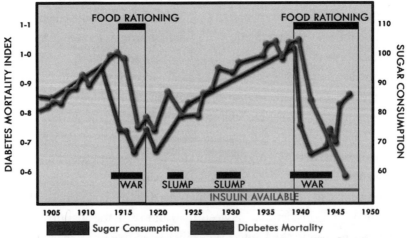

England and Wales. Diabetic Mortality indices. The figures for 1946 and 1947 supplied by Dr. Percy Stocks. Drawn by Thomas L. Cleave in *The Saccharine Disease*.

United States, remarkably had more than four times t,
diabetes than the average rate found in similar-age me,
Japan. For Japanese Americans, the ones who develope
ate the most animal protein and animal fat, each of which ˌ ˌnu
in animal-based foods.[7] These second-generation Japanese Americans
ate a meatier diet with less plant-based food than men born in Japan.
The researchers wrote, "Apparently, the eating habits of Japanese men
living in the United States resemble more the American eating style
than the Japanese." The consequence: four times as much incidence
of diabetes.[8]

The benefits and safety of a plant-source-only diet has been scientifically recognized by the American Dietetic Association (ADA), the
world's largest organization of professional dieticians, published the
following statements in June 2003 on a vegetarian diet and lifestyle:

> Vegetarians have been reported to have lower body mass indices than
> nonvegetarians, as well as lower rates of death from ischemic heart dis-
> ease; vegetarians also show lower blood cholesterol levels; lower blood
> pressure; and lower rates of hypertension, type 2 diabetes, and prostate
> and colon cancer. Well-planned vegan and other types of vegetarian
> diets are appropriate for all stages of the life cycle, including during
> pregnancy, lactation, infancy, childhood and adolescence.
>
> Vegetarian diets offer a number of nutritional benefits. It is the
> position of the American Dietetic Association and Dietitians of Canada
> that appropriately planned vegetarian diets are healthful, nutritionally
> adequate, and provide health benefits in the prevention and treatment
> of certain diseases.[9]

Meat eating is diabetogenic on all accounts, and meat is by no means
an ideal food or protein source for humans. Meat eating creates the preconditions for diabetes and accelerates the complications of the condition once it has manifested. Research cited in *Spiritual Nutrition* shows
that meat protein may even increase insulin resistance, a precondition
for diabetes and the diabetic degenerative process. Let's investigate the
negative aspects of meat eating and consider whether these realities

should be included or excluded from a Culture of Life antidiabetogenic diet and lifestyle designed to completely reverse diabetes.

According to T. Colin Campbell, PhD, numerous studies have shown that vegetarians and vegans are slimmer than their meat-eating counterparts. People in these studies who are vegetarian or vegan are anywhere from 5 to 30 pounds slimmer than their fellow citizens.[10, 11, 12, 13, 14, 15, 16]

Cardiovascular disease is significantly higher in meat eaters. In 1961, the American Medical Association (AMA) stated that 97 percent of heart disease would be eliminated if people gave up eating meat and ate a vegetarian diet.

Udo Erasmus reports in his book *Fats That Heal, Fats That Kill* that several species of fish actually contain toxic fats and oils. An example is the toxic cetoleic fatty acid, found in herring, capelin, menhaden, anchovetta, and even in cod liver oil!

Younger women who regularly eat red meat appear to face an increased risk for a common form of breast cancer, according to a large, well-known Harvard study of women's health published in the *Archives of Internal Medicine* (November 2006). The study of more than 90,000 women found that the more red meat the women consumed in their 20s, 30s, and 40s, the greater their risk for developing breast cancer fueled by hormones in the next 12 years. Those who consumed the most red meat had nearly twice the risk of those who ate red meat infrequently.[17]

Men whose mothers had a low beef intake, compared to men whose mothers with high beef intake, were more virile. Sons of mothers with low beef consumption had sperm concentrations 24.3 percent higher than those of high-beef-consumption mothers. Eighteen percent of sons of mothers with high beef consumption had sperm levels lower than what the World Health Organization considers the lower limit of subfertility; this rate of infertility was three times higher than sons of mothers with low beef consumption. Extrapolating, there are two theoretical potentials: sons of vegan mothers are more virile, and vegan men are more virile. This may seem paradoxical in that beef is a yang (male energy) food, but current agricultural practices involve much feminizing estrogen being added to the cattle intake.

Research has also shown that removing meat from your diet and eating a plant-sourced diet can reduce or eliminate asthma. Thirty-five patients who had suffered from bronchial asthma for an average of 12 years, all receiving long-term medication—20 including cortisone— were put on a plant-source-only diet for one year. In almost all cases, medication was able to be withdrawn or drastically reduced. There was a significant decrease in asthma symptoms. Twenty-four patients (69 percent) fulfilled the treatment. Of these, 71 percent reported improvement at four months and 92 percent at one year.[18]

Osteoporosis is significantly higher in meat eaters or even women who drink three or more glasses of milk per day. Research suggests that the higher amounts of protein in these animal source foods create an acidity that forces the bones to give up calcium to neutralize the acidity. The high phosphorus content in meat also pulls calcium from the bones. In essence, from the perspective of health and diabetes in particular, animal-flesh-sourced protein—fish included—is inferior to vegetable protein as a quality protein source.

According to the Max Planck Institute, cooking coagulates approximately 50 percent of the protein, making the food less digestible, more coarse, and more inflammatory. In essence, cooking meat protein creates a situation in which one actually gets only one-half the protein that is eaten, while the other coagulated half acts as an inflammatory toxin.

The best and most assimilable sources of protein are the algaes, such as spirulina or blue-green algae (which are about 60–70 percent protein and 95 percent assimilable protein); as compared to eggs (which are 44 percent assimilable); meat, chicken, and fish (which are approximately 16–18 percent assimilable); nuts and seeds (which are roughly 20–30 percent protein); and bee pollen (which is 20 percent highly assimilable protein). Other examples of moderate-protein live foods are greens, grains, beans, and avocado, olives, all sprouts (including sprouted grains and beans), green vegetables (especially spinach, watercress, arugula, kale, broccoli, brussels sprouts, collard greens, and parsley), powdered grasses, and green superfood powders.

Environmental Toxicity in Foods Is Linked to Increased Rates of Diabetes

Animals concentrate plant foods to form their tissues. And if there is toxicity in their air, water, and/or food environment—such as chemicals, pesticides, herbicides, larvicides, fungicides, detergents, bleaches, toxic solvents—then these toxins accumulate in the animal. Dairy products contain approximately five-and-a-half times as many pesticides as commercial fruits and vegetables as well as at least 15 times higher radioactive particles. And flesh foods, such as beef, fish or chicken, which are higher up on the food chain, contain 15 times as many pesticide residues as commercial fruits and vegetables and up to 30 times more radioactive particles such as I-131 (and other radioactive particles such as released from Fukashima) and depleted uranium (contained in weapons used by at least 17 nations).

From a practical point of view, eating fish is potentially dangerous because of the widespread, ever-increasing pollution of the waters of the world as well as the recent ongoing radioactive contamination from Fukushima of the ocean waters (directly) and fresh waters (indirectly through the air). The biggest water contaminants are PCBs and mercury. PCBs, along with dioxin, DDT, and dieldrin, are among the most toxic chemicals on the planet. According to John Culhane, in his 1980 article "PCBs: The Poisons That Won't Go Away," only a few parts per billion of these substances can cause cancer and birth defects in lab animals.[19] The tenth annual Council on Environmental Quality, sponsored by the U.S. government, reported PCBs in 100 percent of all human sperm samples. According to a *Washington Post* article in 1979, PCBs are considered one of the main reasons that the average sperm count of the American male is approximately 70 percent of what it was 30 years ago. This same article also points out that 25 percent of college students were sterile at the time as compared to 0.5 percent 35 years earlier. Most toxicity experts agree that the main source of human contamination comes from eating fish from waters in which the PCB levels are high, which today can be almost anywhere. The Environmental Protection Agency estimates that fish can accumulate up to nine million times the level of PCBs in the water in which they live. PCBs have been found in fish from the deepest and most remote parts of the world's oceans.

Fish and shellfish are natural accumulators of toxins because they live and are flushed by the water in which they dwell. Shellfish such as oysters, clams, mussels, and scallops filter 10 gallons of water every hour. In a month, an oyster will accumulate toxins at concentrations that are 70,000 times greater than the water they are living in. The dietary pollution problem isn't solved by not eating fish—after all, half the world's fish catch is fed to livestock. According to *Diet for a New America* by John Robbins, more fish are consumed by U.S. livestock than by the entire human population of all the countries in Western Europe. Periodic testing in the United States has found eggs and chickens highly contaminated with PCBs after being fed fish contaminated with PCBs.

Mercury toxicity from ingesting fish is another well-known source of illness. Two forms of mercury are the most dangerous: quicksilver mercury and methylmercury, which is about 50 times more toxic. Although there is general agreement that mercury in plants is a less toxic form, experts do not agree on whether the mercury in fish is stored primarily in the form of the more toxic methylmercury. In any case, children and adults who ate fish from mercury-contaminated waters in Minamata Bay, Japan, in 1953, along the Agano River in Niigata, Japan, in 1962, and other locations in Iraq, Pakistan, and Guatemala, all have suffered death, coma, or a variety of brain and neurological damages.

Researchers in Taiwan say they have established for the first time that the mercury compound present as a contaminant in some seafood can damage the insulin-producing cells in the pancreas. In their experiments, Shing-Hwa Liu and colleagues exposed cell cultures of insulin-producing beta cells to methylmercury. They used concentrations of methylmercury at about the same levels as people would consume in fish under the U.S. Food and Drug Administration's recommended limits.[20]

Contamination of fish is widespread. According to Rudolph Ballentine, MD, mercury toxicity is being reported with increasing frequency by physicians as well as dentists. The two main contributing factors seem to be a diet high in fish and the common use of silver-mercury amalgams for dental work. Fish consumption alone may be enough to cause mercury toxicity. An article by the Canadian Medical Association in 1976 reported that Indians in Northern Canada, who ate more than a pound of fish per day, had symptoms of mercury poisoning. A 1985 study in West Germany of 136 people who regularly consumed fish from the Elbe River found a correlation between the blood levels of both mercury and pesticides and the amount of fish eaten.

In a study published in the *Diet and Nutrition Letter* of Tufts University, it was reported that the more fish pregnant mothers ate from Lake Michigan, the more their babies showed abnormal reflexes, general weakness, slower responses to external stimuli, and various signs of depression. They found that mothers eating fish only two or three times a month produced babies weighing seven to nine ounces less at birth and with smaller heads.[21] Jacobsen, in a 1986 follow-up study reported in *Child Development*, found that there was a definite correlation between the amount of fish the mothers ate and the child's brain development, even if fish was eaten only once a month. He found that the more fish the pregnant mothers ate, the lower was the verbal IQ of the children.[22] These children also had lower SAT scores 17 to 18 years later. Children are usually the most sensitive to toxins, and they are prime indicators of what may be happening to adults on a more subtle level. A Swedish study in 1983 found that the milk of nursing mothers who regularly ate fatty fish from the Baltic Sea had higher levels of PCBs and pesticide residues than even meat eaters. Lactovegetarians were found to have the lowest pesticide residues in this study, as compared to flesh-food consumers.

Dairy Consumption

> For everyone who lives on milk, being still an infant, is
> unskilled in the word of righteousness. But solid food is for
> the mature, for those whose faculties have been trained by
> practice to distinguish good from evil.
>
> **Hebrews 5:13–14**

Children with diabetic genetic tendencies who drink cow's milk have an 11 to 13 times higher rate of juvenile diabetes than children who are breastfed by their own mothers for at least three months. Although many are not aware of it, as just stated, milk consumption is directly associated with juvenile diabetes. In 1994, the American Academy of Pediatrics decided, based on this data, to strongly encourage families with a diabetic history not to give their children cow's milk or cow's milk products for at least two years. The key to understanding this is that there are more than 100 antigens found in milk. According to a 1999 study reported in the journal *Diabetes* by Outi Vaarala, researchers found up to eight times the number of antibodies against milk protein in dairy-product-consuming children who also developed juvenile diabetes.[23] Finland, which has the world's highest milk consumption, also has the world's highest per capita rate of insulin-dependent Type-1 diabetes.[24] The problem is that the antibodies to the milk antigens cross-react with the beta cells of the pancreas, creating inflammation, beta cell destruction, and scarring. This consequently blocks or destroys beta cell production of insulin.

This is not new information. In 1992, the *New England Journal of Medicine* reported a study done in Finland on children ages 4 to 12. They measured the antibodies in these children against BSA (bovine serum albumin). Of the 142 children with juvenile diabetes, every single one had an antibody titer greater that 3.55 and not one of the 79 nondiabetic children had an antibody titer greater than 3.55. The complete lack of overlap of serum antibodies of these two populations lead to some very productive studies in understanding the relationship of cow's milk intake and incidence of juvenile diabetes. One study in Chile[25] found that genetically susceptible children who were weaned too early onto cow's milk—before three months of age—had a risk factor for juvenile diabetes of 13.1 times greater than children who did not have a genetic proclivity or who were breastfed for at least three months. Another significant study in the United States[26] found that children with a genetic tendency who were weaned onto cow's milk before three months had a Type-1 diabetes incidence 11.3 times greater than those who did not have a genetic tendency and who were breastfed for at least three months. The general statistical view is that anything more than three to four times higher is considered a significant finding.

Charting the degree of milk consumption from birth to age 14 against the onset of Type-1 diabetes reveals the correlation between milk consumption and Type-1 diabetes.[27] It is no accident that Japanese children, who have the lowest milk consumption, have 1/36th the incidence of Type-1 diabetes than do the children from Finland, who had the highest consumption of milk.

CHART 9.3: ASSOCIATION OF COW'S MILK CONSUMPTION AND INCIDENCE OF TYPE 1 DIABETES IN DIFFERENT COUNTRIES

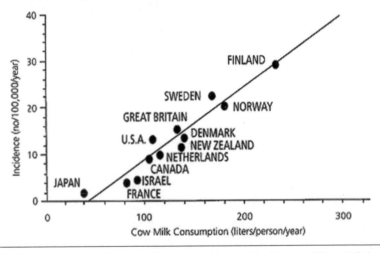

FIGURE 2. Association of cow's milk consumption and incidence of Type-1 diabetes in different countries (Source: T. Colin Campbell, *The China Study*)

When the data for both the genetically susceptible and nonsusceptible are merged, there is an increased risk for children who are weaned and put on cow's milk before three months of approximately 1.5 times, which is approximately a 50 percent increase in incidence of Type-1 diabetes. One additional study in Finland showed that the consumption of cow's milk increased the rate of Type-1 diabetes by 500–600 percent.[28]

The overall results strongly suggest that cow's milk, especially in children who are genetically susceptible and who are weaned before three months, significantly increases the risk of developing Type-1 diabetes. Milk consumption leads to many other health and spiritual problems.

Allergies and Lactose Intolerance

Cow's milk is the number one cause of food allergies among infants and children, according to the American Gastroenterological Association.[29] Most people begin to produce less lactase, the enzyme that helps with the digestion of milk, when they are as young as two years old. This reduction can lead to lactose intolerance.[30] Millions of Americans are lactose intolerant, and an estimated 90 percent of Asian Americans and 75 percent of Native Americans and African Americans suffer from the condition, which can cause bloating, gas, cramps, vomiting, headaches, rashes, and asthma.[31] Studies have also found that autism and schizophrenia in children may be linked to the body's inability to digest the milk protein casein. Symptoms of these diseases diminished or disappeared in 80 percent of the children who were switched to milk-free diets.[32] A UK study showed that people who were suffering from irregular heartbeats, asthma, headaches, fatigue, and digestive problems "showed marked and often complete improvements in their health after cutting milk from their diets."[33]

Osteoporosis

Walter Willett is chairman of the Nutrition Department at the Harvard School of Public Health and coauthored a major study of more than 75,000 American nurses, which found that women with the highest calcium consumption from dairy products actually had substantially more fractures than women who drank less milk. Citing a 1980 study in the journal *Clinical Orthopedics and Related Research*, Mark Hegsted of Harvard University makes the point that people in the United States and Scandinavian countries consume more dairy products than anywhere else in the world, yet they have the highest rates of osteoporosis.[34] As pointed in out in *Conscious Eating* and the *American Journal of Clinical Nutrition*, there is a problem of excessive protein in the diet. This excessive animal protein creates acidity and a high phosphorus content that pulls calcium out of the bones and therefore is a plausible explanation for why those with the highest dairy intake have the highest rates of osteoporosis. A 1985 study in *The American Journal of Clinical Nutrition* suggests that dairy products offer no protection against osteoporosis, probably due to the high protein content of milk.[35]

The bottom line is that calcium deficiency is not a threat to someone eating a plant-source-only cuisine. In fact, inadequate calcium intake appears not to be a problem at all. A scholarly review of the subject in the *Postgraduate Medical Journal* in 1976 revealed that calcium deficiency caused by an insufficient amount of calcium in the diet is not known to occur in humans at all.[36]

Cancers

The general world research, in almost all categories of cancers, suggest that the consumption of flesh food and dairy are associated with higher rates of the main cancers, such as breast, colon, prostate, pancreatic, lymphatic, and ovarian cancers. Plant-source proteins, occurring lower on the food chain, seem to have a lower correlation with cancer. *The China Study* makes the correlation that the people who ate the most plant-based foods were the healthiest and tended to have the least amount of chronic disease. More important, they discovered this by using the findings of other researchers and clinicians worldwide, as the plant-source-only diet has time and again been shown to reverse and/or prevent chronic diseases thought to be activated by high animal-protein consumption.[37]

Lymphoma

In Norway, 15,914 individuals were followed for 11-and-a-half years. Those drinking two or more glasses of milk per day had 3.5 times the incidence of cancer of the lymphatic organs.[38] One of the more thoughtful articles on this subject is from Allan S. Cunningham of Cooperstown, New York, writing in *The Lancet*, November 27, 1976 (page 1184), in an article entitled "Lymphomas and Animal-Protein Consumption." Cunningham tracked the beef and dairy consumption in terms of grams per day for a one-year period, 1955–56, in 15 countries. New Zealand, United States, and Canada had the highest consumption, respectively. The lowest meat and dairy consumption was in Japan. The difference between the highest and lowest was nearly 30-fold: 43.8 grams/day for New Zealanders versus 1.5 for Japan. Cunningham found a highly significant positive correlation between deaths from lymphomas and beef and dairy ingestion in the 15 countries analyzed. The reason for the role of dairy is that the dairy intake creates a chronic immunological stress that tends to cause lymphomas in laboratory animals and also possibly in humans. We know that ingestion of cow's milk can produce generalized lymphopathy, swollen liver, swollen spleen, and significant adenoid hypertrophy. It can be hypothesized that meat protein adds its general carcinogenic effect to the specific carcinogenic effect on the lymph from dairy.

Ovarian Cancer

Drinking more than one glass of milk a day, or its equivalent, has been shown to give women a 3.1 times greater risk of ovarian cancer than nonmilk drinkers. Harvard Medical School did a study and analyzed data from 27 different countries, to find the same increased amount of ovarian cancer associated with dairy.

A positive relationship between ovarian cancer and dairy products was first reported in *The Lancet* by D. W. Cramer et al. in 1989, when it was suggested that lactose consumption may be a dietary risk factor for ovarian cancer.[39] More recently, data collected from the Harvard Nurses

Health Study was used to assess the lactose, milk, and milk product consumption in relation to ovarian cancer risk in more than 80,000 women. Over 16 years of follow-up, 301 cases of one particular type of ovarian cancer were confirmed in this study group. Results showed that women who consumed the most lactose had twice the risk of this type of ovarian cancer than women who drank the least lactose. It was suggested that galactose (a component of lactose) may damage ovarian cells, making them more susceptible to cancer.[40]

In 2004, Susanna Larsson and colleagues of the Karolinska Institute in Stockholm, Sweden, published a study[41] in the *American Journal of Clinical Nutrition* that examined the association between the intake of dairy products and lactose and the risk of ovarian cancer. In this study of 61,084 women, ages 38 to 76, the diet was assessed over three years. After 13.5 years, 266 participants had been diagnosed with ovarian cancer. Results showed that women consuming four or more servings of dairy a day had double the risk of ovarian cancer, compared to those consuming low or no dairy. Milk was the dairy product with the strongest positive association with ovarian cancer.

Lung Cancer

A study by Curtis Mettlin, funded by the American Cancer Society and cited in the *International Journal of Cancer*, April 15, 1989, showed that people drinking three or more glasses of whole milk a day had a twofold increase in lung cancer.[42]

Breast and Prostate Cancers

The journal *Cancer* in 1989 reported that men drinking three or more glasses a day of whole milk were shown to have a 2.49 times increase in prostate cancer.[43] A 2001 Harvard review of the research put a finer point on it:

> Twelve of . . . fourteen case-control studies and seven of . . . nine cohort studies [have] observed a positive association for some measure of dairy products and prostate cancer; this is one of the most consistent dietary predictors for prostate cancer in the published literature

[italics added]. In these studies, men with the highest dairy intakes had approximately double the risk of total prostate cancer, and up to a fourfold increase in risk of metastatic or fatal prostate cancer relative to low consumers.[44]

We see this data corroborated in world data for breast and prostate cancer rates in China, Japan, England, Scotland, and Canada (by the International Agency for Research), and in the United States (by the Surveillance Epidemiology and End Results Program of the National Cancer Institute). Figure 3 illustrates that the lowest rates of breast and prostate cancer are consistently in China and Japan, where dairy and animal meat are rarely consumed. As Jane Plant, PhD, remarks in *The No Dairy Breast Cancer Prevention Program*:

The Japanese cities of Hiroshima and Nagasaki have similar rates of breast cancer: and remember, both cities were attacked with nuclear weapons, so in addition to the usual pollution-related cancers, one would also expect to find some radiation-related cases. If, as a North American woman, one was living a Japanese lifestyle in industrialized, irradiated Hiroshima, you would slash your risk of contracting breast cancer by a half to a third. The conclusion is inescapable. Clearly, some lifestyle factor not related to pollution, urbanization, or the environment is seriously increasing the Western woman's chance of contracting breast cancer.[45]

Looking at Figure 3, one can see that a black man in the United States is 280 times more likely to develop prostate cancer than a man in rural Quidong, China, and 70 times more prone than a man in urban Tianjin, China. Plant continues: "We know . . . that whatever causes the huge difference in breast and prostate cancer rates between Eastern and Western countries, it isn't genetic. Migration studies show that when Chinese or Japanese people move to the West, within one or two generations their rates of incidence and mortality from breast and prostate cancer approach those of their host community."[46]

Over the next couple of years, Plant and her husband Peter examined the results of the China-Cornell-Oxford Project of T. Colin Campbell, and credited the fact that Easterners do not eat dairy products for

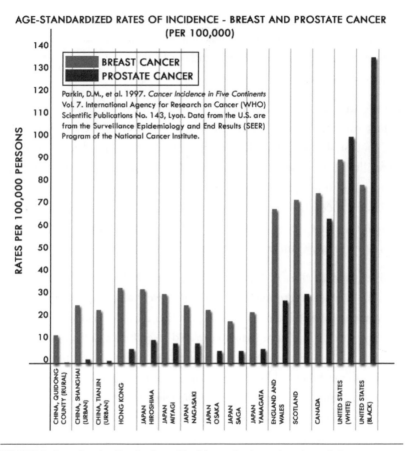

FIGURE 3. Age-standardized rates of incidence for breast and prostate cancer

their low rates of breast and prostate cancer. Pick up an Asian recipe book at the store—you'll find no mention of dairy products.

Pus Cells

One cubic centimeter (cc) of commercial cow's milk is allowed to have up to 750,000 somatic cells (common name, "pus") and 20,000 live bacteria before it is kept off the market. That amounts to a whopping 20 million live bacteria and up to 750 million pus cells per liter. According to Robert Cohen, author of *Don't Drink Your Milk*, the average liter of milk in Florida has 633 million pus cells, the highest in the nation. Montana is the lowest, with 236 million pus cells per liter. This is not a healthy thing, whether it is 236 or 633 million. Besides pus cells and blood, which are now normal in milk produced during machine suckling, the milk is also high in pesticides, herbicides, antibiotics, hormones, radioactive iodine, and disease factors such as mad cow prion and bovine leukemia virus. In addition, research cited by Robert Cohen has made the point that there is up to a gallon of extra mucus in the body created as a result of drinking dairy. The mucus problem is associated with the fact that 87 percent of milk protein is casein, the main ingredient of Elmer's Glue.

High-Stress Lifestyle and Hypertension

When the body is under stress, many hormones are released that indirectly increase insulin excretion and indirectly create insulin resistance—a precursor to a diabetic physiology. These hormones release energy in the form of glucose and fat, which is made available to the cells of the body. This provides fuel for what has been traditionally referred to as the "fight or flight" response. With stress, one sees increases in the secretion of catecholamines (adrenalin and adrenalin-like chemicals), especially from the adrenals, resulting in an increased glucose release from the liver into the blood stream, and glucocorticoid or steroid hormones secreted by the adrenal glands and growth hormone produced by the pituitary gland. Extreme stress for months at a time, as well as depression, has been known to trigger the onset of a diabetic physiology.

In the United States, 62.5 percent of adults with diabetes reported having hypertension. Hypertension is part of the basket of symptoms seen in Syndrome X, discussed later.

Candida

Candida is also commonly associated with diabetes and is a larger symptom of a Culture of Death diabetogenic diet and lifestyle. Candida is a fungal parasite that excretes toxic waste, as mycotoxins, that can get into the bloodstream and cause symptoms of bloating, clouded thinking, depression, diarrhea, exhaustion, halitosis (bad breath), menstrual pains, thrush, unclear memory recall, recurring vaginal or bladder infections, anxiety, constipation, diarrhea (or both), depression, environmental sensitivities, fatigue, feeling worse on damp or muggy days or in moldy places, food sensitivities, insomnia, low blood sugar, mood swings, premenstrual syndrome, ringing in the ears, and sensitivities to perfume, cigarettes, or fabric odors. Diets high in cooked starches (bread, baked potato, cakes, cookies, pasta) and diets loaded with refined or hybridized (seedless) fruit sugars both feed candida. Diabetes with its higher blood sugar levels makes people good candidates for candida.

My book *Rainbow Green Live-Food Cuisine* examines the pathogenic microorganism candida and how its presence in the body pushes the recycling button or "composting button" as the candida functions to recycle the organism it inhabits back to the soil. In essence, candida accelerates the rate of fermentation of the system. At the turn of the nineteenth century, candida yeast was primarily seen in people who were dying of cancer and other very serious diseases. Depending on the degree of toxicity, this composting process leads to chronic disease, misery, and ultimately death. The key to restoring health is minimizing or eliminating the toxic conditions so that the composting button is turned off. A low-sweet, live-food, nonacidic diet and healthy lifestyle are the key factors to reversing the aging-degenerative process of chronic candidiasis. The diet and lifestyle to do this is exactly the antidiabetogenic diet and lifestyle of the Culture of Life that we are outlining in this book.

Depression

According to an evaluation of 20 studies over the past 10 years, the prevalence rate of diabetics with major depression is three to four times greater than in the general population. While depression affects 3–5 percent of the population at any given time, the rate is 15–20 percent in patients with diabetes, according to the American Diabetic Association. Women in particular are at greater risk, according to other studies.[47]

For many years, it has been hypothesized that depression is a diabetic complication, which is almost certain given that the diabetogenic diet and lifestyle is the same diet and lifestyle that creates a biologically altered brain, fatty-acid and amino-acid deficiencies, and toxemia and thus gives rise to depression. More recent research, however, points to depression as a possible cause or trigger for diabetes. Researchers at Kaiser Permanente's Center for Health Research in Portland, Oregon, looked at 1,680 diabetic members of its health maintenance organization. They found that when compared with nondiabetics, those with diabetes were more likely to have been treated for depression within six months before their diabetes diagnosis. About 84 percent of those diabetics also reported a higher rate of earlier depressive episodes than those in the control group. Gregory Nichols, a Kaiser researcher who conducted the study, said the study suggests depression frequently precedes the onset of diabetes, rather than vice versa.[48]

A major study in 2004 by Johns Hopkins and other centers tracked 11,615 initially nondiabetic adults ages 48 to 67 over six years and found that "depressive symptoms predicted incident Type-2 diabetes." In prospective analyses, after adjusting for age, race, sex, and education, individuals in the highest quartile of depressive symptoms had a 63 percent increased risk of developing diabetes compared with those in the lowest quartile.[49]

The good news is that I have developed a five-step program for treating depression naturally that seems to work in about 90 percent of patients. It is detailed in my book, *Depression-Free for Life*.

Metabolic Syndrome (Syndrome X)

Syndrome X was first coined as a term by Gerald Reaven, MD, at Stanford University to describe a group of symptoms that arise from an overall metabolic disorder. These symptoms may include Type-2 diabetes, obesity with an inability to lose weight, high cholesterol, high blood pressure, ovarian cysts, high triglycerides, low HDL cholesterol, and coronary heart disease and are a major subset of CDDS. Some 655,000 people are newly diagnosed each year, and it is estimated that an equal 655,000 cases are not diagnosed. Some estimates cite some 47 million people with the basket of symptoms known as Syndrome X. A classic symptom and hint of the metabolic syndrome is the accumulation of fat in the abdomen and the inability to lose fat and weight. Dr. Simeon Margolis, coauthor of a Johns Hopkins report on Syndrome X, says that abdominal obesity is often the first outward sign of Syndrome X. It seems to be associated with insulin resistance. Some long-term studies have suggested that the higher the fasting blood insulin levels and the greater the amount of abdominal fat, the greater likelihood of death from Syndrome X.

The metabolic disorder that we've created through unnatural ways of living from the lifestyle and diet of the Culture of Death has a significant effect on people's health. Some researchers estimate that we age one-third faster when blood sugar levels are high. Some of the negative impact is related to the glycation process, in which glucose fuses with protein and lipids. It disorganizes the protein and lipid function, creating cross-linkages and disrupting the protein-lipid function in the cell membrane and enzymes. The glycation process also results in greatly increased free radical production. Untreated or even poorly managed Syndrome X and diabetes produce an accelerated aging and death process.

Syndrome X and diabetes also create a chemical change in the nerves. These changes impair the nerves' ability to transmit signals. Symptoms of nerve damage include numbness, tingling, increased sensitivity to touch, insensitivity to pain and temperature, and loss of coordination. The excess sugar also damages blood vessels that carry the oxygen and nutrients to the nerves. People with Syndrome X are more likely to develop obstruction to the arteries and therefore increased or decreased blood flow to the extremities, which creates increased rates of amputations. Up to 70 percent of people with Syndrome X have some form of nerve damage. It is even worse in smokers. Some people feel the metabolic syndrome is not reversible, but with the Dr. Cousens Diabetes Recovery Program—A Holistic Approach, I have seen a high frequency of the reversal of this syndrome, even when it has already progressed to diabetes.

Toxicity of Heavy Metals and Drinking Water

The development of insulin-dependent diabetes mellitus (IDDM) Type-2 is thought to be associated with the pathogenic interaction of environmental toxic agents with the pancreatic beta cells. It is also associated with hyperglycemia and hyperglycemic spikes, as will be explained in Chapter 5.[50]

Just as consuming organic foods is a way to avoid ingesting toxins, becoming aware of the quality of water one drinks and uses is increasingly essential in today's polluted world, since water can be a major source of toxins. According to *Diet for a Poisoned Planet* by David Steinman, less than 1 percent of the Earth's surface water is safe to drink. In some places in the United States and other countries, the term "drinking water" for tap water should be considered nothing more than a euphemism.

The water that the general public uses comes from two sources: underground sources, such as springs and wells, and surface water, such as rivers and lakes. Presently, both these sources are becoming more and more polluted as toxic chemicals, acid rain, raw sewage, agricultural herbicides, pesticide runoff, chlorination, fluoridation, sewage landfills, and radioactive wastes are either dumped into or seep into them. One of the best-known examples of toxic water pollution to date is the infamous Love Canal, where according to the *New York Times* in 1984, thousands of tons of toxic chemicals were dumped, including 60 pounds of the deadly poison dioxin.

The pollution situation is so out of control that in monitoring cancer rates in Philadelphia, one researcher was able to correlate the different rates and types of cancer in the population with the specific river the people lived near. According to Steve Meyerowitz, in his book *Water*, the Environmental Cancer Prevention Center found that residents drinking from the west side of the Schuylkill River had 67 percent more deaths from esophagus cancer than those on the east side. Those drinking from the Delaware River on the east side suffered 59 percent more deaths from cancer of the brain, 83 percent more malignant melanoma, and 32 percent more colorectal cancers than those on the west side. This is just one of many studies linking specific water pollution to an increase in cancer rates.

Medical science has discovered how sensitive the insulin receptor sites are to chemical poisoning. Metals such as cadmium, mercury, arsenic, lead, fluoride,[51] and possibly aluminum may play a role in the actual destruction of beta cells through stimulating an autoimmune reaction to them after they have bonded to these cells in the pancreas. It is because mercury[52] and lead attach themselves at highly vulnerable junctures of proteins that they find their great capacity to provoke morphological changes in the body. Changes in pancreatic function are among the pathogenetic mechanisms observable during lead intoxication.[53]

Cadmium

Cadmium, a widespread heavy metal contaminant found in air, soil, and water, can accumulate in the pancreas and exert diabetogenic effects in animals. In a large cross-sectional study, urinary cadmium levels are significantly and dose-dependently associated with both impaired fasting glucose and diabetes.[54] Such accumulations increase the likelihood of kidney damage and failure, spur free radical activity, and exacerbate neuromuscular complications of Type-2 diabetes.[55, 56, 57, 58] Cadmium sources include tap water, fungicides, marijuana, processed meat, rubber, seafood (cod, haddock, oyster, tuna), sewage, tobacco, colas (especially from vending machines), tools, welding material, evaporated milk, airborne industrial contaminants, batteries, instant coffee, incineration of tires/rubber/plastic, refined grains, soft water, galvanized pipes, dental alloys, candy, ceramics, electroplating, fertil-izers, paints, motor oil, and motor exhaust.

Mercury

Because mercury is increasingly becoming elevated in all forms of life, we can assume that more people will have some defects in pancreatic function. Pancreatic support is increasingly necessary for optimal health.

In August 2006, the American Chemical Society published research that showed conclusively that methylmercury induces pancreatic cell apoptosis and dysfunction.[59] Mercury is a well-known toxic agent that produces various types of cell and tissue damage, yet billions of people are exposed to levels of mercury harmful to pancreatic health. In the case of diabetes, mercury is especially telling, for it affects the beta cells, the insulin itself, and the insulin receptor sites, setting off a myriad of complex disturbances in glucose metabolism.[60]

Mercury leads the pack in the potency of its toxicity and in the pervasiveness of its presence in the environment through fish, air, and water, medicine through vaccines, and dentistry with dental amalgams. Some say we are all receiving, just through our air, water, and food, about a microgram of mercury a day. Sounds like a little until you calculate that a microgram contains 3,000 trillion atoms with each of them holding the potential to deactivate insulin and the receptor sites crucial to their function.[61]

Arsenic

Studies out of Taiwan and Bangladesh show that individuals who are exposed to higher amounts of arsenic—in their soil and/or drinking water—have a higher independent risk of developing Type-2 diabe-tes.[62, 63] Arsenic in tap water is common; this hormone disruptor is sus-pected of playing a role in diabetes. Arsenic interferes with the action of glucocorticoid hormones, which belong to the same family of ste-roid hormones as estrogen and progesterone. Glucocorticoids turn on many genes that help regulate blood sugar and even ward off cancer. Repeatedly drinking water containing certain amounts of arsenic has been linked to increased rates of cancer and diabetes. The underlying mechanism is now thought to be hormone disruption.[64]

Lead

Lead exposure has been associated with an increased risk of hypertension and is a well-established risk factor for kidney disease. Lead either affects blood pressure indirectly through alterations in kidney function or via more direct effects on the vasculature or neurologic blood pressure control. Researchers at Harvard Medical School state: "Our findings support the hypothesis that long-term low-level lead accumulation (estimated by tibia bone lead) is associated with an increased risk of declining renal function particularly among diabetics or hypertensives, populations already at risk for impaired renal function."[65]

Fluoride

"Fluoride in Drinking Water: A Scientific Review of EPA's Standards," made public by the National Research Council in 2006, states the following:

> The conclusion from the available studies is that sufficient fluoride exposure appears to bring about increases in blood glucose or impaired glucose tolerance in some individuals and to increase the severity of some types of diabetes. In general, impaired glucose metabolism appears to be associated with serum or plasma fluoride concentrations of about 0.1 mg/L or greater in both animals and humans. In addition, diabetic individuals will often have higher than normal water intake, and consequently, will have higher than normal fluoride intake for a given concentration of fluoride in drinking water. An estimated 26 million people in the U.S. have diabetes mellitus; therefore, any role of fluoride exposure in the development of impaired glucose metabolism or diabetes is potentially significant.[66]

Filtering Your Water

Compressed, activated, charcoal block filters are an inexpensive way to get approximately 95 percent protection from the carbon-based organic pollution, pesticides, herbicides, insecticides, PCBs (polychlorinated biphenyls), cysts, heavy metals, asbestos, VOCs (volatile organic chemicals), and THMs (trihalomethanes) in our water. They also eliminate chlorine, some fluoride, and foul odors. They do not, however, absorb inorganic mineral salts such as chloride, fluoride, sodium, nitrates, and soluble minerals. For this reason, they are best for city water systems but not for well water systems, which have a potential to be polluted with high amounts of nitrates from agricultural wastes. A concern regarding granular charcoal filters is their tendency to be a gathering ground for bacteria, yeasts, and molds, and their inability to remove pollutants found in some drinking water. Some of the more sophisticated charcoal filters do have a reverse wash system in an attempt to compensate for this. Another problem with charcoal filters is that the charcoal can break down with age or from hot water and release the contaminants back into our drinking water. The best way to avoid this is to pay attention to any change in taste, smell, or color of the water, or a reduction in water flow rate. Duane Taylor, a water expert from North Coast Waterworks in Sonoma County, California, suggested in a personal communication that the main problem with charcoal filters is that the user does not replace the filter often enough. He recommends purchasing a filter unit that will stop the flow to make the user changes the filter when its filtering capacities are used up. If one does not have such a filter, then he recommends changing the filter at 75 percent of the manufacturer's suggested lifetime. If one waits until there is a taste change, decrease in rate of flow, or smell to the water, the filter may already be dumping contaminants back into the water. Activated carbon is rated on its ability to remove iodine and phenols. The iodine number should be greater than 1,000 on the measuring scale, and the phenol number should be 15 or less. Another important consideration for carbon filter effectiveness is the contact time of water with the filter. The slower the flow rate and the more carbon there is in the filter, the better job the filter does.

Reverse osmosis (RO) is one of the best methods to get pure water without using up a lot of energy. RO units remove 97–99 percent of contaminants. They remove bacteria, viruses, nitrates, fluorides, sodium, chlorine, particulate matter, heavy metals, asbestos, organic chemicals, and dissolved minerals. They do not remove toxic gases, chloroform, phenols, THMs, some pesticides, and low-molecular-weight organic compounds. When combined with an activated carbon filtration system, however, they can remove the entire spectrum of impurities from the drinking water, including organic and inorganic chemicals. Many RO units now have pre- and postfilters to take care of any residual impurities that the RO unit does not remove.

In RO, the water to be filtered is forced through a semipermeable membrane by the moving elements from more-concentrated to less-concentrated solutions. The membrane is permeable to pure water but not to most of its impurities. If conditions are right for sufficient water pressure and the water is not excessively hard, almost no energy is needed for the operation of RO systems. A pressure pump is needed if the total dissolved solids are greater than one thousand parts per million. The water is as pure as distilled, yet it is not heated as in distilled water and therefore not destructured, which is a great advantage in one way. Sometimes a pressure pump is needed for extremely hard water, and this does require electrical energy. The main problem with an RO unit is the fragility of the semipermeable membrane. Some membranes can be destroyed by chlorinated water, highly alkaline water, or temperatures above 100°F. If the water is chlorinated, a cellulose membrane is needed. A polymer membrane can be used if the water is not chlorinated.

Some people have had the membrane break in less than the expected three years. For this reason, it is good to check the water purity regularly. Newer and stronger membranes are now available on the market, but we are still in the habit of checking the water purity every four months and/or whenever there is a change in the taste. While RO units are similar in appearance and claimed performance, there are many complex, interdependent choices regarding pretreatment, membrane selection, and posttreatment. To select a system that fits your water filtration needs and to develop the best maintenance plan, it is best to talk with someone who has in-depth knowledge of the many factors involved. If properly selected and maintained, an RO unit may be the most energy-efficient and best way to protect your water. In the past, RO units required a lot of water to work properly, which is a disadvantage, particularly during times of drought. Some of the newer models have been designed to operate with minimal water usage.

Water distillers, although generally slightly more expensive, remove up to 99.99 percent of contaminants from water, including bacteria, fluoride, nitrates, radionuclides, and/organic and inorganic toxins, as well as heavy metals such as lead, mercury, and cadmium, and soluble minerals such as calcium and magnesium. Some toxic organic compounds, such as THMs and dioxin, have a boiling point that is the same as or lower than water and therefore are not filtered out by the distillation process. The heating of the water also disrupts potential homeopathic patterns of toxins that are left in the water in reverse osmosis filtration. Some of the more expensive distillers have built-in preboiler or postboiler filters as options to eliminate this problem.

There are two major drawbacks to water distillers: One is that they are energy-intensive and relatively more expensive (unless one has a solar water distiller). The other problem is that distilled water is dead, unstructured water so foreign to the body that one actually gets a temporarily high white blood cell count in response to drinking it. It is, however, possible to revive this dead, destructured water by the use of a product called Crystal Energy, and procedures I have outlined in detail in my book *Spiritual Nutrition*. I feel that the water distiller is the safest way to approach the water toxicity problem and have outlined in detail how to reactivate distilled water in *Spiritual Nutrition*.

Vaccinations and Increased Juvenile Diabetes Rates[67]

In the May 24, 1996, *New Zealand Medical Journal*, J. Bart Classen, MD, a former researcher at the National Institutes of Health, reported a 60 percent increase in Type-1 diabetes following a massive campaign in New Zealand from 1988 to 1991 to vaccinate babies six weeks of age or older with hepatitis B vaccine. His analysis of a group of 100,000 New Zealand children followed since 1982 showed that the incidence of diabetes before the hepatitis B vaccination program began in 1988 was 11.2 cases per 100,000 children per year, while the incidence of diabetes following the hepatitis B vaccination campaign was 18.2 cases per 100,000 children per year.[68]

In the October 22, 1997, *Infectious Diseases in Clinical Practice*, Dr. Classen presented more data further substantiating his findings of a vaccine-diabetes connection. He reported that the incidence of diabetes in Finland was stable in children younger than four years of age until the government made several changes in its childhood vaccination schedule. In 1974, 130,000 children ages three months to four years were enrolled in a vaccine experimental trial and injected with hepatitis B vaccine or meningococcal vaccine. Then, in 1976, the pertussis vaccine used in Finland was made stronger by adding a second strain of bacteria. According to the National Vaccine Information Center's (NVIC) report, "Juvenile Diabetes and Vaccination: New Evidence for a Connection," during the years 1977–79, there was a 64 percent increase in the incidence of Type-1 diabetes in Finland compared to the years 1970–76.[69]

Doctors started reporting in the medical literature as early as 1949 that some children injected with pertussis (whooping cough) vaccine (now part of the DPT or DTaP shot) were having trouble maintaining normal glucose levels in their blood. Lab research has confirmed that pertussis vaccine can cause diabetes in mice.

As diabetes research progressed in the 1960s, 1970s, and 1980s, there were observations that viral infections may be a cofactor in causing diabetes. The introduction of live virus vaccines, such as the live MMR (measles, mumps, rubella) vaccine made from weakened forms of the live measles, mumps, and rubella viruses, has raised questions about whether live vaccine virus could be a cofactor in causing chronic auto-immunological diseases such as Type-1 diabetes.

In 1982, another vaccine was added to the childhood vaccination schedule in Finland. Children ages 14 months to 6 years were given the live MMR vaccine. This was followed by the injection of 114,000

Finnish children three months and older with another experimental Hib vaccine. In 1988, Finland recommended that all babies be injected with the hepatitis B vaccine.

The introduction of these new vaccines in Finland was followed by a 62 percent rise in the incidence of diabetes in the zero-to-four-years age group and a 19 percent rise of diabetes in the five-to-nine-years age group between the years 1980 and 1982 and 1987 and 1989. As shown in the NVIC report, Classen concluded,

> The net effect was the addition of three new vaccines to the 0–4 year old age group, and a 147 percent increase in the incidence of IDDM. The addition of one new vaccine to the 5–9 year olds resulted in a 40 percent rise in diabetes incidence. With no new vaccines added to the 10 to 14 year olds, a rise in the incidence of IDDM was seen by only 8 percent between the intervals 1970–1976 and 1990–1992. The rise in IDDM in the different age groups correlated with the number of vaccines given.[70]

The CDC published data supporting a link between timing of immunization and the development of diabetes.[71] The data from the CDC's preliminary study supports published data that immunization starting after two months is associated with an increased risk of Type-1 diabetes. The U.S. government study showed that hepatitis B immunization starting after two months was associated with an almost doubling of the risk of IDDM Type-1.

Caffeinated Beverages

Researchers at Queen's University in Ontario investigated the effect of caffeine ingestion on insulin sensitivity in sedentary lean men and obese men with and without Type-2 diabetes. They also examined whether chronic exercise (a three-month aerobic exercise program) influences the relationship between caffeine and insulin sensitivity in these individuals. Their results showed that caffeine ingestion was associated with a significant reduction in insulin sensitivity by a similar magnitude in the lean (33 percent), obese (33 percent), and diabetic (37 percent) groups in comparison with those given placebo. After exercise training, caffeine ingestion was still associated with a reduction in insulin sensitivity by a similar magnitude in the lean (23 percent), obese (26 percent), and Type-2 diabetic (36 percent) groups in comparison with those given placebo.

Figure 4 shows that with exercise, insulin sensitivity did go up, but in all groups, whether lean, obese, or Type-2 diabetic, caffeine intake significantly reduced insulin sensitivity. The researchers concluded that caffeine consumption is associated with a substantial reduction in insulin-mediated glucose uptake independent of obesity, Type-2 diabetes, and chronic exercise.[72]

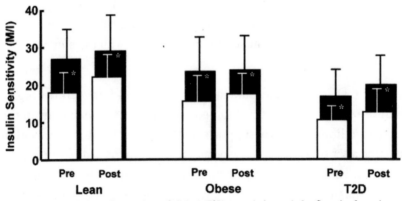

Insulin sensitivity in the lean, obese, and type 2 diabetic (T2D) groups before and after 3 months of exercise. Insulin sensitivity is expressed as the ratio of the amount of glucose metabolized to the prevailing plasma insulin levels [M (mg · kgSM−1 · min−1)/I (µU/ml) x 100] during the last 30 min of the euglycemic clamp. *Glucose uptake is significantly lower (P < 0.05) in the caffeine trial (black bar) compared with the placebo trial (white bar), independent of group and exercise training.

Source: SoJung Lee, PHD1, Robert Hudson, MD, PHD2, Katherine Kilpatrick, MD3, Terry E. Graham, PHD4 and Robert Ross, PHD. "Caffeine Ingestion Is Associated With Reductions in Glucose Uptake Independent of Obesity and Type 2 Diabetes Before and After Exercise Training." Diabetes Care 28:566-572, 2005

FIGURE 4. Insulin sensitivity in lean, obese, and Type-2 diabetic groups with and without caffeine intake, before and after three months of exercise

Thank You for Not Smoking

According to the CDC, 17.7 percent of U.S. adults with diabetes smoke, and the dangers are very real for diabetics. Smoking affects both carbohydrate and lipid metabolism. In one study of diabetics, 114 smokers were compared to 49 nonsmokers. The smokers had a 15–20 percent higher insulin requirement and serum triglyceride concentration. In heavy smokers, the insulin requirement was 30 percent higher. Researchers have found that chronic smokers were likely to be more insulin resistant, hyperinsulinemic, and dyslipidemic compared to matched groups of nonsmokers. It is believed that catecholamines, a type of hormone, are produced in greater quantity in smokers and act as an antagonist to insulin action.[73] A study of 40 patients with Type-2 diabetes found insulin resistance was markedly aggravated among those who smoked.[74]

A contributing factor to insulin resistance is nicotine-containing products. Please understand that insulin resistance is a precursor to diabetes, so anything that contributes to insulin resistance encourages a move from prediabetes to diabetes or makes an existing diabetic condition worse. Chronic cigarette smoking has been found to markedly aggravate insulin resistance for Type-2 diabetics.[75] Lack of exercise certainly helps to activate the expression of Type-2 diabetes.[76] The good news is that even mild exercise can help stave off cigarette cravings and withdrawal symptoms as well as decrease a smoker's chance of reaching for a cigarette, according to a study published in the journal *Addiction*. Researchers from the University of Exeter and the University of Toronto reviewed 14 previously published studies and compared the results. They found that 12 of the studies demonstrated that a session of exercise caused a rapid decrease in cigarette cravings, withdrawal symptoms, and other negative effects of cigarette addiction. As little as five minutes of simple exercises such as walking, isometrics, or muscle flexing proved as effective as a nicotine patch in decreasing an immediate craving.[77] Not only does exercise reduce cravings for cigarettes, but it seems to dramatically improve endurance and fitness, decreases body fat stores, and decrease insulin resistance.

A prospective study of Japanese men concluded that age of smoking initiation and number of cigarettes smoked were major risk factors for developing diabetes.[78] Similarly, data from the U.S. Cancer Prevention

Study found that as smoking increased so the rate of diabetes increased for both men and women.[79]

Nicotine has also been associated with decreasing peripheral circulation and thus increasing the tendency for amputation. Smoking increases adrenaline secretions by 23 percent and thus increases blood sugar. Obviously, smoking decreases lung function and therefore oxygen in the system, and this lack of oxygenation to the tissues decreases peripheral circulation and leads to a greater tendency for gangrene and amputation. Smoking is a documented risk factor for both the development and progression of various types of neuropathy (damage to the peripheral nervous system). A retrospective study of Type-1 and Type-2 diabetic patients found that current or ex-smokers were significantly more likely to have neuropathy than individuals who never smoked (64.8 percent compared to 42.8 percent).[80] A later study found that cigarette smoking was associated with a twofold increase in risk.[81] Studies also show that smoking increases the chances of developing gum disease, a contributing factor in poor glycemic control. In fact, smokers are five times more likely than nonsmokers to have gum disease. For smokers with diabetes, the risk is even greater. If you are a smoker with diabetes, age 45 or older, you are 20 times more likely than a person without these risk factors to get severe gum disease.[82]

Diabetes as an Accelerated Aging

Often diabetes doesn't get diagnosed until its complications begin to arise. Major chronic complications include retinopathy, which leads to blindness; neuropathy, degeneration of the nervous system; nephropathy, or kidney disease; atherosclerotic coronary disease; and atherosclerotic vascular disease. About 85 percent of all diabetics develop retinopathy, 20–50 percent develop kidney disease, and 60–70 percent have mild to severe forms of nerve damage. Diabetics are two to four times more likely to develop cardiovascular disease (which is a factor in 75 percent of diabetes-related deaths) and two to four times more likely to suffer stroke. Multiple studies show that insulin resistance doubles the risk of heart attack as early as 15 years before diabetes is diagnosed, along with risk of stroke. Middle-age people with diabetes have death rates and a heart disease rate two times higher than those without diabetes. Diabetics are also three to four times more likely to develop clinical depression than nondiabetics.

The National Institute of Diabetes and Digestive and Kidney Diseases (NIDDK) reported in 1993 that diabetes is the leading cause of new cases of blindness among adults 20 to 74. Somewhere between 12,000 and 24,000 new cases of blindness per year are caused by diabetic retinopathy. About 60–70 percent of the people with diabetes have mild symptoms to severe forms of diabetic nerve damage. Neuropathy is the major cause of nontrauma lower limb amputation, and studies suggest that as many as 70 percent of amputees die within five years.[83] Many people with diabetes have a "slow stomach" or gastric paresis. These conditions all seem to be associated with hyperinsulinemia (high blood insulin) and hyperglycemia (high blood sugar).

Diabetes and CDDS, in essence, are an accelerated aging. Hyperglycemia and hyperglycemic spikes and the associated hyperinsulinemia, which is a key diagnostic picture in diagnosing CDDS, become a part of the continuum for assessing developing diabetes. It is a tip-off point before we get to diagnosable diabetes and the accelerated aging pattern known as chronic disease. Hyperinsulinemia is telling us that we have a higher risk of developing chronic degenerative diseases. In this context, maintaining a healthy carbohydrate metabolism requires attention and is one of the most important life-extension factors. The diet and lifestyle I am suggesting helps one maintain healthy blood sugar levels.

Proper management of carbohydrate metabolism is key to a healthy life and longevity. A normal FBS, according to ADA data, is 100. However, the latest research shows that if one has a blood sugar of 86 to 99, one is already entering into the first stages of an abnormal metabolism and an accelerated aging process and is beginning to lose control of a healthy carbohydrate metabolism.

A major 12-year study at Harvard University of 42,500 male health professionals ages 40 to 75 who did not initially have diabetes, cardiovascular disease, or cancer found two dietary patterns. One diet was characterized as prudent, with medium to higher concentrations of vegetables, fruit, fish, poultry, and whole grains. The other, characterized as Western, had a high consumption of red meat, processed foods, fat, dairy products, refined grains, sweets, and desserts. The researchers found that the Western dietary pattern was associated with substantially increased risk of Type-2 diabetes. They found that high blood sugar levels led to complications such as blindness, kidney failure, and heart disease. The key factors were being overweight and physically inactive, as well as having a diet that was not prudent. They concluded that all three were important, and it was difficult to separate the risk of diet from the risk of being overweight and physically inactive. The study made crystal clear the importance of all three in creating Type-2 diabetes.[84]

Hyperinsulinemia, a metabolic time bomb, is associated with a whole series of chronic degenerative diseases. It is not only a major risk factor for coronary heart disease but also linked with the rise in plasma-free radicals associated with oxidative stress, which contributes to heart disease and actually decreased brain function. Cell damage resulting from elevated insulin and blood sugar levels can also lead to degenerative diseases such as hypertension and cancer.

Chronically elevated blood sugar also contributes to the formation of advanced glycation end products, also known as AGEs. These result from the nonenzymatic glycosylation of proteins and lipids. Once the proteins and lipids become glycosylated, they lose their function and contribute further to chronic disease, including atherosclerotic cardiovascular disease (ASCVD) and renal failure. They cause part of what we call cross-linkages, which are, in essence, an accelerated aging process. They are evidenced by wrinkles in the skin, which are cross-linkages in the connective tissues. This glycosylation also produces sugar alcohols. The AGEs in sugar alcohols are also associated with nerve damage to blood vessels, kidneys, lenses of the eyes, and the pancreas, and generally accelerate the aging process. The sugar alcohol formation is associated with cataract development and diminished nerve function.

Therefore, at a minimum, what one wants to do is to try to control the high blood sugar.

Genetics

Type-2 has a much stronger genetic component than Type-1. A lot of research on diabetes was done in England, where they have 1.9 million diabetics. In Type-2 diabetes, family histories of diabetes and obesity are major risk factors for the condition. One genetic mutation has been identified as a possible cause of Type-2 diabetes. The mutation was a particular zinc transporter, known as SLC 30 A8, which is involved in regulating insulin secretion.

In another genetic study, a UK team found that people with two copies of the mutant TCF7L2 gene were twice as likely to develop Type-2 diabetes.[85] According to Professor Stephen Humphries, the gene "seems to be causing as many cases of diabetes in the UK as obesity." The researchers discovered that those who carry one variant of the TCF7L2 gene were 50 percent more likely to develop Type-2 diabetes. But those men who carried two copies of the gene were 100 percent more likely to develop diabetes. Professor Humphries, lead researcher on the study for the University College of London Center for Cardiovascular Genetics, said, "Although being overweight is a major risk factor for the development of diabetes, it is clear that an individual's genetic makeup has a big impact on whether or not they will develop diabetes." Professor Humphries said 40 percent of the population carries one mutation of the gene while 10 percent carry both. Again, the message is clear: The genes load the gun, and our lifestyle pulls the trigger. One is not determined by one's genes, although one is affected by one's genes. Genes have a certain tendency to increase susceptibility to one's lifestyle. It is one's lifestyle that makes the difference.

Another gene, ENPP-1, disrupts the way the body stores energy and handles sugar by blocking the hormone insulin. Research by a French and UK team showed that children with a faulty version of ENPP-1 often were obese as young as five years old.

The gene called SUMO-4 helps regulate the body's immune system, which defends against infection. It was found in the United States at the Medical College of Georgia. The gene enables more cytokines to be made and directs the revved-up immune response in the cells of the pancreas that make insulin. In other words, it amplifies inflammation.

Although the evidence strongly shows that there is a genetic component, I do not suggest using that as an excuse and moving into fatalism. One has control of one's destiny and one needs the courage to live a lifestyle that protects oneself from diabetes. That is what this book and chapter is about.

Type-2 diabetes, which we have been describing, is self-inflicted, manifesting in an ever-increasing proportion of young people. Because of poor diet and lifestyle, we are seeing Type-2 diabetes in more and more 5- and 10-year-olds. The Culture of Death diet and lifestyle is obviously accelerating the expression of a poor genotypic tendency for diabetes. In Type-1 diabetes, 85 percent of the people do not have a genetic predisposition, but a genetic predisposition still does play some role. The Type-1 diabetes is called insulin-dependent diabetes mellitus (IDDM) because the beta cells of the pancreas are destroyed by some sort of autoimmune inflammatory process. Research has suggested that 75–90 percent of the people with Type-1 diabetes have abnormally raised antibody titer against their own beta cells. These B-cell antibodies seem to be associated with drinking cow's milk. Two specific proteins in the milk cause the cross-reaction with the beta cells of the pancreas. The drinking of cow's milk in the first few months of life has been associated with 11 to 13 times higher rates of Type-1 diabetes in children who are weaned before three months, compared to those people who don't drink milk.

The symptoms of Type-1 diabetes may come on very quickly. High levels of sugar in the blood and urine, frequent urination, and/or bed-wetting may be seen readily in children. Other symptoms include extreme hunger, extreme thirst, weight loss, weakness, tiredness, irritability, mood swings, and nausea. Type-1 has also been associated with a variety of viral infections. This is in contrast to Type-2 diabetes, which is slow to develop with many of the same symptoms, but with hard-to-heal infections, blurred vision, itchy skin, candida, and the mind not working so clearly. Cases of Type-1 can arise from exposure to viruses, including measles, mumps, infectious mononucleosis, infectious hepatitis, Coxsackie virus, and cytomegalovirus. These viruses cause an immune inflammation response that destroys the beta cells of the pancreas in an infant or an adult. Infant research suggests that exposure to German measles in the womb may have a 40 percent greater chance of developing Type-1 diabetes.

Type-1 diabetes can run in families, but there is a weak association. About 85 percent of people who develop Type-1 diabetes do not have an immediate family member who is diabetic. If you're a twin with diabetes, you have a one-in-three risk factor for Type-1. Figure 5 shows the risk factors associated with other family member diabetics.

Family Risk Factors for Type-1 Diabetes	
If:	Your risk factor is:
Your twin has diabetes	1 in 3
Your sibling has diabetes	1 in 14
One parent has diabetes	1 in 25
Your mother has diabetes	1 in 40–50
Your father has diabetes	1 in 20
No relative has diabetes	1 in 500

FIGURE 5. Family risk factors for diabetes (Source: Rotter, J I, Anderson, C E, Rubin, R, Congleton, J E, Terasaki, P I, and Rimoin, D L. "HLA genotypic study of insulin-dependent diabetes the excess of DR3/DR4 heterozygotes allows rejection of the recessive hypothesis." *Diabetes*, February 1983, 32(2): 169–174.)

Type-2 Diabetes Cometh

In the early stages, Type-2 diabetics or non-insulin-dependent diabetes mellitus (NIDDM) diabetics, do produce insulin, but the cells are unable to use it properly as they are resistant to the signaling of the insulin and leptin. Normal insulin production is below units per day.

In insulin-resistant diabetes, the pancreas may overwork to produce levels of as much as 114 units of insulin in an effort to overcome insulin resistance.[86] The underlying cause of insulin resistance is a breakdown in the communication between the insulin, a chemical messenger, and the receivers of that signal, a significant amount of which are called GLUT-4 transporters. GLUT-4 transporters are proteins within the cell that rise to the cell's membrane, take hold of the glucose, and bring it inside the cell. Insulin resistance means that the cells do not receive the insulin signaling message clearly and do not respond accurately. Because the cells are not hearing the message from the insulin and thus able to take in the sugar, blood glucose levels remain high, causing the pancreatic beta cells to pump out more insulin to "knock" louder on the cell walls. Early in this disease process, the glucose is let in, even with insulin resistance. This is called compensated insulin resistance, as the pancreas has put out more insulin and glucose levels stabilize for a while. As this continues, over time the beta cells of the pancreas are destroyed and/or inflame and wear out from producing up to four times the normal insulin levels. Glucose levels remain elevated in this state of uncompensated insulin resistance, and over time the person experiences an advanced case of Type-2 with beta cell destruction, inflammation, and eventually "beta cell burnout." About 30 percent of the people with Type-2 diabetes do inject insulin daily because their insulin-producing cells become destroyed. Then these Type-2 (NIDDM) diabetics become insulin-dependent diabetics (IDDM).

There are multiple reasons for insulin resistance. Insulin receptors on the outside of the cells may not accept insulin, or there may be too few receptors as the glucose enters the cells, or the cells may not use it properly, or excess dietary fat may accumulate in the cell and disrupt glucose absorption. Part of the issue is that the ability to move from glycogen to glucose is blocked within the cells and there is a backup.

This whole complex insulin resistance mechanism is somewhat affected by free radical production associated with hyperinsulinemia. This elevated free radical production activates nuclear factor kB (NFkB), which is a DNA regulator that acts within the cell nucleus. NFkB

activation intensifies inflammatory responses, resulting in more production of free radicals and eventually beta cell death. So we begin to see
that diabetes is also associated with inflammation, which I later discuss
as para-inflammation. In essence, para-inflammation occurs, not only
through the autoimmune inflammation that we get in Type-1 but also
as the more chronic low-level para-inflammation we may see in Type-2.

N-acetyl cysteine is a precursor to glutathionine (GSH) and is a
powerful antioxidant to moderate cell metabolism and gene expression.
GSH is thought to prevent the oxidation that causes beta cell damage,
and it does this by inhibiting NFkB activation. So it's possible that the
inflammation from the NFkB activation plays an important role in the
development of diabetes. And if that's the case, n-acetyl cysteine, which
inhibits NFkB activation, has the potential to prevent or delay the onset
of the disease. In the presence of other oxidants, NFkB can activate the
vascular cell adhesion molecules (VCAM-1). This molecule helps these
plasma cells attached to the endothelium and therefore creates more
clogged arteries. The VCAM-1 increase has been shown to be one of
the most important events initiating atherosclerosis. Type-2 diabetes
and glucose intolerant hypertensive patients have been found to have
elevated levels of plasma VCAM-1.[87] In diabetics, n-acetyl cysteine may
synergize with the antioxidant vitamins C and E; these three together
seem to reduce blood glucose levels in mice. They also increase beta
cell mass and preserve insulin content.

Diabetes in Children

Type-1 diabetes is rising alarmingly worldwide, at a rate of 3 percent
per year. Some 70,000 children ages 14 and under develop Type-1 diabetes annually.

Increasingly, children are also developing Type-2 diabetes, in both
developed and developing nations, with reports of Type-2 diabetes in
some children as young as 8 years old. Approximately two million children ages 12 to 19 have a Type-2 diabetic condition directly related to
obesity and inactivity.

In a study reported in the November 2005 issue of *Pediatrics*, based on data involving 950 children in a 1999–2000 national health survey, researchers found that among roughly 177,000 Americans under age 20, incidences of both Type-1 and Type-2 have increased. About 25 percent of the diabetic children now have Type-2, compared with just 4 percent 10 years ago. Approximately 7 percent of the children in the study were prediabetic—that translates to two million children. About 16 percent of the kids in the study were obese. The study supports the idea that our children are heading more seriously in the direction of a diabetes disaster.

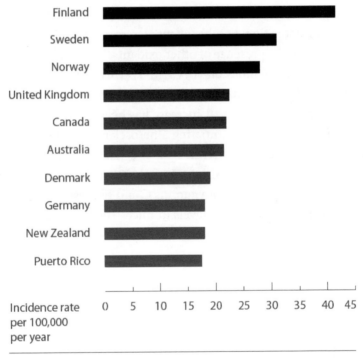

Only countries where studies have been carried out in that country have been included

FIGURE 6. Top 10 countries for incidence rate of Type-1 diabetes in children, up to 14 years old (Source: International Diabetes Federation, *Diabetes Atlas,* 3rd ed., 2006)

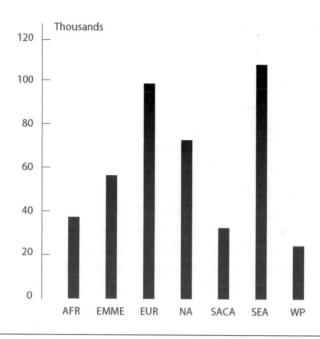

FIGURE 7. Estimated number of prevalent cases of Type-1 diabetes in children, up to 14 years old, by region (Source: International Diabetes Federation, *Diabetes Atlas*, 3rd ed., 2006)

About five million children are overweight in the United States. Overweight is being described as a new epidemic in the American pediatric population, with an overall 33 percent increase in diabetes incidence and prevalence seen in the last 10 years. Type-2 diabetes has changed from a disease of our grandparents and parents to a disease of our children. In 1994 Type-2 diabetes accounted for 16 percent of new cases of pediatric diabetes, and by 1999, it accounted for 8 percent to 45 percent, from state to state.[88] In Ohio and Arkansas, African American children with Type-2 diabetes represented 70–75 percent of new pediatric diabetes cases.[89] In Ventura, California, 31 percent of new adult-onset diabetes involved Mexican American youths. Among the Pima tribe, pediatric diabetes is seen in 20 to 40 individuals per thousand. Unlike Type-1 diabetes, most children with Type-2 diabetes have a family member with Type-2 diabetes; 45 to 80 percent have a parent with

Type-2 diabetes,[90] and 70 to 90 percent report at least one affected first- or second-degree relative. Up to 60 to 90 percent of youth who develop diabetes have ancanthosis, a thickening and hyperpigmentation of skin at the neck. This seems to be associated with insulin resistance. Once Type-2 diabetes is established, the persistence of obesity exacerbates the complications of hypertension, dyslipidemia, atherosclerosis, and polycystic ovarian syndrome, which start to appear despite the fact that these patients are still young.[91]

Investigators reviewed national health surveys of more than 6,000 U.S. children ages 6 to 18 between 1988 and 1994. They also looked at the data from 3,000 children in China and 7,000 in Russia. In the United States about 11 percent of the children were obese and slightly more than 14 percent were overweight, compared to 6 percent in Russia obese and 10 percent overweight; in China only 3.6 percent were obese and 2.4 percent were overweight.[92] In contrast to the United States and England, the Chinese and Russian children from the wealthiest families tended to be heavier.

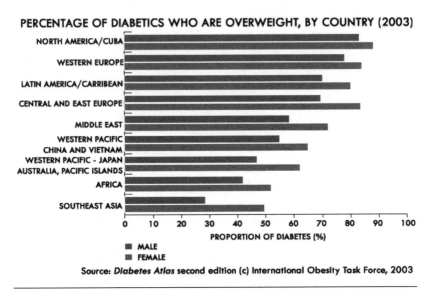

PERCENTAGE OF DIABETICS WHO ARE OVERWEIGHT, BY COUNTRY (2003)

Source: *Diabetes Atlas* second edition (c) International Obesity Task Force, 2003

FIGURE 8. Overweight and obesity among school-age children, 5 to 17 years old, worldwide (Source: International Obesity Task Force, *Diabetes Atlas*, 2nd ed., 2003)

Our children are fed daily propaganda to eat foods that are causing them harm. A Kaiser Family Foundation study analyzed more than 8,000 advertisements using detailed data about the viewing habits of children in three age groups. Researchers found that children of all ages are bombarded with promotions for fast food, junk food, and soda, with 8- to 12-year-olds seeing the most food advertisements. This market, the "tweens," is especially important to advertisers because it encompasses the ages at which youngsters typically begin to make some of their own buying decisions. According to Dr. Susan Linn of the Campaign for a Commercial-Free Childhood (CCFC), "We know that marketing is a factor in the childhood obesity epidemic. It is unconscionable that 8–12-year-olds see, on average, more than 7,600 food commercials a year—the vast majority for candy, snacks, cereals, and fast food."[93]

We understand that overweight is a risk factor for heart disease in adults, but the situation is more ominous still. Autopsy data from the conflicts in Korea[94] and Vietnam,[95] the Bogalusa study,[96] and the PDAY Study[97] all testify to the ubiquitous nature of the disease in young Americans. The 1992 Bogalusa Heart Study examined autopsies performed on children killed in accidental deaths. Researchers found the initial stages of atherosclerosis in the form of fatty plaques and streaks in most children and teenagers.[98]

Diet and Type-2 Diabetes Prevention and Reversal for Children

Research by Dr. Milagros G. Huerta has suggested that magnesium deficiency is related to Type-2 diabetes in obese children, who are more likely to have insulin resistance.[99] This study was performed to see if obese children get enough magnesium in their diets and if a lack of magnesium can cause insulin resistance and thus Type-2 diabetes. Researchers found that 55 percent of obese children did not get enough magnesium from the foods they ate, compared with only 27 percent of lean children. The results showed that obese children got 14.4 percent less magnesium from the foods they ate than lean children, even though obese and lean children ate about the same number of calories per day. Children with lower magnesium levels had a higher insulin resistance. In addition to not eating enough foods rich in magnesium, obese children seem to have problems using magnesium from the foods they eat. Extra body fat can prevent the body's cells from using magnesium to break down carbohydrates.

Characteristic signs of Type-2 diabetes in children include overweight, early stages of heart disease, magnesium deficiency, and insulin resistance. Chlorophyll through a plant-sourced diet is high in magnesium. Chlorophyll is an amazing food that is essential for humans, and at the center of the chlorophyll molecule is the element magnesium. Plant blood (chlorophyll) and human blood (hemoglobin) are not so different, as shown in Figure 9.

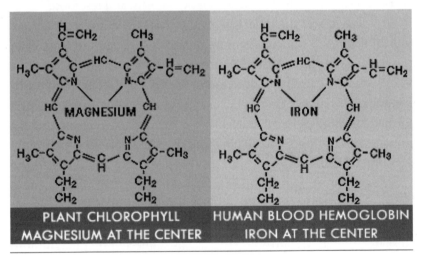

FIGURE 9. Plant chlorophyll and human blood hemoglobin

Magnesium is 17 times as prevalent in the human heart as any other tissue in the body. Famous research scientist Dr. Max Oskar Bircher-Brenner called chlorophyll "concentrated sun power" and said, "Chlorophyll increases the functions of the heart, affects the vascular system, the intestines, the uterus, and the lungs. It raises the basic nitrogen exchange and is therefore a tonic which considering its stimulating properties cannot be compared with any other."[100]

One of the reasons chlorophyll is so effective may be its similarity to hemin. Hemin is part of hemoglobin, the protein fraction of human blood that carries oxygen. Studies done as long ago as 1911 show that the molecules of hemin and chlorophyll are surprisingly alike, with the difference being that chlorophyll is bound by an atom of magnesium and hemin is bound by iron.[101] Experiments have shown that severely anemic rabbits make a rapid return to a normal blood count once chlorophyll is administered.[102] Although the exact details of chemical transaction have not been mapped out, the human body seems to be able to substitute iron and rebuild the blood. It is as if the anemic patient has had a transfusion.

Understanding Insulin Resistance

The diagnosis of insulin resistance is not the same as diabetes. It is associated with CDDS, prediabetes, and exists in many Type-2 diabetics. Insulin resistance, which starts before diabetes, is a whole metabolic shift. About 25 to 35 percent of the population have a degree of insulin resistance and suffer from the health consequences of hyperglycemia.[103] Insulin resistance, which is activated in CDDS, is a common feature of, and possibly contributing factor to, a variety of interlinking health problems including diabetes mellitus,[104] polycystic ovarian syndrome,[105, 106, 107] dyslipidemia,[108] hypertension,[109, 110] cardiovascular disease,[111, 112, 113, 114, 115] sleep apnea,[116] certain hormone-sensitive cancers,[117, 118, 119] and obesity.[120, 121, 122, 123] One key sign to diagnose Type-2 is called abdominal obesity, which is almost a clinical marker for this metabolic dysregulation.

Magnesium deficiency is very common in my clinical experience and is found in about 90 percent of people with diabetes. Insulin resistance is also associated with hypertension. Experimental work with magnesium deficiency showed that giving magnesium increases tissue sensitivity to insulin. If the diet is depleted in potassium, it can also lead to insulin resistance at postreceptor sites.[124] Zinc and chromium play a role in decreasing insulin resistance, as well as does vanadium. Biotin does appear to decrease insulin resistance according to research.[125]

Vitamin E plays a role. About 600 milligrams was all that was needed to make a difference in insulin resistance.

Taurine and glutathione all seem to decrease insulin resistance. CoQ10, which seems to be quite good for this, also results in improvements in blood sugar, blood pressure, and uptakes of C, E, and beta-carotene. Alpha-lipoic acid is specifically good for improving insulin resistance (sensitivity). Fiber creates an improved insulin resistance. Saturated fats make the insulin resistance worse. Vegetables decrease fasting insulin. Vitamin-A-rich foods decrease insulin resistance.

Stress also plays a role at the insulin resistance level. Acute stress seems to be clearly associated with severe, although reversible, insulin resistance.[126] We should pay attention to stress and the treatment of stress.[127] A study by Nelson showed that psychosocial stress played a role in the chronic elevation of cortisol, which results in increased plasma insulin levels. The fatty tissues secrete a hormone called leptin. High leptin levels appear to act on the hypothalamus to decrease body fat. But as the percentage of body fat increases, even high levels of leptin are unable to stimulate the metabolic processes. So, in obesity, we have a leptin resistance.[128] Leptin resistance decreases as a person becomes more sensitive to insulin.

In summary, factors that may contribute to insulin resistance and thus to diabetes include a diet high in simple and complex carbohydrates, which includes high-glycemic meals filled with refined sugar and starches; deficiencies of the omega-3 and omega-6 fatty acids; low fiber intake; stress; deficiencies of the minerals calcium, magnesium, chromium, vanadium, potassium, and zinc; deficiency of carotenoids; low intake of vegetables; lack of exercise; watching television; fluoride, pesticide, herbicide, and heavy metal exposure; nicotine and caffeine; and a diet high in cooked animal tissue and trans fats.

Gestational Diabetes

Gestational diabetes mellitus (GDM) is a third major category of diabetes that needs to be addressed. It occurs in at least 5 to 14 percent of pregnant women. It is important to diagnose this effectively and treat it because it plays a big role in the onset of Type-2 diabetes 5 to 10 years later. Half of women who've had GDM eventually develop Type-2.[129] It is associated with the metabolic changes that take place during a normal pregnancy. To conserve sugar for the baby, mom's placenta produces hormones naturally increase insulin resistance, thus rerouting some of the sugar to her fetus that before pregnancy would have gone to her cells. Early in pregnancy, maternal estrogen and progesterone increase and promote pancreatic beta cell hyperplasia and increased insulin release.[130]

This rise in insulin increases peripheral glucose utilization and glycogen storage and lowers glucose levels, but this shifts as the pregnancy progresses. There are increased levels of human chorionic gonadotropin (HCG), which also leads to insulin resistance. Cortisol, which has the highest diabetic creating potency, peaks at 26 weeks. Progesterone, with anti-insulin qualities, peaks at 32 weeks. These two milestones, 26 and 32 weeks, encompass an important time during which the pancreas releases 1.5 to 2.5 times more insulin to respond to the resistance.[131]

The Diabetogenic Potency of Hormones in Pregnancy		
Hormone:	Peak elevation (weeks):	Diabetogenic potency:
Prolactin	10	Weak
Estradiol	26	Very weak
HCG	16	Moderate
Cortisol	26	Very strong
Progesterone	32	Strong

FIGURE 10. The diabetogenic potency of hormones in pregnancy

GDM is the most common medical complication in pregnancy. Women who have it face a significantly greater risk of developing diabetes later in their life. It may be immediate or long term, in terms of complications. Statistically associated with GDM is an increase in preeclampsia and resulting increased C-sections. A study of postpartum eclampsia women by Coustan and associates showed that 6 percent were found to have an irregular glucose tolerance at zero to two years postpartum; 13 percent had irregular blood sugars at three to four years; 15 percent at five to six years; and 30 percent at 7 to 10 years postpartum.[132] Other studies have documented Type-2 diabetes at three to five years postpartum in 30 to 50 percent of the women. Repeated insulin resistance physiologies, due to additional pregnancies, lead to an increase in the rate of developing Type-2 diabetes postpregnancy. The relative risk for Type-2 diabetes was 1.95 for each 10 pounds gained during pregnancy. This is also associated with greater risk for developing hypertension, hyperlipidemia, EKG changes, and mortality.[133] Women with GDM had higher triglycerides and fatty acids, beta hydroxy butyrate, and LDL, and lower HDL cholesterol than women without GDM. Their children have an increased rate of perinatal mortality and morbidity. One study showed a fourfold increase in perinatal mortality in pregnancies complicated by improperly managed GDM.[134] Other studies have suggested an increased rate in stillbirths associated with GDM.

Maternal hyperglycemia leads to fetal hyperglycemia and fetal hyperinsulinemia with increases in fetal growth. Growth is bigger in the fatty and the liver tissues.

In studies of children of women with pregestational diabetes and GDM, they found that irregular glucose tolerance was 13 times higher than in controls. It appears that children of mothers with GDM have a higher incidence of obesity. The research shows that Type-2 diabetes occurred in 8.6 percent of children with prediabetic mothers and 45 percent of infants with diabetic mothers.[135]

Alzheimer's Associated Diabetes

Approximately 4.5 million Americans have Alzheimer's disease, and that figure may triple in less than 50 years, according to the Alzheimer's Association. More than 65 percent of Americans are overweight or obese, and the CDC estimates that some 51 million people are considered prediabetic, which implies a hyperglycemic dysregulation that greatly increases the chance of developing diabetes, obesity, heart disease, and, according to new research, Alzheimer's. This hyperglycemic link could foretell a dramatic increase in Alzheimer's cases, unless dietary and lifestyle interventions are made now.[136]

Researchers are beginning to connect Alzheimer's with diabetes, obesity, and heart disease. It is such a strong connection that Alzheimer's is being referred to by scientists at Brown Medical School as Type-3 diabetes.[137] A variety of studies have shown that people with Type-2 diabetes have about double the average incidence of Alzheimer's. One study out of the Karolinska Institute in Sweden found that even people with borderline diabetes, meaning people with high blood sugar but not in the diabetic range, had a 70 percent greater risk of developing Alzheimer's.[138] Apparently the risk of dementia rises in people with high blood sugar. The current theories are that the poor brain circulation caused by diabetes is a primary factor as well as insulin resistance in the areas of the brain associated with memory and cognition, such as the limbic system, hippocampal, cortical, and precortical areas. An eight-year study out of Kaiser Permanente tracked 22,582 patients ages 50 or above with Type-2 diabetes and found that diabetic individuals with high blood sugar experience an increased risk of dementia and Alzheimer's. Compared to those with normal glycosylated hemoglobin levels (HgbA1c less than 5.7), those with HgbA1c levels greater than 12 were 22 percent more likely to develop dementia, and those with HgbA1c levels above 15 were 78 percent more likely to develop dementia. As with peripheral vascular disease going to amputations, there may be a vascular dementia that is triggered by low blood flow to the brain.

New research linking diabetes and Alzheimer's suggests that the high blood sugar of diabetes can lead to the formation of advanced glycation end products, or AGEs.[139] AGEs are sugar-derived substances that form in the body through an interaction between carbohydrates and proteins, lipids, or nucleic acids such as DNA. AGEs adversely affect the structure and function of proteins and the tissues that contain proteins.[140] Recent studies have shown that both the formation and accumulation of AGEs are enhanced in diabetes.[141] AGEs become even more destructive when coupled with free radicals formed during cellular energy production. These highly reactive agents produce oxidative stress that can cause cellular damage. Oxidative stress is more and more associated with the causative formation of AGEs, which in turn may induce even more oxidative stress. New evidence shows that oxidative stress may be an important causative factor in both insulin resistance and Type-2 diabetes.[142, 143]

Brain autopsies of Alzheimer's patients find signs of significant oxidative damage by free radicals, and new research indicates that AGEs may initiate this damage.[144] It is the oxidative damage and the accumulation of AGEs in both diabetes and Alzheimer's that is the biochemical similarity between these two diseases.

We do have nutritional protection against oxidative stress of this kind. Studies show that alpha-lipoic acid helps protect the brain against damage caused by free-radical-induced oxidative stress, which has important implications for its potential role in protecting against Alzheimer's disease.[145, 146]

Other good news is that the high blood sugar of diabetes and the increased risk for Alzheimer's is more related to consumption of processed high-glycemic foods than natural foods. New research suggests that antioxidants in fruit and vegetable juices may lower the risk of Alzheimer's disease. The Kame Project, a long-term study of more than 1,800 Japanese Americans conducted in Seattle, began in 1992–94 to study participants who had no dementia and averaged 71 years of age. The group was followed through 2001. During that time, 81 cases of probable Alzheimer's were diagnosed in participants who had completed the food surveys. Those who reported drinking fruit or vegetable juices at least three times per week were 73 percent less likely to have developed Alzheimer's as those who drank juice less than once a week.[147] This is great news, as the Culture of Life antidiabetogenic diet includes ample amounts of fresh vegetable juice.

Cancer Associations

In addition to diabetes, there is a strong link between high insulin levels and some types of cancer. In one study, 10 postmenopausal women with endometrial cancer had significantly higher fasting serum insulin levels than the controls. Researchers found insulin receptors in the postmenopausal ovaries, which is a unique place to find them.[148] In a study of 752 women with endometrial cancer and 2,606 controls, an association was confirmed between NIDDM and an increased risk of endometrial cancer.[149] Insulin is thought to affect the development of endometrial cancer through its hormonal stimulating properties. In 22 endometrial cancer patients in one study, those with high hyperinsulinemia had significantly more steroid hormone receptors in the tumor area, compared with patients with low insulin anemia.[150, 151] Researchers also discovered a link between colon cancer and insulin levels, and this may be associated with insulin's role as a growth factor in the colon, as in excess it will stimulate excess colon cell growth, which may turn into cancer. In 102 cases of colorectal cancer, researchers found that those with the highest level of fasting glucose had almost twice the increased risk of colon cancer. Those with the highest fasting insulin levels also were associated with the increased risk of colon cancer.[152]

A recent study in the *American Journal of Clinical Nutrition* has shown that people who consume a large amount of processed sugar each day are at a much higher risk for pancreatic cancer, which kills about 30,000 Americans each year. Of nearly 80,000 men and women whose diets were studied during 1997–2005, 131 developed pancreatic cancer. Those who drank carbonated or corn-syrup laden drinks even twice a day were 90 percent more likely to contract pancreatic cancer than those who never drank them. Those who added sugar to their foods or beverages at least five times daily had a 70 percent higher risk of developing pancreatic cancer than those who did not.[153] Clearly, increased insulin demand due to high sugar consumption burdens the pancreas and increases pancreatic cancer risk.

Chapter 2 Summary

In Chapter 1 overwhelming data was presented that diabetes is a world-wide pandemic. In Chapter 2 the reader can see that by living in the Culture of Death (expressed by a diet and lifestyle high in carbohydrates and especially highly refined carbohydrates, dairy products, processed white flour, processed white sugar, cooked animal flesh, trans fats, nicotine, caffeine, commercial foods high in agrochemicals, heavy metal toxicity, vaccinations, poor air and water quality, and high stress), we have created the pandemic of diabetes. In other words, diabetes is a symptom of the Culture of Death.

I believe that these healthy results can be repeated in all indigenous cultures that choose to give up white flour, white sugar, and cooked hydrogenated and animal fats and return to the land and their indigenous diets and lifestyles.

Economic Status Is Not a Diabetes Causal Factor for Those Determined to Live a Healthy Life

In Western societies, a lower-class economic status does not sentence individuals or families to a cheap, highly processed diet that brings diabetes, although it does make it harder to change the diabetic trend. Being empowered by the message of this book to eat organic, whole, live foods, of which you only need to eat half as much to get the nutrients as compared with cooked food, can prevent and reverse diabetes. I have yet to find a person, no matter how difficult their economic status, who could not switch over to this Culture of Life diet and lifestyle if seriously motivated. And the exciting thing about this in our advanced Western culture is that one is able to acquire foods and food concentrates that are allowing one to access more powerful forms of nutrition than our ancestors ever dreamed possible. This means that one can do even better than just achieve a nondiabetic physiology—one can achieve a postdiabetic physiology in which their health is better than it was before the diabetes and better than most people in the world who have never developed diabetes.

Even in developing societies, where urbanization with its diet and lifestyle has increased rates of diabetes, moving back to a rural agrarian lifestyle can make accessible the indigenous diets, which for centuries have protected people from having diabetes. I have already initiated programs in Mexico, Ghana, Ethiopia, Cameroon, and Nigeria based on this insight. It is useful to remind the reader that the Pima Indians, who are now suffering from an estimated 90 percent rate of diabetes, had only one single documented case of diabetes by 1920 when they were still living on their land and eating their indigenous diet. Their cousins, the Tarahumaras, who have maintained their natural diet and remained on their land, have only 6 percent incidence of diabetes.

In addition to the Culture of Death, tendencies that aggravate and pull the trigger on the loaded gun of genetic propensities, there are also economic considerations. Those people living in weaker economic conditions seemed to be more susceptible, with the exception of China, Russia, and India, where those of greater affluence have more access to junk foods and are running higher rates of obesity, which is associated with diabetes.

In general, what I am saying is that it is the modern world diet and lifestyle that is a Crime Against Wisdom. The point is clear. The reader is given the option to choose the Culture of Life over the Culture of Death. Chapters 3 through 6 of this book give you the knowledge and wisdom to no longer suffer the Crimes Against Wisdom of the Culture of Death. These chapters will show how to do this in a straightforward, uncomplicated way that enables you to live a life of abundance, free of diabetes.

Chapter 3 Preview

In Chapter 3 I will be discussing a preliminary theory of the causes of diabetes that will give you more insight into how to effectively manage your metabolism. This is a theory that begins to explain the effectiveness of the clinical results. As a scientist, one understands that, as with all theories, they must be proven. Theories give us a way to investigate what is going on. Further research is then needed to disprove or prove them. In the fifth chapter of this book I will present a comprehensive theory based on the last 120 clients I have seen in my Dr. Cousens's Diabetes Recovery Program—A Holistic Approach. The key is that there are potentially significant results. In this next chapter I will be presenting a beginning theory that helps to develop and understand the rationale for the Dr. Cousens's Diabetes Recovery Program—A Holistic Approach for healing diabetes, especially Type-2 and gestational, as well as providing a path for future research. The beautiful thing is that my approach is both safe and outstanding for developing high-level wellness in general, as well as for reversing diabetes. It is a win-win proposition.

Notes

1. Hu, F B, Li, T Y, Colditz, G A, Willett, W C, and Manson, J E. "Television watching and other sedentary behaviors in relation to risk of obesity and type 2 diabetes mellitus in women." *JAMA*, 2003, 289: 1785–91.

2. Olshansky, S J, Passaro, D J, Hershow, R C, et al. "A potential decline in life expectancy in the United States in the 21st century." *New Eng J Med*, March 17, 2005, 352(11): 1138–45. http://content.nejm.org/cgi/content /abstract/352/11/1138?ck=nck.

3. Pollan, M. "You are what you grow." *New York Times*, April 22, 2007.

4. Whitaker, J D. *Reversing Diabetes*. New York: Warner Books, 2001, p. 116.

5. Wolfe, D. *Eating for Beauty*. San Diego: Maul Brothers, 2002, pp. 33–38.

6. Snowdon, D A, and Phillips, R L. "Does a vegetarian diet reduce the occurrence of diabetes?" *American Journal of Public Health*, 1985, 75: 507–12.

7. Tsunehara, C H, Leonetti, D L, and Fujimoto, W Y. "Diet of second-generation Japanese American men with and without NIDDM." *Am J Clin Nutr*, 52 (1990): 731–38.

8. Ibid.

9. Mangels, A R, Messina, V, and Melina, V. "Position of the American Dietetic Association: Vegetarian diets." *J Am Diet Assoc*, June 2003, 103(6): 748–65.

10. Ellis, F R, and Montegriffo, V M E. "Veganism, clinical findings and investigations." *Am J Clin Nutr*, 1970, 23: 249–55.

11. Berenson, G, Srinivasan, S, Bao, W, Newman, W P, Tracy, R E, and Wattigney, W A. "Association between multiple cardiovascular risk factors and atherosclerosis to children and young adults. The Bogalusa Heart Study." *New Eng J Med*, 1998, 338: 1650–56.

12. Key, T J, Fraser, G E, Thorogood, M, et al. "Mortality in vegetarians and nonvegetarians: Detailed findings from a collaborative analysis of 5 prospective studies." *Am J Clin Nutri*, 1999, 70(suppl.): 516S–524S.

13. Bergan, J G, and Brown, P T. "Nutritional status of 'new' vegetarians." *J Am Diet Assoc*, 1980, 76: 151–55.

14. Appleby, P N, Thorogood, M, et al. "Low body mass index in nonmeat eaters: The possible roles of animal fat, dietary fibre, and alcohol." *Int J Obes*, 1998, 22: 454–60.

15. Dwyer, J T. "Health aspects of vegetarian diets." *Am J Clin Nutr*, 1988, 48: 712–38.

16. Key, T J, and Davey, G. "Prevalence of obesity is low in people who do not eat meat." *BMJ*, 1996, 313: 816–17.

17. Stein, R. "Breast cancer risk linked to red meat, study finds." *The Washington Post*, November 14, 2006. http://www.washingtonpost.com /wp-dyn/content/article/2006/11/13/AR2006111300824_pf.html.

18. Lindahl, O. "Vegan regimen with reduced medication in the treatment of bronchial asthma." *Journal of Asthma*, 1985, 22: 44.

19. Culhane, J. "PCBs: The poison that won't go away." *Reader's Digest*, December 1980, pp. 112–16.

20. International Medical Veritas Association. "Diabetes and mercury poisoning." October 2006. http://www.flcv.com/diabetes.html.

21. Robbins, J. *Diet for a New America*. Tiburon, CA: H J Kramer, 1987, p. 333. Cited in "Infant abnormalities linked to PCB contaminated fish." *Vegetarian Times*, November 1984, p. 8.

22. Robbins. *Diet for a New America*. p. 334. Cited in Jacobsen, S. "The effect of intrauterine PCB exposure on visual recognition memory." *Child Development*, 1985, vol. 56.

23. Vaarala, O, et al. "Cow's milk formula feeding induces primary immunization to insulin in infants at genetic risk for Type-1 diabetes." *Diabetes*, 1999, 48: 1389–94.

24. LaPorte, R E, Tajima, N, Akerblom, H K, et al. "Geographic differences in the risk of insulin-dependent diabetes mellitus: The importance of registries." *Diabetes Care*, 1985, 8(suppl. 1): 101–7.

25. Perez-Bravo, F, Carrasco, E, Gutierrez-Lopez, M D, et al. "Genetic predisposition and environmental factors leading to the development of insulin-dependent diabetes mellitus in Chilean children." *J Mol Med*, 1996, 74: 105–9.

26. Kostraba, H N, Cruickshanks, K J, Lawler-Heavner, J, et al. "Early exposure to cow's milk and solid foods in infancy, genetic predisposition, and risk of IDDM." *Diabetes*, 1993, 42: 288–95.

27. LaPorte, Tajima, Akerblom, et al. "Geographic differences in the risk of insulin-dependent diabetes mellitus."

28. Virtanen, S M, Laara, E, Hypponen, E, et al. "Cow's milk consumption, HLA-DQB1 genotype, and Type-1 diabetes." *Diabetes*, 2000, 49: 912–917.

29. "American Gastroenterological Association medical position statement: Guidelines for the evaluation of food allergies." *Gastroenterology*, 2001, 120: 1023–25.

30. National Digestive Diseases Information Clearinghouse. "Lactose intolerance." *National Institute of Diabetes and Digestive and Kidney Diseases*, March 2003.

31. Taylor, C. "Got milk (intolerance)? Digestive malady affects 30–50 million." *The Clarion-Ledger*, August 1, 2003.

32. "Cow's milk protein may play role in mental disorders." *Reuters Health*, April 1, 1999.

33. Carrell, S. "Milk causes serious illness for 7M Britons. Scientists say undetected lactose intolerance is to blame for chronic fatigue, arthritis and bowel problems." *The Independent*, June 22, 2003.

34. Lewinnek, G E, Kelsey, J, White, A A III, et al. "The significance and a comparative analysis of the epidemiology of hip fractures." *Clin Ortho Rel Res*, 1980, 152: 35–43.

35. Recker, R R, and Heaney, R P. "The effect of milk supplements on calcium metabolism, bone metabolism and calcium balance." *Am J Clin Nutr*, 1985, 41: 254–63.

36. Patterson, C R. "Calcium requirements in man: A critical review." *Postgraduate Medical Journal* 54 (April 1978): 244–48.

37. Campbell, T C. *The China Study*. Dallas: Benbella Books, 2004, p. 7.

38. Ursin, G, Bjelke, E, Heuch, I, et al. "Milk consumption and cancer incidence: A Norwegian prospective study." *Br J Cancer*, 1990, 61: 456–59.

39. Cramer, D W, Harlow, B L, Willett, W C, Welch, W R, Bell, D A, Scully, R E, Ng, W G, and Knapp, R C. "Galactose consumption and metabolism in relation to the risk of ovarian cancer." *The Lancet*, 1989, 2(8654): 66–71.

40. Fairfield, K M, Hunter, D J, Colditz, G A, Fuchs, C S, Cramer, D W, Speizer, F E, Willett, W C, and Hankinson, S E. "A prospective study of dietary lactose and ovarian cancer." *Intl J Cancer*, 2004, 110(2): 271–77.

41. Larsson, S C, Bergkvist, L, and Wolk, A. "Milk and lactose intakes and ovarian cancer risk in the Swedish Mammography Cohort." *Amer J Clin Nutr*, 2004, 80(5): 1353–57.

42. Mettlin, C. "Milk drinking, other beverage habits, and lung cancer risk." *Intl J Cancer*, April 15, 1989, 43(4): 608–12.

43. Mettlin, C, Selenskas, S, Natarajan, N, et al. "Beta-carotene and animal fats and their relationship to prostate cancer risk. A casecontrol study." *Cancer*, 1989, 64: 605–12.

44. Chan, J M, and Giovannucci, E L. "Dairy products, calcium, and vitamin D and risk of prostate cancer." *Epidemiol Revs*, 2001, 23: 87–92.

45. Plant, J A. *The No-Dairy Breast Cancer Prevention Program*. New York: St. Martin's Press, 2001, p. 74.

46. Plant. *The No-Dairy Breast Cancer Prevention Program*. p. 75. Cited in Kliewer, E V, and Smith, K R. "Breast cancer mortality among immigrants in Australia and Canada." *J Natl Cancer Inst*, 1995, 87(15): 1154–61. See also Cancer Research Campaign. "Factsheet 6.2, Breast Cancer—UK." 1996.

47. McManamy, J. "Depression and diabetes." http://www.mcmanweb.com /article-42.htm.

48. "Scientists examine link between diabetes, depression." *San Antonio Express News*, June 16, 2000.

49. Golden, S H, Williams, J E, Ford, D E, et al. "Depressive symptoms and the risk of Type 2 diabetes." *Diabetes Care*, 2004, 27: 429–35.

50. Yoon, J W, et al. "Effects of environmental factors on the development of insulin-dependent diabetes mellitus." *Clin Invest Med*, September 1987, 10(5): 457–69.

51. Banu Priya, C A Y, et al. "Toxicity of fluoride to diabetic rats." *Fluoride*, 1997, 30(1): 51–58. http: //www.fluoride-journal.com/97-30-1/301-51. htm.

52. Trakhtenberg, I M. *Chronic Effects of Mercury on Organisms*. Washington, DC: GPO, 1974.

53. Timoshina, I V, Liubchenko, P N, and Khzardzhian, V G. "Functional state of the pancreas in workers exposed to the long-term action of lead." *Ter Arkh*, 1985, 57(2): 91–95. (Article in Russian.)

54. Schwartz, G G, Il'Yasova, D, and Ivanova, A. "Urinary cadmium, impaired fasting glucose, and diabetes in the NHANES III." *Diabetes Care*, February 2003, 26 (2).

55. Satarug, S, Haswell-Elkins, M R, and Moore, M R. "Safe levels of cadmium intake to prevent renal toxicity in human subjects." *Br J Nutr*, December 2000, 84(6): 791–802.

56. Fahim, M A, Hasan, M Y, and Alshuaib, W B. "Cadmium modulates diabetes-induced alterations in murine neuromuscular junction." *Endocr Res*, May 2000, 26(2): 205–17.

57. Jin, T, Nordberg, G, Sehlin, J, Wallin, H, and Sandberg, S. "The susceptibility to nephrotoxicity of streptozotocin-induced diabetic rats subchronically exposed to cadmium chloride in drinking water." *Toxicology*, December 1999, 142(1): 69–75.

58. Gumuslu, S, Yargicoglu, P, Agar, A, Edremitlioglu, M, and Aliciguzel, Y. "Effect of cadmium on antioxidant status in alloxane-induced diabetic rats." *Biol Trace Elem Res*, May 1997, 57(2): 105–14.

59. Chen, Y W, Huang, C F, Tsai, K S, Yang, R S, Yen, C C, Yang, C Y, Lin-Shiau, S Y, and Liu, S H. "Methylmercury induces pancreatic beta-cell apoptosis and dysfunction." *Chem Res Toxicol*, August 2006, 19(8): 1080–85.

60. International Medical Veritas Association. "Diabetes and mercury poisoning."

61. Ibid.

62. Tseng, C H, et al. "Long-term arsenic exposure and incidence of noninsulin- dependent diabetes mellitus: A cohort study in arseniasishyper-endemic villages in Taiwan." *Environ Health Perspect*, September 2000, 108(9): 847–51.

63. Rahman, M, et al. "Diabetes mellitus associated with arsenic exposure in Bangladesh." *Am J Epidemiol*, 1998, 148(2): 198–203.

64. Berkson, L. *Hormone Deception*, New York: Contemporary Books, 2000, p. 312.

65. Shirng-Wern Tsaih, et al. "Lead, diabetes, hypertension, and renal function: The normative aging study." *Environmental Health Perspectives*, 2004, 12(11).

66. National Research Council. *Fluoride in Drinking Water: A Scientific Review of EPA's Standards*. Washington, DC: National Academies Press, 2006.

67. The information in this section is gathered from the National Vaccine Information Center (NVIC), a national, nonprofit educational organization founded in 1982. NVIC is the oldest and largest consumer organization advocating for vaccine safety and informed consent protections in the mass vaccination system.

68. National Vaccine Information Center. "Juvenile diabetes and vaccination: New evidence for a connection." http://www.nvic.org/vaccines-and-diseases/Diabetes/juvenilediabetes.aspx.

69. Ibid.

70. Ibid.

71. Centers for Disease Control. *Pharmacoepidemiology and Drug Safety*, 1998, 6(2): S60.

72. So Jung Lee, et al. "Caffeine ingestion is associated with reductions in glucose uptake independent of obesity and Type 2 diabetes before and after exercise training." *Diabetes Care*, 2005, 28: 566–72.

73. Meister, K. *Cigarettes: What the Warning Label Doesn't Tell You*. New York: The American Council on Science and Health, 1996.

74. Targher, G, Alberiche, M, Zenere, M B, et al. "Cigarette smoking and insulin resistance in patients with non-insulin dependent diabetes mellitus." *J Clin Endocrinol Metab*, 1997, 82: 3619–24.

75. Targher, et al. "Cigarette smoking and insulin resistance."

76. Kelley, D E, Goodpaster, B, Wing, R R, and Simoneau, J A. "Skeletal muscle fatty acid metabolism in association with insulin resistance, obesity, and weight loss." *Am J Physiol*, 1999, 277: E1130–E1141.

77. Gutierrez, D. "Exercise shown to powerfully decrease cigarette cravings." April 4, 2007. http://www.newstarget.com/021769.html.

78. Kawakami, N, et al. "Effects of smoking on incidence of non-insulin dependence diabetes mellitus." *Am J Epidemiology*, January 15, 1997, 145(2): 103–9.

79. Will, J C, et al. "Cigarette smoking and diabetes mellitus: Evidence of a positive association from a large prospective cohort study." *Int J Epidemiol*, 2001, 30: 554–55.

80. Mitchell, B, Hawthorne, V, and Vinik, A. "Cigarette smoking and neuropathy in diabetic patients." *Diabetes Care*, 1990, 13: 434–47.

81. Sands, M, et al. "Incidence of distal symmetric (sensory) neuropathy in NIDDM: The San Luis Diabetes Study." *Diabetes Care*, 1997, 20: 322–29.

82. "Diabetes and periodontal disease fact book." http://www.healthnewsflash.com/conditions/diabetes_and_periodontal_disease.php.

83. Klienfield, N R. "Diabetes and its awful toll quietly emerge as a crisis." *New York Times*, January 9, 2006. http://query.nytimes.com/gst/fullpage.html?res=9907e2da1f30f93aa35752c0a9609c8b63&pagewanted=all.

84. *Annals of Internal Medicine*, 136(3): 130.

85. Humphries, S E, Gable, D, Cooper, J A, et al. "Common variants in the

TCF7L2 gene and predisposition to type 2 diabetes in UK European whites, Indian Asians and Afro Caribbean men and women." *J Molecular Medicine*, December 2006, 84(12): 1005–14.

86. Murray, M, and Pizzorno, J. *Encyclopedia of Natural Medicine*, Rocklin, CA: Prima, 1998.

87. De Mattia, G, Bravi, M C, Laurenti, O, Cassone-Faldetta, M, Proietti A, De Luca, O, Armiento, A, and Ferri, C. "Reduction of oxidative stress by oral N-acetyl-L-cysteine treatment decreases plasma soluble vascular cell adhesion molecule-I concentrations in non-obese, nondyslipidaemic, normotensive, patients with non-insulin-dependent diabetes." *Diabetologia*, 1998, 41(11): 1392–96.

88. Kaufman, F R. "Type diabetes in children and young adults: A 'new epidemic.'" *Clinical Diabetes*, 2002, 20: 217–18.

89. Ibid.

90. Ibid.

91. Ibid.

92. Wang, Y. "Cross-national comparison of childhood obesity: The epidemic and the relationship between obesity and socioeconomic status." *Intl J Epidemiology*, October 2001, 30: 1129–36.

93. Adams, M. "Campaign for commercial-free childhood blasts TV promotion of junk foods to children." http://www.newstarget.com/021835.html.

94. Enos, W F, Holmes, R H, and Beyer, J. "Coronary disease among United States soldiers killed in action in Korea." *JAMA*, 1953, 152: 1090–93.

95. McNamara, J J, Molot, M A, Stremple, J F, and Cutting, R T. "Coronary artery disease in combat casualties in Vietnam." *JAMA*, 1971, 216: 1185–87.

96. Berenson, et al. "Association between multiple cardiovascular risk factors."

97. Strong, J P, Malcolm, G T, McMahan, C, Tracy, R, Newman, W, Hederick, E, and Cornhill, J. "Prevalence and extent of atherosclerosis in adolescents and young adults." *JAMA*, 1999, 281: 727–35.

98. Berenson, et al. "Association between multiple cardiovascular risk factors."

99. Huerta, M G, et al. "Magnesium deficiency is associated with insulin resistance in obese children." *Diabetes Care*, 2005, 28: 1175–81.

100. Bircher-Benner, M. *Food Science for All and a New Sunlight Theory of Nutrition: Lectures to Teachers of Domestic Economy*. London: C. W. Daniel & Company, 1939.

101. Wigmore, A. *The Hippocrates Diet and Health Program*. Wayne, NJ: Avery Press, 1984.

102. Hughes, J H, and Latner, A L. "Chlorophyll and hemoglobin regeneration after hemorrhage." *Journal of Physiology*, University of Liverpool, 1936, 86, 388.

103. Grimm, J J. "Interaction of physical activity and diet: implications for insulin-glucose dynamics." *Public Health Nutr*, 1999, 2: 363–68.

104. Moore, M A, Park, C B, and Tsuda, H. "Implications of the hyperinsulinaemia-diabetes-cancer link for preventive efforts." *Eur J Cancer Prev*, 1998, 7: 89–107.

105. Arthur, L S, Selvakumar, R, Seshadri, M S, and Seshadri, L. "Hyperinsulinemia in polycystic ovary disease." *J Reprod Med*, 1999, 44: 783–87.

106. Pugeat, M, and Ducluzeau, P H. "Insulin resistance, polycystic ovary syndrome and metformin." *Drugs*, 1999, 58: 41–46.

107. Baranowska, B, Radzikowska, M W, et al. "Neuropeptide Y, leptin, galanin and insulin in women with polycystic ovary syndrome." *Gynecol Endocrinol*, 1999, 13: 344–51.

108. Kotake, H, and Oikawa, S. "Syndrome X." *Nippon Rinsho*, 1999, 57: 622–26. (Article in Japanese.)

109. Watanabe, K, Sekiya, M, Tsuruoka, T, et al. "Relationship between insulin resistance and cardiac sympathetic nervous function in essential hypertension." *J Hypertens*, 1999, 17: 1161–68.

110. Lender, D, Arauz-Pacheco, C, Adams-Huet, B, and Raskin, P. "Essential hypertension is associated with decreased insulin clearance and insulin resistance." *Hypertension*, 1997, 29: 111–114.

111. Stubbs, P J, Alaghband-Zadeh, J, Laycock, J F, et al. "Significance of an index of insulin resistance on admission in nondiabetic patients with acute coronary syndromes." *Heart*, 1999, 82: 443–47.

112. Lempiainen, P, Mykkanen, L, Pyorala, K, et al. "Insulin resistance syndrome predicts coronary heart disease events in elderly nondiabetic men." *Circulation*, 1999, 100: 123–28.

113. Misra, A, Reddy, R B, Reddy, K S, et al. "Clustering of impaired glucose tolerance, hyperinsulinemia and dyslipidemia in young north Indian patients with coronary heart disease: A preliminary casecontrol study." *Indian Heart J*, 1999, 51: 275–80.

114. Davis, C L, Gutt, M, Llabre, M M, et al. "History of gestational diabetes, insulin resistance and coronary risk." *J Diabetes Complications*, 1999, 13: 216–23.

115. Despres, J P, Lamarche, B, Mauriege, P, et al. "Hyperinsulinemia as an independent risk factor for ischemic heart disease." *N Engl J Med*, 1996, 334: 952–57.

116. Tiihonen, M, Partinen, M, and Narvanen, S. "The severity of obstructive sleep apnea is associated with insulin resistance." *J Sleep Res*, 1993, 2: 56–61.

117. Moore, Park, and Tsuda. "Implications of the hyperinsulinaemia-diabetes-cancer link."

118. Pujol, P, Galtier-Dereure, F, and Bringer, J. "Obesity and breast cancer risk." *Hum Reprod*, 1997, 12: 116–25.

119. Stoll, B A. "Essential fatty acids, insulin resistance, and breast cancer risk." *Nutr Cancer*, 1998, 31: 72–77.

120. Grundy, S M. "Hypertriglyceridemia, insulin resistance, and the metabolic syndrome." *Am J Cardiol*, 1999, 83: 25F–29F.

121. Belfiore, F, and Iannello, S. "Insulin resistance in obesity: Metabolic mechanisms and measurement methods." *Mol Genet Metab*, 1998, 65: 121–28.

122. Samaras, K, Nguyen, T V, Jenkins, A B, et al. "Clustering of insulin resistance, total and central abdominal fat: Same genes or same environment?" *Twin Res*, 1999, 2: 218–25.

123. Benzi, L, Ciccarone, A M, Cecchetti, P, et al. "Intracellular hyperinsulinism: A metabolic characteristic of obesity with and without type 2 diabetes: Intracellular insulin in obesity and type 2 diabetes." *Diabetes Res Clin Pract*, 1999, 46: 231–37.

124. Norbiato, G, Bevilacqua, M, Meroni, R, et al. "Effects of potassium supplementation on insulin binding and insulin action in human obesity: Protein modified fast and refeeding." *Eur J Clin Invest*, 1984, 14: 414–19.

125. Reddi, A, DeAngelis, B, Frank, O, et al. "Biotin supplementation improves glucose and insulin tolerances in genetically diabetic KK mice." *Life Sci*, 1988, 42: 1323–30.

126. Brandi, L S, Santoro, D, Natali, A, et al. "Insulin resistance of stress: Sites and mechanisms." *Clin Sci (Colch)*, 1993, 85: 525–35.

127. Nilsson, P M, Moller, L, and Solstad, K. "Adverse effects of psychosocial stress on gonadal function and insulin levels in middle-aged males." *J Intern Med*, 1995, 237: 479–86.

128. Hamann, A, and Matthaei, S. "Regulation of energy balance by leptin." *Exp Clin Endocrinol Diabetes*, 1996, 104: 293–300.

129. *Alternative Medicine*, February 2007, p. 61.

130. Kuhl, C, and Holst, J J. "Plasma glucagon and insulin: Glucagon ratio in gestational diabetes." *Diabetes*, 1976, 25: 16.

131. Freinkel, N. "Banting lecture 1980: Of pregnancy and progeny." *Diabetes*, 1980, 29: 1023–35.

132. Coustan, D R, Carpenter, M W, O'Sullivan, P S, and Carr, S R. "Gestational diabetes mellitus: Predictors of subsequent disordered glucose metabolism." *Am I Obstet Gynecol*, 1993, 168: 1139–45.

133. O'Sullivan, J B. "Subsequent morbidity among GDM women." In *Carbohydrate Metabolism in Pregnancy and the Newborn*, ed. Sutherland, H W, and Stowers, J M. New York: Churchill Livingstone, 1984.

134. O'Sullivan, J B, Charles, O, Mahan, C M, and Dandrow, R V. "Gestational diabetes and perinatal mortality rate." *Am I Obstet Gynecol*, 1973, 116: 901–4.

135. Screening for gestational diabetes is technical and should be done with your doctor, who knows how to do it, but it is usually performed with a 50 gram oral glucose dose given between 20 and 28 weeks, followed by a one-hour venous glucose dose. A test result of above 140 at one hour suggests a gestational diabetes problem.

136. Rosick, E R. "The deadly connection between diabetes and Alzheimer's." *LE Magazine*, December 2006. http://www.lef.org /magazine/mag2006/dec2006_report_alzheimer_02.htm.

137. Rivera, E J, Goldin, A, Fulmer, N, Tavares, R, Wands, J R, and de la Monte, S M. "Insulin and insulin-like growth factor expression and function deteriorate with progression of Alzheimer's disease: Link to brain reductions in acetylcholine." *J Alzheimers Dis*, December 2005, 8(3): 247–68.

138. "Alzheimer's disease." *Alternative Medicine*, February 2007, p. 66.

139. Takeuchi, M, Kikuchi, S, Sasaki, N, et al. "Involvement of advanced glycation end products in Alzheimer's disease." *Curr Alzheimer Res*, February 2004, 1(1): 39–46.

140. Rosick, E R. "The deadly connection between diabetes and Alzheimer's." *Life Extension*, December 2006, pp. 33–41.

141. Ramasamy, R., Vannucci, S J, Yan, S S, et al. "Advanced glycation end products and RAGE: A common thread in aging, diabetes, neurodegeneration, and inflammation." *Glycobiology*, July 2005, 15(7): 16R–28R.

142. Opara, E C. "Oxidative stress, micronutrients, diabetes mellitus and its complications." *J R Soc Health*, March 2002, 122(1): 28–34.

143. Houstis, N, Rosen, E D, and Lander, E S. "Reactive oxygen species have a causal role in multiple forms of insulin resistance." *Nature*, April 2006, 440(7086): 944–48.

144. Moreira, P I, Smith, M A, Zhu, X, et al. "Oxidative stress and neurode-generation." *Ann NY Acad Sci*, June 2005, 1043: 545–52.

145. Arivazhagan, P, and Panneerselvam, C. "Alpha-lipoic acid increases Na+K+ATPase activity and reduces lipofuscin accumulation in discrete brain regions of aged rats." *Ann NY Acad Sci*, June 2004, 1019: 350–54.

146. Lovell, M A, Xie, C, Xiong, S, and Markesbery, W R. "Protection against amyloid beta peptide and iron/hydrogen peroxide toxicity by alpha lipoic acid." *J Alzheimer's Dis*, June 2003, 5(3): 229–39.

147. Hitti, M. "Fruit, veggie juices may cut Alzheimer's risk. Antioxidants may be the key, say researchers." WebMD Medical News. June 20, 2005. http://my.webmd.com/content/Article/107/108607.htm.

148. Nagamani, M, Hannigan, E V, Dinh, T V, and Stuart, C A. "Hyperinsulinemia and stromal luteinization of the ovaries in post-menopausal women with endometrial cancer." *J Clin Endocrinol Metab*, July 1988, 67(1): 144–48.

149. Parazzini, F, La Vecchia, C, Negri, E, Riboldi, G L, Surace, M, Benzi, G, Maina, A, and Chiaffarino, F. "Diabetes and endometrial cancer: An Italian case-control study." *Int J Cancer*, 1999, 81(4): 539–42.

150. Nagamani, et al. "Hyperinsulinemia and stromal luteinization."

151. Vishnevsky, A S, Bobrov, J F, Tsyrlina, E V, and Dilman, V M. "Hyperinsulinemia as a factor modifying sensitivity of endometrial carcinoma to hormonal influences." *Eur J Gynaecol Oncol*, 1993, 14(2): 127–30.

152. Schoen, R E, Tangen, C M, Kuner, L H, Burke, G L, Cushman, M, Tracy, R P, Dobs, A, and Savage, P. "Increased blood glucose and insulin, body size, and incident colorectal cancer." *J Natl Cancer Inst*, 1999, 91(13): 1147–54.

153. Larsson, S C, Bergkvist, L, and Wolk, A. "Consumption of sugar and sugar-sweetened food and the risk of pancreatic cancer in a prospective study." *Am J Clin Nutr*, November 2006, 84(5): 1171–76.

CHAPTER 3

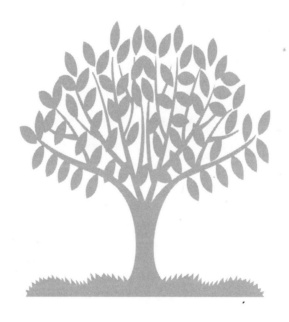

A Preliminary Theory of Diabetes

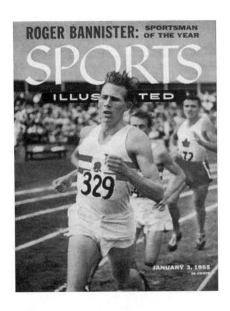

No longer conscious of my movement, I discovered a new unity with nature. I had found a new source of power and beauty, a source I never dreamt existed.

Roger Bannister, on breaking the four-minute mile

When Roger Bannister broke the four-minute mile in 1954, no one believed that humans had the physiological capacity to run that far that fast. When Bannister clocked 3:59.4, that presumption was dissolved and with it the conventional paradigm and belief system limitations. Now it is commonplace for high school milers to run a mile in less than four minutes. This book announces that the four-minute mile of diabetes has been broken and there is the capacity to completely reverse both non-insulin-dependent diabetes mellitus (NIDDM) and insulin-dependent diabetes mellitus (IDDM) Type-2 diabetes, and most dramatically, Type-1 diabetes.

By developing a preliminary theory of the causative level of diabetes, one becomes significantly empowered to develop an overall approach for the reversal of diabetes. The word *reversing* is different from ameliorating, modifying, or decreasing the amount of medication needed.

I am not talking about managing Type-1 or Type-2 diabetes, which is the old paradigm, exemplified by a belief system stated in the *New York Times* and backed by most doctors treating diabetes: "Diabetes has no cure. It is progressive and fatal." I have developed the knowledge, clinical know-how, and experience to completely reverse Type-2 diabetes. (I will address a more complete theory for healing Type-1 diabetes in Chapter 5.) The four-minute mile of diabetes has been broken. All that is needed is to let go of our belief that diabetes cannot be reversed—then we are free to cultivate the understanding of what is possible.

Actually, doctors have been using live foods to reverse diabetes as far back as 1920, when Dr. Max Gerson healed Dr. Albert Schweitzer of Type-2 diabetes with live-food nutrition. For the last 30 years, after turning to live foods in my own life and in using it as a baseline for all healing as a holistic physician, this strategy has been reversing Type-2 diabetes regularly. With the energy released by this understanding comes the determination to change our lifestyle and dietary patterns to achieve this result. The mythology supported by the allopathic treatment approach, which has indeed not been particularly successful, is that diabetes is a one-way, downhill road to death involving multiple complications. The statistics show that diabetes, as currently approached, will steal 10 to 19 years from a person's life. When one is freed from the lifestyle of the Culture of Death and transitions to the Culture of Life, the current pattern of irreversibility shifts to one of reversibility.

Type-2 diabetes is a disease of both a complex and simple etiology. Based on clinical experience, as well as world research, the number one culprit is the huge increase in intake of processed white sugar, white bread, and refined carbohydrates, as well complex natural carbohydrates such as grains. The breakthrough in understanding the primary cause of diabetes was found in Dr. Thomas Cleave's 1975 book *The Saccharine Disease: Conditions Caused by the Taking of Refined Carbohydrates* (such as sugar and white flour), which showed that within 20 years after processed white flour and sugar are introduced into a culture, there is an "outbreak" of diabetes. His statistical analysis showed processed sugar rather than fat as the primary cause.

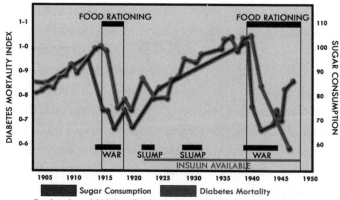

England and Wales. Diabetic Mortality indices. The figures for 1946 and 1947 supplied by Dr. Percy Stocks. Drawn by Thomas L. Cleave in *The Saccharine Disease*.

According to Dr. Cleave, until 1955 the primary cause of diabetes was thought to be related to fat consumption. This was because of a paper presented in 1949 by H. P. Himsworth,[1] who made the correlation that during World War II diabetes mortality fell in direct relationship to the fall in fat consumption.

Dr. Cleave showed that when diabetes mortality was charted against the consumption of refined carbohydrates—white sugar and white flour—rather than total consumption of carbohydrates (both complex and refined), there was a much closer statistical correlation between refined carbohydrate consumption and diabetes mortality. This correlation was greater for refined carbohydrates with diabetes than for fat consumption. Dr. Cleave also showed that the increase in fat consumption from 1900 to 1960 was minor compared with the increase in consumption of refined carbohydrates during this same time period, when diabetes moved from twenty-seventh in the list of causes of death to seventh by the 1960s. Only the dramatic increase in the consumption of refined carbohydrates matched the dramatic increase in diabetes mortality. This point was made clearer by the fact that in communities where refined carbohydrates were not introduced, and where a high consumption of complex carbohydrates was avoided, there was not a significant increase in diabetes.

Therefore, Dr. Cleave concluded, as I have, that the introduction of refined carbohydrates into a culture was the primary, but not sole, cause of the dramatic increase in diabetes. Other contributing underlying causes include increased consumption of cooked animal flesh and trans fats; a diet high in junk, processed, and GMO foods; heavy metals; agrochemicals; vitamin D deficiencies; mineral and vitamin deficiencies in general resulting from a diet of nutrient-poor processed foods; and hormonal imbalances and deficiencies such as a deficiency in testosterone. Lifestyle habits also play a role—obesity, emotional stress, inadequate sleep, television viewing, and lack of exercise. Dr. Cleave's cross-cultural work, however, highlighted the main issue, which was an excess increase in the consumption of white sugar and white flour.

In 1959 G. D. Campbell[2] also showed that there seemed to be a period of 20 years from the time refined carbohydrates (white sugar and white flour) are introduced into a culture and an outbreak of diabetes. His research on the urban Zulu was published in the *South African Medical Journal* in 1960.[3] V. Albertson also confirmed this "20-year rule" in Iceland studies. In Iceland around the 1850s, the diet was 85 percent protein and fats with no refined carbohydrates,[4] but with the introduction of refined carbohydrates, protein and fats were reduced to 45 percent, and following the 20-year rule, there was an outbreak of diabetes.

A. M. Cohen's 1960 study of Yemenite Jews showed a low incidence of diabetes in Yemen with a general diet that was high in fat and protein and with one of the two lowest sugar intakes in the world.[5] When these Yemenite Jews moved to Israel, there was a marked increase in white sugar consumption, and Yemenite Jews in Israel, from a culture in which diabetes was unknown, became equal for the incidence of diabetes to that of the Israeli culture.

The Canadian Eskimos also had a high raw-animal-fat diet. After refined carbohydrates were introduced, their cultures were also found to have an increased incidence of diabetes within 20 years. Dr. Cleave wrote, "With the greater availability of sugar and white flour, the consumption of the former substance amongst Canadian Eskimos has now risen to over 100 lb. per head per year and, with the expiring of the 20-year incubation period already discussed, diabetes is now commonly occurring amongst them."

Evidence from studies in India of rural and urban groups of the same culture showed their diabetes incidence being significantly higher in the urban setting, with its much higher consumption of refined carbohydrates. It is not reasonable to relate it to the consumption of fats, as those cultures have only one-half the fat consumption that is needed for good health.

In the United States, Cherokee Indians also followed the pattern of high refined carbohydrate intake associated with high diabetes incidence. In the Natal Indians of the Zulu tribe, an increase in diabetes incidence was directly related to refined carbohydrate consumption. Dr. Cleave's data suggest that there is now no country where the incidence of diabetes cannot be directly related to increased refined carbohydrate intake. Similar findings were found for all indigenous groups migrating to urban environments, such as Kurdish immigrants. Similar data have been gathered from Australian Aborigines,[6] New Guinea aboriginal groups,[7] and Polynesians in general.[8]

In summary, cross-cultural studies show that the primary cause of Type-2 diabetes is the introduction of refined carbohydrates into cultures that previously had low incidences of diabetes, whether on a low-protein-and-fat and high-complex-carbohydrate diet or a high-fat and protein diet. The main environmental cause of the worldwide pandemic of Type-2 diabetes is the introduction of white sugar, white flour, and white rice into these cultures, resulting in an "outbreak" of Type-2 diabetes 20 years later. It is obvious that a successful program for healing diabetes must eliminate all refined and junk food carbohydrates from the diet.

Dr. Cleave's book synthesized and tabulated the cross-cultural studies and showed that the introduction of refined carbohydrates into the cultures with a previously low incidence of diabetes saw an outbreak of diabetes within 20 years. This indicates that the main dietary cause of diabetes is processed sugar. In my clinical experience I have found that even moderate- to high-glycemic fruits and/or grains in the diet raise the blood glucose levels of those with prediabetes and diabetes. While limited amounts of these foods may be acceptable for those not in a pre-diabetic or diabetic physiology, I do not recommend them until people are maintained in a healthy physiology (optimally a fasting blood sugar [FBS] of 70–85 for at least six months to a year but minimally an FBS of less than 100 for three months). At that time, it is most prudent to introduce only low-glycemic berries, cherries, citrus, and some occasional whole grains in the maintenance diet. Reversing and healing the diabetic, physiological pathology takes stronger and more focused approach than an ongoing maintenance and/or prevention program.

Cooked Animal Flesh and Trans-Fatty Acids

Another contributor to the onset of diabetes is a diet high in cooked animal flesh and trans-fatty acids. An excess of animal flesh and trans-fatty acids is associated with increased diabetes, cancer of the breast and prostate, immune dysfunction, and infertility. Dr. Walter Willett and Dr. Alberto Ascherio of the Harvard School of Public Health have estimated that 30,000 premature deaths each year are attributable to our consumption of trans fats.[9] Foods high in trans-fatty acids include margarine, commercial peanut butter, and prepackaged baked goods, cakes, pies, and cookies. Naturally occurring trans fats can also be found in some animal products such as dairy products and beef fat, since the trans isomer is produced by bacteria in the gastrointestinal tract of cattle and other ruminants. These naturally occurring trans fats may account for as much as 21 percent of the food sources for American adults, according to the U.S. Food and Drug Administration.[10] Trans-fatty acids disrupt cell membrane function because they change fat molecular structures from a cis fatty acid to a trans-fatty acid, or from a curved shape to a straight shape; their actual molecular structure is thus changed and decreases the function of the cell membrane, which some people theorize is the actual brain of the cell and certainly critical for efficient movement of glucose into the cell. The partially hydrogenated fats are high in trans-fatty acids and are detrimental to cell membrane function.

It is important to understand that not all fats are harmful. The omega-3 fatty acids and monounsaturated fats improve insulin function. One study of 86,000 women followed over 16 years, in the Nurses Health Study, found that those who consumed one ounce of nuts five times per week decreased their risk of Type-2 diabetes by 27 percent. Evidence suggests that a raw, plant-source-only diet, moderately high in walnuts and almonds, may be helpful in the prevention of diabetes and in regulating glycemic control. This may be because the omega-3 and 6 fatty acids in proper 1:2 ratio and the monounsaturated fats act to strengthen and repair the cell membrane structure and function. The wrong types of fats in our diets create an abnormal cell membrane structure, leading to impaired action of insulin. A poorly functioning cell membrane decreases cellular viral immunity, creates low-grade inflammation, and makes us susceptible to the development of chronic disease.

Achieving Normal Blood Sugar Levels

In the Dr. Cousens's Diabetes Recovery Program—A Holistic Approach, it is common to see Type-2 diabetics shift from blood sugars of 300–400 while on medication to safe or normal FBSs, being taken off all medications, including insulin, within one to four days. Within one to three weeks many have their FBS go down to the optimum of 85. Some people, particularly those with Syndrome X (also known as metabolic syndrome, an advanced form of chronic diabetes degenerative syndrome [CDDS], which is essentially prediabetes or diabetes) may take three or four weeks or even a year to heal. Psychological stresses, as we pointed out, create elevated cortisol, which increases inflammation and undermines our ability to control insulin and glucose. Whether it takes four days to a few weeks, or a month, or even two months isn't the point, so much as that we have the capacity within us to return to a healthy physiology, with an FBS that is consistently below 100.

Diabetes is a complicated metabolic imbalance of carbohydrates, lipids, and proteins made worse with inflammation, heavy metal toxicity, nutritional deficiencies, and other hormonal imbalances. Complications involve free radical damage, sorbitol buildup in the tissues and organs, and a glycosylated protein/lipid buildup. All these greatly accelerate the aging process. Diabetes in this context can be considered a sign of accelerated aging.

Diabetes is a symptom of the Culture of Death, which now appears in the world population as a pandemic. We have the opportunity to return to a world Culture of Life and live a lifestyle that naturally protects us against diabetes, as was done by indigenous groups for thousands of years. With that in mind, we are going to take a look at the physiology of Type-1, Type-2, and gestational diabetes. Although different, there are significant overlaps. First, let us look at blood glucose levels and their impact on our health.

What Are Healthy Blood Glucose Levels?

What are conventionally considered "normal" glucose levels are actually unhealthy. The newer research now suggests that the optimal FBS, which is one's blood glucose first thing in the morning, should be at 70–85. Accelerated aging begins with an FBS of 86 or greater, and with that come an increased risk of premature death. We have just begun to recognize that even a high normal glucose can eventually become a serious threat to our health. The point is we need to understand the complex toxic effects that high blood sugar or hyperglycemia creates in the body. It should be clear at this point that a high blood sugar damages cells through multiple mechanisms and accelerates all elements of aging.

The following list shows the potential problems that can arise from a high-glycemic diet. Items marked with an asterisk (*) were compiled and listed by Nancy Appleton, PhD, author of *Lick the Sugar Habit*, and published in *Health Freedom News*, June 1994.

> Acidic stomach*
> Alcoholism*
> Anxiety*

Appendicitis*
Arthritis*
Asthma*
Atherosclerosis*
Cancer of the breast, ovaries, intestines, prostate, and
    rectum*
Candida and other fungal infections*
Cataracts*
Changed structure of protein*
Chromium deficiency*
Copper deficiency*
Decreased growth hormone secretion*
Depletion and imbalancing of neurotransmitters
Depression
Diabetes*
Disorganizing of the minerals in the body*
Drowsiness and decreased activity in children*
Eczema in children*
Elevated glucose and insulin responses in oral contraceptive
    users*
Elevation of low-density lipoproteins (LDL, the "bad"
    cholesterol)*
Emphysema*
Food allergies*
Gallstones*
Gastric or duodenal ulcers*
Heart disease*
Hemorrhoids*
Hypertension*
Hyperactivity, anxiety, difficulty concentrating, and
    crankiness in children*
Hypoglycemia
Impaired structure of DNA*
Increase in AGEs, or advanced glycation end products,
    which accelerate aging

Increase in triglycerides*
Increased cholesterol*
Increased fasting levels of glucose and insulin*
Increased free radicals in the bloodstream*
Increased inflammatory prostaglandins*
Increased risk of Crohn's disease and ulcerative colitis*
Insulin resistance*
Interference with absorption of calcium and magnesium*
Interference with the absorption of protein*
Kidney damage*
Loss of teeth calcium as a result of calcium being pulled
    from normal blood and bone by sugar combining with it
Lowered enzymes' ability to function*
Malabsorption in those with functional bowel disease*
Migraine headaches*
Multiple sclerosis*
Obesity*
Osteoporosis*
Periodontal disease*
PMS (up to 275 percent increase)
Raised adrenaline levels in children*
Reduction of high-density lipoproteins (HDL, the "good"
    cholesterol)*
Saliva acidity*
Skin aging, due to changes in the structure of collagen*
Syndrome X
Tooth decay*
Varicose veins*
Weakened eyesight*
Weakened immune system*

The key to healing diabetes is eating and living in a way that creates an FBS of less than 100 and optimally between 70 and 85. A potent means of achieving this is associated with caloric restriction.

This information comes from animal studies and our clinical experience, where caloric restriction induced significant reductions in blood glucose levels.[11, 12, 13] The message is *the less we eat, the longer we live, and the better control we have over blood glucose.* By decreasing caloric intake, our risk of age-related diseases is diminished, and a slowing of aging is activated.[14, 15, 16, 17, 18, 19, 20, 21, 22] When people eat too much in general, their blood sugar often rises. On a restricted-calorie diet, their blood sugar is more likely to stay at normal levels. This observation is from my clinical experience in watching people I call the "canaries in the mine." These are people with Type-1 diabetes or sensitive Type-2s. I would ask them to try a particular food or to watch when they over-ate and observe their blood glucose levels. This is not as scientifically accurate as double-blind studies, but it certainly has pointed me in the right direction. With age, fasting glucose levels increase either as health decreases or, as I will discuss later, the enzyme glucose-6-phosphatase becomes dysregulated.

To further illustrate this point, a study of 2,000 men over a 20-year period showed that those with fasting glucose levels over 85 had a 40 percent increased risk of death from cardiovascular disease.[23] With this kind of data, one should not be surprised that I would define an FBS above 85 as a beginning stage of glucose toxicity. The researchers concluded that "fasting blood glucose values in upper normal range appeared to be an important independent predictor of increased cardiovascular death and nondiabetic middle aged men."

How did researchers decide that a blood glucose of 85 was the upper limit? The pancreas is key for regulating glucose, by releasing insulin into the system when there is an excess of glucose in the blood. In this way, high insulin levels contribute to obesity because insulin brings glucose as fat into the cells. For this reason, hyperinsulinemia is associated with being overweight, as well as Type-2 diabetes, cardiovascular disease, kidney disease, and certain types of cancer. In a normal person, the pancreas stops secreting insulin when the glucose levels drop below 83 mg/dl.[24, 25, 26] This fact is key to our understanding of what is a healthy blood glucose. Previously allopathic medicine waited until reaching an

FBS of 109 before a prediabetic condition was suspected. Now we are looking at this in a much different way. Insulin continues to be secreted when blood glucose levels are above 83. So the body is telling us that the pancreas wants to keep the glucose levels down to a safer range than what allopaths currently consider safe or convenient. Dr. Roy Walford's work on calorie restriction showed that restricting caloric intake lowers fasting glucose by 21 percent on average from 92 to 74 in humans. Dr. Walford was the one who found that people who practiced caloric restriction also had a 42 percent reduction in fasting insulin.[27] Before the pancreas eventually gets exhausted, overweight and obese people were found to have very high insulin levels, which is a result of insulin resistance.[28, 29] This research supports the teaching of "the less we eat, the longer we live." This assumption also is supported by the major long-lived human cultures averaging about 1,500 calories/day as compared to our Western culture's intake of 3,000–3,800 calories/day. My clinical observations have also been that blood sugar increases when diabetics overeat, even if it is the overeating of healthy foods.

I am recommending a range of 70 to 85 as the optimal FBS. I consider borderline impaired fasting glucose tolerance to be an FBS of 86 to 99 (a precursor for prediabetes); and an FBS at 100 to 125 and over is considered prediabetes by my standards. An FBS of 99 or less is considered normal by allopathic standards and thus nondiabetic, which is why I use this standard for considering someone healed as it is generally accepted in the medical community as nondiabetic. *Healed*, however, does not mean *optimal*. This is significantly different from the current assumptions. On October 24, 2003, the scientific committee of the American Diabetes Association actually did create a new and better definition of prediabetic or impaired glucose tolerance of a blood glucose of 100 or greater. They lowered the breakpoint from 109 to 100 mg/dl, which now means that the value of 100 or more would lead to a diagnosis of impaired fasting glucose or prediabetes. According to the general scientific literature, those who fall into the prediabetic range would probably develop diabetes within 10 years.

Glycemic Index and Insulin Index

Another approach that helps lower blood glucose is decreasing the intake of high-glycemic-index foods and high-insulin-index foods. The glycemic index (GI) is a measure of what happens to your blood sugar when you consume particular foods. GI numbers show how much one helping (50 grams) of a particular food raises your blood sugar.

Although useful, the GI does not provide a complete and accurate understanding of the full range of foods and their effect on glucose metabolism. In some instances, a food has a low GI rating but a high insulin index rating. Another vantage point at understanding how diet affects insulin levels has been proposed by Susanne H. A. Holt, Janette C. Brand Miller, and Peter Petocz.[30] They state that the GI concept does not consider insulin responses to particular foods. Their research proposes a method for obtaining a more accurate assessment of dietary factors to insulin response, based on a more realistic isoenergetic basis. The insulin index is based on the insulin response to various foods, and certain foods (such as lean meats or proteins) seem to cause an increased insulin response despite there being no carbohydrates

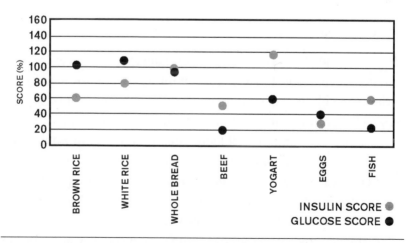

FIGURE 1. Insulin and glucose scores of selected foods (Source: Holt, Miller, and Petocz, "An insulin index of foods: the insulin demand generated by 1000-kJ portions of common foods." *Am J Clin Nutr*, 1997, 66: 1264-76.)

present. Additionally, other foods seem to cause a disproportionate insulin reaction for the carbohydrate load. Holt and her colleagues have noted that glucose and insulin scores are mostly highly correlated, but high-protein foods and bakery products (rich in fat and refined carbohydrates) "elicit insulin responses that were disproportionately higher than their glycemic responses." In other words, a number of factors other than carbohydrate content mediate in stimulation of insulin secretion. For example, protein-rich foods or the addition of protein to a carbohydrate-rich meal can stimulate a modest rise in insulin secretion, without increasing blood glucose concentration.

From these data, we can at least theorize that some complex carbohydrates do not produce insulin responses much greater than protein-rich foods such as beef or fish. Perhaps surprisingly, the insulin levels for beef and fish are greater than their glucose levels, and the glucose level for yogurt is higher than the insulin levels or glucose levels of carbohydrate-rich foods such as brown rice, white rice, and bread. Hopefully this will lay rest to the myth that protein-rich animal foods do not cause a significant rise in insulin when compared to carbohydrate-rich foods.

Satiety Index

The satiety index (SI) is a relatively new concept[31] that measures how full or satiated people feel after consuming a given calorie load from a variety of foods. It is measured by asking people to rate how satiated they feel after a meal and by how much food they eat after a two-hour delay after consuming the test food. Thus a high-SI food would leave people more satisfied after eating a set amount of calories, and they would also eat less two hours later when given something else to eat, presumably because they are still less hungry. It seems likely that a diet made up of higher-SI foods would likely lead to less hunger and a lower calorie intake. High-fructose corn syrup is a concern because it brings high amounts of sugar into the system but does not activate a feeling of being satiated; thus people are more likely to keep eating. High-fructose corn syrup sweeteners have been implicated in the epidemic of obesity.

Glycation

Associated with a high blood sugar is the destructive effect of the glucose as it links with protein and lipids in a process called *glycation*: the higher the blood glucose, the more severe the destructive glycation process. When the glucose nonenzymatically links with protein or lipid molecules, it results in the formation of nonfunctioning structures in the body. This results in poorly functioning enzymes, poorly functioning cell membranes, and cross-linkages of proteins in all tissues. Two extracellular proteins, collagen and elastin, are particularly affected, and one sees it in the skin as wrinkles. The formation of AGEs throughout the body is an accelerated aging process, hence the apt abbreviation of glycosylation or glycation as AGEs. AGE-related changes to collagen and elastin are believed to contribute to the stiffness of blood vessels and the urinary bladder, as well as impaired functioning of the kidneys, heart, retinas, and other organs and tissues. Moreover, damaging glycation reactions trigger inflammatory signaling, which scientists believe could provoke tissue damage and cancers.[32] As we will learn shortly, inflammation is the fourth of the Seven Stages of Disease, and it is followed by ulceration (Stage 5) and fungation (Stage 7, cancer). In diabetes, the rapid formation and accumulation of AGEs contribute to complications of disease, including injury to small blood vessels (microangiopathy) that impairs kidney and eye health.

In addition to those formed in the body, AGEs can also be introduced by external sources. For example, tobacco smoke contains precursors to advanced glycation end products, which increase AGE levels in the body. Foods that have been subjected to processing and heat also act as sources of AGEs.[33] This actually includes baby foods, as will be discussed later. I concur with Julian Whitaker, MD, that fructose is a "highly reactive molecule that readily attaches to proteins, changing their structure and interfering with normal activity. Studies show that fructose accelerates glycosylation, damaging proteins to a significantly greater degree than sucrose or glucose."[34] Our most prominent source of this damaging sugar is high-fructose corn syrup in soft drinks, which, according to the USDA Economic Research Service, comprised more than 25 percent of the beverages consumed by Americans in 1997. A 2005 study found that the low AGE content of a vegan diet could benefit diabetics.[35] The Culture of Life antidiabetogenic diet I employ is unprocessed, unheated, plant-source-only foods, and moderately low-glycemic, meaning that the AGE issue is minimized. It is thus optimal for reducing and eliminating diabetes and its complications.

Oxidative Stress

A higher blood glucose creates an oxidative stress as well. Research has clearly shown that the antioxidants vitamin C and E inhibit the formation of AGEs[36] and have been shown to reduce protein glycosylation both in vivo and in vitro,[37, 38] with beneficial results in the treatment of Type-2 diabetes. Vitamins C and E also act as scavengers of free radicals generated by the glycosylated proteins.[39] Davie, Gould, and Yutkin supplemented 12 nondiabetic subjects with 1 gram daily of vitamin C and demonstrated significant decreases of glycosylated hemoglobin of 18 percent and glycosylated albumin of 33 percent over a three-month period.[40] Jain, McVie, and Jaramillo found a significant reduction in glycosylated hemoglobin as well as a lowering of triglycerides in 35 Type-1 diabetics supplemented with 100 IU d-alpha tocopherol for three months.[41] The use of these incredible antioxidants will be discussed at greater length in Chapter 4.

Fasting Blood Sugar: Under 85

Glycosylation and oxidative stress are major reasons for why keeping an FBS of 85 and below is so important. Any FBS above 85 suggests that there is a metabolic disturbance, which is what I am describing as part of CDDS and diabetes. This metabolic disturbance leads to general degeneration. In a later chapter, I will discuss the physiology of this. So as we look at this process in terms of the carbohydrates, we can understand full well that all carbohydrates are not all the same. Simple carbohydrates—anything with white sugar, white bread, or high-fructose corn syrup—are more pathogenic than complex carbo-hydrates. An interesting cultural study conducted 50 years ago that makes this point is that of the O'Odham people of Southern Arizona, historically known as the River Pima and Papago, who had almost no diabetes. Now they have one of the highest levels of diabetes in the world, and some Native Americans are estimating about 90 percent incidence. Before the introduction of a processed diet, the Pimas were involved in desert farming and wild food gathering, which included complex carbohydrates and insulin-laden foods that protected them. Such foods had lower GIs, including lima beans, velvet mesquite pods, nopal cactus, and nonbitter emery oak acorns. These foods had significantly lower glycemic ratings. Their diet was historically based on legumes and some corn. Some of these foods were actually high in insulin as well and also high in gum pectins and complex carbohydrates. These desert plants, used to capture and store life-giving water, also contain the same agents that make beans, mesquite, plantago, belotas, chia seeds, nopalitos, and prickly pear fruit effective regulators of blood sugar. Because of the Pimas interface with Western culture and diet, and certain shifts that limited their access to antidiabetogenic foods, they shifted to a high-refined-sugar and cooked-animal-flesh diet, resulting in high rates of diabetes.

Most foods high on the glycemic and insulin indexes greatly accelerate the metabolic imbalance. If you have a blood sugar that is 180–200 mg/dl after eating, or actually at any time of day, that is considered diagnostic of diabetes. If your FBS is 126 or higher on two separate occasions, it supports a presumptive diagnosis of diabetes and merits further testing.

The glucose tolerance test is a very sensitive test for diabetes. The classic amount is 75 grams of glucose dissolved in 300 ml of water, and if your blood glucose value is 180 to 200 or above two hours later, it is diagnostic of diabetes. Two hours after drinking the glucose, the normal value should be less than 140; anything between 140 and 180 is prediabetes. Levels above 180 in the first hour or 200 at the end of the first hour indicate diabetes. At the Tree of Life, we only use 40 grams of glucose in a five-hour test because the sugar is such a stress on the system. We find clinically that our results have been highly sensitive and accurate at this amount. Another test for diabetes is the glycosylated hemoglobin (HgbA1c), which is not as specific or sensitive as the glucose tolerance test but a lot easier to do. A value of 5.7 or less suggests there is no diabetes. The glycosylated hemoglobin test has to do with how much protein hemoglobin in the red blood cells is glycosylated. One can use it to monitor the diabetic process every three to four months.

There is also the fructosamine test, which can be done as frequently as a monthly basis. I like to test both glycosylated hemoglobin and fructosamine before the program and at 3 months, but for research purposes I have done it after the 21-day program cycle. These tests can be thrown off by any occasion that creates an impaired glucose tolerance, including use of medications such as diuretics, glucocorticoids, and nicotinic acid. One is going to have more accuracy in monitoring the healing of diabetes by using the two tests rather than one.

Dietary Fat and Diabetes

The role of high cooked-animal-fat and trans-fat intake in diabetes has been suspected since the early twentieth century. As far back as the 1920s, Dr. S. Sweeney produced reversible diabetes in all of his medical school students by feeding them a high vegetable-oil diet for 48 hours. None of the students had previously been diabetic.[42] However, overloading a system like in this experiment is not a natural situation, as normal levels may actually be healing because they create optimal cell membrane composition versus an overload in a laboratory experiment. I make the suggestion, however, that fat in the system may be biphasic, meaning that at one level it may be healthy and antidiabetic and at an excess level, like in Dr. Sweeney's research, it would be diabetogenic. In the summary chapter this will be further discussed. The role of animal fats and protein, which research suggests is a secondary causative factor in diabetes, does increase the Type-2 diabetes incidence on the average by about 35–50 percent. This will be discussed in Chapter 5. A key distinction to be made in the fat discussion is that not all fats are equal. Cooked animal fats and trans fats seem to be detrimental and pathological for diabetes, but uncooked, live, plant-source-only fats in moderation seem to be both protective and healing.

In Japan, Thailand, other Asian countries, and Africa, people on the traditional diet had a low incidence of diabetes. As soon as people from these cultures moved away from their natural complex-carbohydrate diet of rice, leafy greens, starchy vegetables, beans, and noodles toward white flour and white sugar, they immediately began to develop increased rates of diabetes. With this understanding, it is best for one to be conscious when we use the word *carbohydrate*. Leafy greens, high-fiber vegetables, and sprouts, which are the primary complex carbohydrates I recommend, do not cause diabetes. These foods are also rich in fiber and, coupled with a high-fiber diet, give us a slow rate of breakdown of glucose into the system and therefore do not significantly tax or stress the system glycemically. These foods have a low to moderate GI and a low insulin index. When people from these indigenous cultures hit the Western diet of pathological carbohydrates, white sugar, white flour, and processed junk foods, rates of Type-2 diabetes soar.

Trans-fatty acids and cooked saturated animal fats, which contain trans-fatty acids, tend to block and disorganize the cell membranes in a way that disrupts the insulin receptors in the cells. This clinical experience gives us an insight into fat metabolism: that we should be removing these specific fats—animal fats and trans fats—off our plate as much as possible.

Dr. Barnard performed a 12-week study on the impact of a healthy vegan diet on diabetes. It showed that the average person on a no animal fat intake, high-complex-carbohydrate, and moderate- and low-protein diet lost 12 pounds, with FBS dropping 28 percent. There was a 46 percent drop in diabetic medication usage.[43] This study was interesting because there were no limits on calories or amounts of carbohydrates, and there was no change in exercise regime. The next study he did was one that included women who were moderately or severely overweight but didn't have the diagnosis of diabetes. They were put on a diet that contained no animal fat and was low in vegetable oils. A control group was on a cholesterol-lowering diet. The vegetarian group lost about a pound per week, and the control group lost about eight pounds in total per person.[44] The study group's body cells became more and more sensitive to insulin; at 14 weeks their insulin sensitivity had improved by 24 percent. From these results, he theorized that a no animal and low-moderate plant-source-only plant fat diet activated the natural ability to open the insulin receptors in the cells to allow glucose into the system. In another study, he observed 99 people over 22 weeks. Forty-nine were on a vegan moderate low-fat diet with no animal products or junk, processed carbohydrates, or other junk foods, and no limits on complex carbohydrates. The remaining 50 people were on the basic American Diabetes Association (ADA) diet. The ADA diet reduced glycosylated hemoglobin by 0.4 percent. The vegan diet was three times more effective, reducing the HgbA1c by 1.2 percentage points (one point being considered 1 percent). So the average value of glycosylated hemoglobin fell from 8 percent to 6.8 percent during the 22 weeks. One diabetes study in the UK showed that a one-point drop in glycosylated hemoglobin with Type-2 diabetes reduces the risk of kidney or eye complications by 37 percent.[45] The diet designed by Dr. Dean Ornish in his famous work in 1990 supports this general idea. His diet was low fat (a 10 percent fat intake) with no junk carbohydrates; processed, GMO foods; or trans fats. After about one year, the angiograms showed that 82 percent of the people who started with significantly blocked coronary arteries were starting to open up their arteries. In addition, people exercised, meditated, and had no smoking.[46] As to be further discussed in Chapter 5, both Dr. Ornish's and Dr. Barnard's results may be more related to eliminating white flours, white sugar, junk foods, and cooked animal fats.

A study[47] reported in the February 2004 *New England Journal of Medicine* tested young people whose parents or grandparents had Type-2 diabetes. These were healthy people but were found to have a certain amount of excess fat in their cells, called *intramyocellular fat*. Their intramyocellular fat was up to 80 percent higher than normal. In some cases, the excess fat was beginning to block insulin function. It is interesting that one newer theory of cell function, developed by Dr. Bruce Lipton and described in his book *The Biology of Belief*, considers the cell membrane the brain of the cell. The cell membrane is greatly affected by extracellular signaling, and insulin and glucose are extracellular signalers; consequently, both influence intracellular signaling by their action on the cell membrane. These genetically predisposed people had a much higher level of intramyocellular lipids, which seems to be significant. Intramyocellular fat accumulates to a certain extent and tends to interfere with insulin's intracellular signaling process. The mitochondria, which burn fat and produce energy for the cells, were unable to keep up with metabolizing the accumulated fat. The study showed that limiting the fat intake helped to decrease the insulin resistance. The researchers also saw that those people with Type-2 diabetes appeared to have far too much fat in their cells and less than normal amounts of mitochondria. On another level, people with diabetes seem to have less mitochondria than needed to burn up the accumulated fat. As will be discussed later, the endoplasmic reticulum in the mitochondria seem to be an interface where the body tries to cope with the worldwide problem of overnutrition, which results in para-inflammation, insulin resistance, and the consequent rising tide of Type-2 diabetes in the world. Another study[48] was done on people following a plant-source-only diet, and they found that the vegan participants had 30 percent lower intramyocellular lipid levels in their calves, compared to the omnivores. This suggests that a vegan diet makes one less susceptible to activating the diabetic intracellular fat accumulation genes. In the case of fat, the accumulation of excess fat in the cells weakens intracellular signaling of insulin. This appears to be less a diabetogenic force in those on a plant-source-only (vegan) diet, even with a plant-source-only fat intake of 25–45 percent, as Type-2 diabetics are rapidly healing with this percentage of plant fat in the diet.

Researchers at the Pennington biomedical research center in Baton Rouge, Louisiana, studied 10 young men who were in reasonably good health, putting them on an animal-based, high-fat diet. What they found is that in only three days the men accumulated significantly more intramyocellular fat. The first point this makes is that it's really easy to build up intramyocellular fat on a high-fat diet. But more important, they tested the genes associated with the mitochondria and their energy production and found that the fatty foods these volunteers ate actually turned off the genes that affected the cells' ability to burn fat. The genes that produce mitochondria seemed to be disabled. The implication fits with my larger theory that excessive cooked animal fat and trans fat interferes with the normal workings of the cells, including the ability to adequately respond to the intracellular signaling of insulin. With the excessive intracellular animal- and trans-fat accumulation, the glucose cannot be properly metabolized. Whether it is because it can't move from glycogen to glucose and therefore creates a glucose backup or because glucose cannot get into the cell, the detrimental animal fatty foods seem to either disable the genes so they are not able to produce more mitochondria or eliminate the fat. Most likely, both mechanisms occur. Theoretically, the point is that a high-saturated-cooked-animal-fat, high-trans-fatty-acid, high-refined-carbohydrate diet decreases and disrupts the healthy antidiabetes gene expression and contributes to the onset of Type-2 diabetes. Animal-based fatty foods in this category seem to have a disabling effect on the gene, meaning that our DNA goes to a lower phenotypic expression, and so they are not able to produce more mitochondria or eliminate the fat. The basic point is that what we eat speaks to our genes—and a high animal fat and trans-fatty acid intake gives a negative message to the genes, activating increased insulin resistance and the CDDS/diabetic process. Based on these theoretical understandings, the key to diabetes reversal is to activate an upgrade of the antidiabetic phenotypic gene expression. As no clear research has been done with raw, unprocessed plant fats but has been done with cooked, processed trans and animal fats, it would be rather unscientific to expand the diabetogenic problem to be associated with raw plant fats. My research with 120 diabetics, showing their dramatic improvement and healing, strongly suggests that at least a 25–45 percent raw plant-source-only fat intake is at least neutral to the antidiabetes healing process and most likely helpful to the healing process and to the building of the deep primordial healing life force. This will be explained in more depth in Chapter 5.

After working with diabetes since 1973, and as a consumer of live-food, plant-source-only cuisine since 1983, I have gained certain insights about what is a healthy fat and the role of healthy fats in creating health. I have observed different things in relationship to different amounts of fat. One of the possible problems that I have seen in long-term use of a 10-percent-fat diet is the higher percentage of omega-3 and cholesterol deficiencies in people on such a diet, which create significant symptoms and pathologies and compromise overall health. Omega-3 and cholesterol deficiencies result in less effective cell-membrane function, nerve transmission, serotonin production, and other neurotransmitter production, transmission, and neuroreceptor site functions in the cells. These deficiencies may result in serious clinical symptoms. This will be discussed in more detail in Chapter 5.

The quality of the fat is far more significant than the amount of fat, although both are important. Studies by Dr. Edward Howell on the Eskimos showed that when they ate high amounts of raw blubber, they did not develop heart disease, high blood pressure, or any significant morbidity. When they began cooking their blubber, they began to develop heart disease and high blood pressure. Specific data on diabetes before and after the change from raw blubber to cooked are not available, but since the switch to the Western cooked-animal-fat diet, which also includes white sugar and white flour, there certainly has been a significant increase in Type-2 diabetes in this and all indigenous tribal groups that have deviated from their natural indigenous diet and gone to white sugar, white flour, and cooked animal flesh. The additional message here is that cooking destroys enzymes and alters the structure of the fat from cis to trans. When you cook or fry saturated fat, it becomes unhealthy. In addition, the processing of fats through hydrogenation changes them from a cis structure to a trans structure. In other words, there is actually a physical change in the structure of the fat molecule when cooked or hydrogenated.

Unfortunately, there is not as much data on the subject as I would like. At temperatures of 320–428°F, depending on the oil being cooked, the production of trans-fatty acids as well as more immediately harmful free-radical products starts deleterious chain reactions in the fat molecules. The antioxidants in the oil, such as beta-carotene and vitamin E, are used up as well. Also, the lipases that are in the raw blubber, needed for healthy fat metabolism, are destroyed. The hydrogenation process used to turn oils into semisolid or solid fats requires temperatures up to 428°F for several hours. This produces high amounts of trans-fatty acids, which are more solid than cis fatty acids. The process of physically changing the cis fat structure to a trans-fatty acid creates a pathogenic molecule that negatively affects every single cell membrane in the body. The defense systems of the cell membranes are minimized, the immune system of the cell is lowered, and the ability of the cell membrane to do cell signaling is compromised. The cell membrane can no longer act effectively as the brain of the cell and consequently all levels of health are impaired.

In making this scientifically based distinction between cooked trans fats and raw, uncooked plant cis fats, the question was, do raw fats impair the healing of diabetes or actually cause diabetes? Research shows that five ounces a week of nuts drops the incidence of Type-2 diabetes by 27 percent. The next consideration is the effect of raw plant fats on the healing of diabetes. This is answered at the Tree of Life Rejuvenation Center, where I have found dramatic positive results in healing diabetes by putting people on live foods with a live-moderate-fat diet. Because of our unmatched results, I am now recommending a 25–45 percent uncooked, plant-source-only fat intake, depending on a person's constitution. Plant-source food has no cholesterol, so the cholesterol levels tended to go to normal in my clients. Because of this, I am not convinced that all fat in general is the problem, so much as whether it is cooked, animal based, and/or hydrogenated

CIS- STRUCTURE TRANS- STRUCTURE

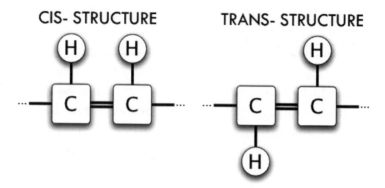

fat, in which the actual structures have changed. Changes in the cell membrane have a possible consequent compromise in cell signaling. Plant-source-only, live-food fats, such as those in almonds and walnuts, have actually been shown in published studies to lower cholesterol and help with the healing of diabetes. The people in my study on a 25-45 percent fat diet experienced a 44 percent average decrease in their LDL cholesterol in 21–30 days. Most of these people went to an LDL of approximately 82, which is significantly positive for the prevention of heart disease.

Some research[49, 50, 51] shows there are abnormal membrane phospholipid profiles in cooked fat, which is of major significance in both Type-1 and Type-2 diabetes. Insulin stimulates and glucagon inhibits a particular enzyme, which influences the availability of polyunsaturated fats for membrane incorporation. This is another aspect of the effect of insulin on the fat metabolism and how the fatty acid composition of the membrane lipids affects the function of insulin. Research shows that increasing membrane fluidity by taking in higher levels of dietary polyunsaturated fatty acids, especially the omega-3s, actually increases the number of insulin receptors, therefore increasing insulin activity.

Research[52, 53] suggests that there is hyperinsulinemia and insulin resistance in approximately 75 percent of Type-2 diabetics in the initial phases. The elevated levels of insulin happen because insulin signaling is not being heard.[54] Later on, there is more of a para-inflammatory burnout and actual cell dysfunction and death of the overworked pancreatic beta cells—hence insulin production goes down. The inability of Type-2 diabetic cell membranes to process insulin is not necessarily a result only of insulin and glucagon influences but, as I pointed out earlier, is due to leptin and insulin resistance that results in high concentrations of insulin, which because of its biphasic nature, can actually turn off receptor function at high concentrations. I remind the reader that this supports my theory that the diabetic onset of Type-2 may be associated in some way with cell membrane abnormalities. One study comparing 575 diabetics with 319 nondiabetics showed there was a problem incorporating polyunsaturated fatty acids into the cell membrane for the diabetics.[55] All the diabetic red blood cell membranes were lower in polyunsaturated fatty acids. Plasma phospholipids, triglycerides, and cholesterol esters were also affected, suggesting there is an impairment of polyunsaturated fatty acid metabolism in diabetes. This suggests that in NIDDM impaired insulin activity may be both a cause and an effect of membrane polyunsaturated fatty acid composition.

In summary, although it is complicated, the point is to make the strong suggestion that Type-2 diabetes, from a fat perspective, is associated primarily with dysfunctional fat metabolism and secondarily with a high animal-fat and trans-fat intake. A moderate fat diet of 25–45 percent raw plant-source fats does not seem associated or causally connected with Type-2 diabetes.

Research has also shown that the omega-6 to omega-3 ratios are generally not in balance in Type-2, being too high in omega-6. This imbalance is made worse with the intake of approximately 13.3 grams per person per day of trans-fatty acids, as documented in the United States.[56] Research has shown that diets relatively high in saturated fat and trans-fatty acids, such as we see with flesh foods and hydrogenated fats, can significantly affect insulin efficiency and glucose response. When we increase the percentage of omega-3 fatty acids in the diet, insulin resistance can be improved or prevented.[57, 58, 59] It is highly suggestible that a disordered polyunsaturated fatty metabolism has some role in NIDDM.

Research does show that when you increase the ratio of polyunsaturated fatty acids to saturated fatty acids, there is an improved insulin binding.[60] Rats fed high-fat diets became insulin resistant. Saturated fatty acids caused the most deterioration. Linolenic acid caused the least problem. The use of omega-3 from flaxseed oil normalized insulin function in the high saturated-fatty-acid group. Research has also shown that the higher the amount of saturated fatty acids in the cell membrane, the more insulin resistance there is.[61, 62]

In individuals with abdominal obesity, it is worth suspecting hyperinsulinism. People with hyperinsulinism may have a diminished ability to utilize glucose peripherally; they may also have increased circulating free fatty acids, affecting glucose metabolism and creating a decline in insulin receptors.[63] The South Asian Indians and the Pima Indians have a genetic predisposition to NIDDM, but it didn't really manifest until they switched in the 1940s to a Western diet. The epidemic of NIDDM in these groups seems to be directly related to the dramatic increase in white sugar, white flour, junk food, and processed foods, which include an overall total calories excess of refined carbohydrates and total fat and unbalanced omega-6 versus omega-3 ratios.

In summary, trans-fatty acids are indeed a diabetogenic problem, causing imbalances in omega-6 versus omega-3 ratios of fatty acids. This evidence suggests that a diet that is relatively low in cooked animal and trans fats, relatively high in raw omega-3 fatty acids, and free of high-density refined carbohydrates would be very helpful for the indigenous people worldwide and for everyone, in preventing and reversing NIDDM. It is highly possible that some of the confusion about fat intake and any sort of linkage to Type-2 diabetes is directly related to people not understanding the significant difference between the pathological quality of trans, hydrogenated, and cooked animal fats and the healthy moderate intake of raw, uncooked, plant-source-only fats. In other words, not all fats are created equal. Some fats are healthy, and others are pathogenic.

Type-1 Diabetes (IDDM)

The cause of Type-1 diabetes is different than Type-2. Its genetic component is not as direct, but transmission is believed to be an autosomal dominant, recessive, or mixed chromosome, although no mechanism is proven. The genetic research does suggest that if a first-degree relative has IDDM, a child has a 5–10 percent chance of developing Type-1 diabetes.[64]

Research has been pretty detailed on the diabetes genes for Type-2. It is believed that the susceptibility gene resides in the sixth chromosome and the major alleles that suggest risk are HLA-DR3, HLA-DW3, HLA-DR4, HLA-DW4, HLA-B8, and HLA-B15. The genes do play a role. The onset of Type-1 seems to be linked with an environmental insult, an allergen such as cow's milk, or a virus that initiates this process in genetically susceptible people.

These insults create an inflammation response, called *insulinitis*. What happens is that the activated T-lymphocytes infiltrate the islet cells in the pancreas. Macrophages and T-cells appear to be involved in the destructive cycle as they release cytokines that create free radical damage. This free-radical-induced islet beta cell death involves breaks in the DNA strands. The enzyme to repair the DNA free-radical damage requires large amounts of NAD-plus. This creates a depletion of the intracellular NAD pools, and that leads to islet cell death.[65] Type-1

PATHOGENESIS OF TYPE-1 DIABETES MELLITUS

EVENT	AGENT OR RESPONSE
Genetic susceptibility ↓	HLA-DR3, DR4, DW3, DW4, B8, B15
Environmental Event ↓	Virus, Cow's milk protein ingested by mother *or child*
Insulitis ↓	Infiltration of activated T lymphocytes
Activation of autoimmunity ↓	Self ⟶ non-self transition
Immune attack on pancreatic beta cells ↓	Islet cell antibodies, cell mediated immunity
Diabetes Mellitus Type-1	>90% of beta cells destroyed
	Source: *Harrison's Principles of Internal Medicine*

FIGURE 2. Pathogenesis of Type-1 diabetes mellitus

is primarily an inflammatory response from an autoimmune reaction from antibodies being made against the beta cells.

Certain viruses seem to attack and destroy the pancreatic beta cells directly, rather than through an autoimmune reaction.[66] Mumps, prior to the onset of diabetes, was found in 42.5 percent of the subjects versus 12.5 percent in the control group.[67] In some of the para-inflammatory, autoimmune cases, there are also elevated levels of Coxsackie virus IGM antibodies.[68] Exposure to virus infections in utero or during childhood may initiate beta cell damage.[69] Rubella and chickenpox don't seem to make any significant differences.[70]

There is a significant correlation between antibodies to cow's milk protein, particularly to bovine serum albumin, in the onset of IDDM.[71,72,73,74] Some studies have found that somewhere between 75 and 90 percent of the cases of Type-1 have antibodies against the beta cells of the pancreas, compared to 0.5 to 2 percent in normal cases.[75]

Cow's milk seems to be strongly linked to the onset of Type-1. Those with Type-1 diabetes were more likely to have been breastfed for less than three months and exposed to cow's milk before four months. Research has also shown that children who consumed pasteurized cow's milk before the age of three months were 11 times more likely to develop Type-1 diabetes.[76] In 1992, Canadian and Finnish researchers reported in the *New England Journal of Medicine* their examination of blood from 142 children, newly diagnosed with Type-1 diabetes. They found that in those children, a high percentage of them had antibodies against certain proteins in cow's milk. These antibodies cross-reacted with beta cells of the pancreas.[77] One study in Finland, Sweden, and Estonia identified 242 newborns at risk for developing Type-1 because each had a first-degree relative with the condition. They encouraged the mothers to breastfeed, and when weaning their babies, some mothers used a specifically modified baby formula in which the dairy proteins were broken up into individual amino acids. The other mothers were allowed to use regular cow's milk. The children who were fed the specific formula were much less likely to develop the antibeta cell antibodies; their risk was cut by 62 percent.[78] In 2002, in a study involving families in 15 countries, researchers found that large proteins can pass through the Peyer's patches in the small intestine and into the system, even in adults. This study suggests that even mothers who drink cow's milk could be passing on the antigen of the cow's milk to their infants. In 1991 researchers did indeed find that cow's milk's proteins ingested by a nursing mother end up in her breast milk.[79] In 1994, the American Academy of Pediatrics issued a report after looking into the matter of antibodies to cow's milk protein in association with the onset of Type-1 diabetes in children. Based on more than 90 studies, the American Academy of Pediatrics agreed that, indeed, the risk of diabetes could likely be reduced if infants are not exposed to cow's milk protein early in life.[80]

So if we really want to protect our kids, we must not expose them directly to cow's milk; mothers should also refrain from drinking cow's milk to prepare for or to support breastfeeding. The good news here is multifold: mothers' breast milk is best, and we can also feed our children nut and seed mylks made at home to provide superior nutrition at no risk to their health. These mylks, found in the recipe section of this book, are desirable for the mother as well, before, during, and after pregnancy to support her nutritional needs.

Type-2 Diabetes (NIDDM)

In Type-2 diabetes, also called non-insulin-dependent diabetes mellitus (NIDDM) or insulin-dependent Type-2 (IDDM), obese people in the early diabetic stages secrete as much as 114 units of insulin, which is more than 9 times the 10 units of insulin that I suggest are within normal limits. (Standard, normal, allopathic limits are higher.) In this context, there seem to be two major stages in Type-2 diabetes: First, there is hyperglycemia, which with blood glucose above 110 has actually been shown to kill beta cells. Then there is a hyperinsulin stage for the majority. As this process continues, the beta cells of the pancreas begin to inflame; they get exhausted, scar, and create a shift from hyperinsulinemia to a state of insulin dependence. Therefore, it is very important to maintain an FBS of 85 or lower to keep pancreatic cells from wearing out and creating a hypoinsulin stage. Individuals with Type-1 usually have a fasting insulin of 0 to 2 units. I consider optimal fasting insulin to be between 4 and 6 units.

Chronic Complications

> And we have made of ourselves living cesspools and driven
> doctors to invent names for our diseases.
>
> > **Plato**

The chronic complications of diabetes take us into another level of understanding about the seriousness of diabetes. First I am going to focus on Type-1 and then the long-term complications that apply both to Type-1 and Type-2. In Type-1, you may accidentally get excess exogenous insulin, which may cause insulin shock. You have the issue of diabetic ketoacidosis, which is primarily a Type-1 diabetic problem, where fat is broken down for energy and ketones create acidity. You also have what is called nonketogenic hyperosmolar syndrome, with rapid dehydration because you have so much sugar that your body is attempting to get rid of excess sugar and you lose large amounts of water through the urine, which is called polyuria. The hyperosmolar syndrome can be a serious problem. It can also be activated by medical problems such as pneumonia, burns, stroke, and use of certain drugs such as glucocorticoids and diuretics. Fasting can also set all of these off, and this is why I do not encourage Type-1 diabetics to fast.

Chronic complications in both Type-1 and Type-2 diabetes are similar. They emerge from the same causal pathways. They include two main metabolic problems: the glycosylated protein/lipids and the intracellular accumulation of sorbitol. The glycosylated proteins lead to changes in the structure and function of almost all the protein systems in the body, significantly affecting protein metabolism, enzyme function, and virtually all the tissues. An example of problems caused by glycosylation would be glycosylated low-density concentrated

lipoproteins (LDL). LDL is usually at high levels in diabetics. The glycosylated LDL molecules don't bind to the LDL receptors and are thus
unable to shut off the endogenous cholesterol synthesis. The result is
that you tend to get more cholesterol than your body needs. Excessive
glycosylation also occurs in red blood cells, in the lenses of the eye, and
in the myelin sheath of the nerves. This glycosylation creates deacti-
vation of enzymes, inhibition of regulatory molecule binding, cross-
linking of glycosylated proteins, trapping of soluble proteins by the
glycosylated extracellular matrix, abnormalities in nucleic acid function, altered molecular recognition, and increased immunogenicity.[81]
All this accelerates the aging process.

Sorbitol buildup inside the cells is another major serious metabolic
problem. Sorbitol is a by-product of glucose metabolism that takes
place in the cells with the action of the enzyme aldose reductase. In
a normal physiology, once the sorbitol is formed, it is metabolized by
polyol dehydrogenase to fructose. This conversion to fructose allows
it to be excreted from the cell. In the diabetic with high blood sugars,
the sorbitol accumulates and plays a major role in the development of
secondary complications. The sorbitol is involved in a variety of ways,
but the basic mechanism can be seen in cataracts, as an example. High
blood sugar, either from an inability to metabolize the sugar or by
eating too much sugar, results in the shunting of glucose to the sorbitol pathway, which is a secondary pathway. But since the lens of the
eye is impermeable to sorbitol, the lack of the polyol dehydrogenase
enzyme occurs from excess demand, and the sorbitol accumulates to
high concentrations. It persists even if glucose levels go to normal. This
accumulation creates an osmotic gradient that draws water into the
cells to maintain the osmotic balance in the eye cells. Associated with
this osmotic process, the cells release small molecules such as inositol,
glutathione, niacin, vitamin C, magnesium, and potassium to maintain
the osmotic balance. These compounds are needed to protect the lens
from damage but are being lost because of the excess sorbitol; the loss
makes the lens cells susceptible to further damage. The result is that
the delicate protein fibers in the lens become opaque.

This intracellular accumulation of the sorbitol is a major factor in many complications of diabetes. It is found in the lens of the eye, the Schwan cells of the peripheral nerves, the papillae of the kidney, the Islets of Langerhans in the pancreas, and the Murel cells of the blood vessels. This tells us that it seems to be associated with almost every tissue, and though its exact function is not clear, it is associated with these complications.

Cardiovascular Disease

People who have diabetes are two to four times more likely than non-diabetics to develop heart disease or have a stroke, and three-fourths of all diabetics (77,000 annually) ultimately die from heart disease.[82] Deaths from heart disease in women with diabetes have increased 23 percent over the past 30 years, compared to a 27 percent decrease in women without diabetes. Deaths from heart disease in men with diabetes have decreased by only 13 percent, compared to a 36 percent decrease in men without diabetes. Diabetics with renal disease have a cardiovascular disease risk that is sevenfold higher than diabetics without renal disease.

Mainly, it seems, it is our Culture of Death diet and lifestyle that create cardiovascular disease.[83] Dr. Ornish's famous 1990 study of 28 subjects on a 10 percent low-fat, primarily vegetarian diet, which documented a reversal to some extent of arteriosclerotic cardiovascular disease (ASCVD), supports the importance of lifestyle and diet in ameliorating ASCVD. Dr. Esselstyn's pilot study of 11 cardiac patients also supports the healing and ASCVD-reversing power of a vegan diet and lifestyle.[84] He fully monitored patients for five years on a vegan, 10 percent low-fat diet. In slightly more than half of the cases, there was a partial reversal of some of the ASCVD plaques, and there were no cardiovascular deaths. Unfortunately, Dr. Esselstyn gave statins to all his patients, so one cannot make a full causal dietary statement, as statins also decrease heart pathology, but one cannot deny a healthy diet is associated in some way with improved cardiovascular status. Over the last 40 years, my approach has been an 80–100 percent raw, organic, plant-source-only diet, with no white sugar, white flour, trans-fatty acids, junk carbohydrates, processed foods, or GMOs, and I have never had a client die of heart disease—a fact that also supports the importance of diet and lifestyle in heart-disease prevention. It is also interesting that those in my study had significantly lower triglycerides and the cholesterols were lower than those in Ornish's 10 percent low-fat study. It is interesting that all three studies share in common no white sugar, white flour, or junk foods. This suggests that perhaps the primary secret to all our cardio-protective results may be the power of a natural, unprocessed, organic diet without trans fats, white sugar, white flour, or processed or junk food; and also suggests the 10 percent or 25–45 percent plant-fat content in the diet is not the only factor that is creating this result.

Another doctor supporting the case for diet as the underlying cause or prevention for heart disease is *Eat to Live*'s author, Dr. Joel Fuhrman. I have included here a figure he uses to demonstrate this principle,

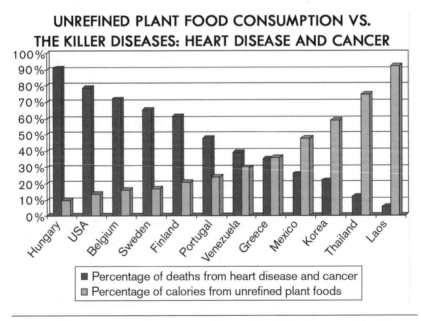

FIGURE 3. Unrefined plant food consumption and the killer diseases, heart disease, and cancer

based on data from the World Health Organization and the UN Food and Agriculture Organization (Figure 3).[85]

Populations with low death rates from the major killer diseases are populations that almost never have overweight members and consume more than 75 percent of their calories from unrefined plant foods. They consume at least 10 times more unrefined plant-source food than the average American.[86]

Even having diabetic parents can increase your risk of developing heart disease. A new study reported in the June 20, 2006, issue of the *Journal of the American College of Cardiology* showed that the blood vessels of people whose parents both have Type-2 diabetes, even if they do not have diabetes themselves, do not respond as well to changes in blood flow as those of people without a family history of diabetes. None of the 38 adults (in their mid to late 30s) in this study had diabetes, but half of them were the offspring of two diabetic parents. The scientists restricted blood flow in the arms of the participants using a blood pressure cuff. Then, using ultrasound, they compared how blood vessels in the arms of participants responded to the surge in blood flow when the cuff was released. Blood vessel responsiveness was impaired in all 19 participants (9 men and 10 women) whose parents had diabetes. Allison B. Goldfine, MD, from the Joslin Diabetes Center and Brigham and Women's Hospital in Boston, Massachusetts, said, "Persons whose parents both have Type-2 diabetes have endothelial dysfunction. This predisposition to atherosclerosis is present even when the offspring do not have diabetes themselves. Insulin resistance has been suggested to be important to both the development of diabetes and cardiovascular disease in large populations. However, in this high-risk group, even the most insulin sensitive offspring had diminished endothelial function."[87]

Hypertension

We are looking at a target blood pressure of 130/80 mm Hg. According to the U.S. Centers for Disease Control (CDC), about 73 percent of adults with diabetes have blood pressure greater than or equal to 130/80 or use prescription medications for hypertension.

Dental Disease

Periodontal (gum) disease is more common among people with diabetes. Among young adults, those with diabetes have about twice the risk of those without diabetes. Almost one-third of people with diabetes have severe periodontal diseases with loss of attachment of the gums to the teeth measuring five millimeters or more. Improving your dental health can also help with glycemic control. Researchers at the State University of New York, Buffalo, treated a group of 113 Pima Indians for periodontal disease and measured their glycemic control three months later. They found improved glycemic control along with a reduction in the bacteria that cause periodontal disease.[88]

Diabetic Neuropathy and Foot Ulcers

Neuropathy is associated with decreased sensory and nerve conduction velocities. Diabetic neuropathy also seems to be associated with sorbitol accumulation.[89, 90] Sorbitol accumulation leads to myoinositol loss. Inositol helps create healthy nerve conduction. Typically, this peripheral neuropathy is associated with paresthesias, hyperesthesias, and pain. On the neurological exam, almost every diabetic I see has some level of a poor vibratory sense, altered pain and temperature sense, and poor deep tendon reflexes. Often within the 21-day program, these symptoms are partially or fully reversed. Recent research also using a vegan diet supports our results. Researchers in California studied 21 people with Type-2 diabetes and neuropathy and, using a vegan diet combined with exercise, found that in only two weeks, 17 of the 21 reported a complete cessation of symptoms and the final four had noticeable improvement.[91]

Diabetic foot complications are the most common cause of nontrauma-based lower-extremity amputations in the industrialized world. Neuropathy, a major etiologic component of most diabetic ulcerations, is present in more than 82 percent of diabetic patients with foot wounds.[92] The incidence of gangrene is 20 times higher as compared to nondiabetics, and the risk of lower-extremity amputation is 15 to 46 times higher in diabetics than in those who do not have diabetes mellitus.[93, 94] Each year, more than 82,000 amputations are performed among people with diabetes. Furthermore, foot complications are the most frequent reason for hospitalization in patients with diabetes, accounting for up to 25 percent of all diabetic admissions in the United States and Great Britain. With ulcers, one must stop all smoking, because nicotine causes arterial constriction, and this further decreases peripheral circulation.

Diabetic Retinopathy

Diabetic retinopathy is another serious complication and is the leading cause of blindness. In diabetic retinopathy, the retinal vessels in the eye weaken and develop microaneurisms that leak blood plasma out of the capillaries. This results in scarring in the eye, which leads to gradual blindness. As the figure shows, it is related to the glycosylated hemoglobin and seems to increase when the glycosylated hemoglobin goes above 6.0.

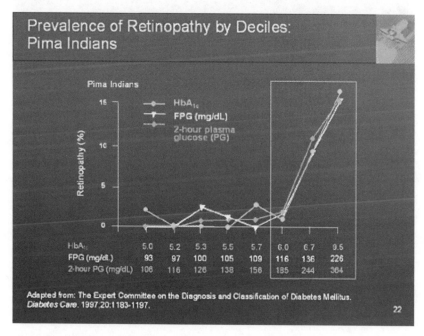

FIGURE 4. Prevalence of retinopathy by deciles (Source: NHANES III)

This National Health and Nutrition Examination Survey (NHANES) III data were derived from looking at retinopathy against fasting, two hours postprandial, and HgbA1c. In retinopathy, pathology presents and increases at a specific point. That point is a HgbA1c of 6.0 percent, an FBS of 110 mg/dL, and a two-hour value of 154 mg/dL. Is this unique to the NHANES data? Well, if you look at Pima Indians and Egyptian studies, you see the exact same thing. When one's HgbA1c goes above the normal range, one starts to develop complications.

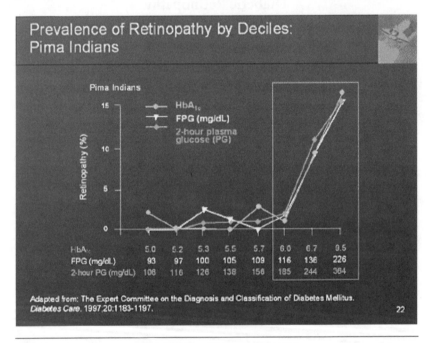

FIGURE 5. Prevalence of retinopathy by deciles: Pima Indians

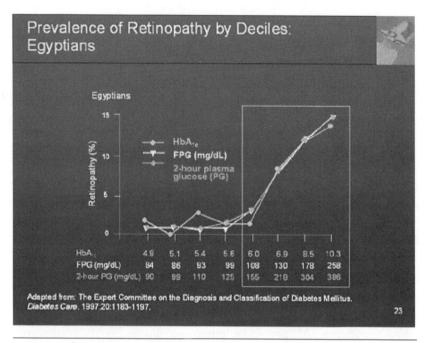

FIGURE 6. Prevalence of retinopathy by deciles: Egyptians

These are important data, because they suggest a finer gauge on why we are encouraging an HgbA1c level of less than 6.0, not 6.5 or 7.0.

Diabetic Nephropathy

Diabetic nephropathy, another serious complication, is the most common cause of chronic kidney failure and end-stage kidney disease in the United States. It is a common cause of high rates of dialysis and death. Once people begin kidney dialysis, they usually die within five years. The diabetic process affects the kidneys in a few ways: glomerulosclerosis, an arteriosclerosis of the entering and leaving renal arteries; arteriosclerosis of the renal artery and its interrenal branches; and deposits of glycogen, fat, and glycopolysaccharides around the tubules. Early on, nephropathy has no symptoms, but as it advances we see edema (swelling, particularly around the eyes), nausea, fatigue, headache, and generalized itching. This also has the potential to be slowly reversed on this program, before they go on dialysis. So far, not one of the 120 people have had to go to dialysis, more than a few came to the program in near renal failure, and all returned to normal kidney function values by the end of the 21-Day program.

The following table summarizes the complications associated with diabetes.

The Spectrum of Glucose Toxicity	
Eyes	Retinopathy (microaneurysms, hemorrhages, exudates, neovascularization)
Kidneys	Nephropathy (albuminuria, nephrotic syndrome, hypo reninemic hypoaldosteronism, end-stage renal disease)
Nerves	Neuropathy (distal sensory and/or motor neuropathy, mononeuritis multiplex, autonomic neuropathy, amyotrophy, chronic demyelinating immune polyneuropathy)
Skin and mucus	Microvascular lesions, necrobiosis lipoidica diabeticorum, staphylococcus/streptococcus infection/cellulitis, fungal membranes infections
Fetus	Macrosomia, congenital anomalies (neural tube defects), shoulder dystocia
Pancreas	Endocrine (decreased insulin secretion, ß-cell failure), exocrine (decreased digestive enzyme synthesis and secretion)
Insulin target	Insulin resistance symptoms in fat deposits especially in tissues, lower abdomen, muscle, and liver
Vascular system	Atherosclerosis, endothelial cell dysfunction (decreased vasodilatation), restenosis

Subtle Insulin Physiology

The physiology of insulin as a hormone is something worth attempting to understand. It is interesting that insulin is biphasic. Hyperinsulinemia results in a biphasic glucose response to epinephrine, first at low levels, then at high levels. Our emotions play an important role in insulin sensitivity or insulin resistance. Part of my treatment may include the use of homeopathic insulin to moderate the communication between the pancreas and the nervous system.

In the 1950s, scientists used the phrase *insulin dependent* to mean that muscles and fat require insulin to take in glucose. Newer research tends to suggest a slightly different physiology. Glucose is transferred into the cells with or without insulin to some extent. In many tissues, there are enough GLUT-4 transporters in cell membranes to guarantee adequate glucose uptake to meet the demands of cellular respiration, even without insulin. For example, insulin is not necessary for glucose to enter the cells of certain parts of the brain or kidneys. Red blood cells are also able to utilize sugar without the assistance of insulin. Furthermore, when you are exercising, the muscle cells can extract glucose from the blood without insulin, using special proteins called GLUT-4 transporters.[95] Although this may be true, Type-1 diabetics who do not receive insulin usually die, so the picture is more complicated. It also has been shown that adipose sites cannot take glucose without insulin.[96] It is interesting that in our limbic system, the area of the brain that affects our memory, sense of safety, survival instincts, eating, appetite drives, and learning contains a high density of insulin receptors.[97, 98] As a physician with a homeopathic training, I have explored the use of homeopathic insulin, and there seem to be positive effects using it, including psychological improvement, perceptual calmness, lower blood glucose, improved elimination and metabolism, reduced metabolic wasting, and reduced development of diabetic complications. This suggests a function of insulin as a signaling molecule.

There is also a relationship between growth hormone and insulin, which is counterregulatory. If one is high in concentration, then the other is low. Muscle protein synthesis is regulated by human growth hormone, and insulin acts to prevent muscle breakdown. Insulin physiology is not exactly the way we have previously conceptualized it. Insulin is a biphasic signaling protein. It both stimulates and inhibits activities in a nonlinear curve.[99] Too much insulin can actually inhibit glucose uptake. The relationship between insulin concentration and protein synthesis suggests that most of insulin's stimulatory effect occurs at low concentrations, while high insulin concentrations may have an opposite effect. Insulin has been shown to mediate lipid, protein, and carbohydrate metabolism, converting nutrients into energy and maintaining cellular identity and replication. Insulin has been found to stimulate DNA, RNA, and protein synthesis. Yet it inhibits these same biological functions at concentrations that are too high and gives us another insight into the problem of hyperinsulinemia, which is seen in insulin resistance. High concentrations of insulin can result in central nervous system and circulatory depression from its inhibitory affects on glucose metabolism.

Lindsay Berkson writes in *Hormone Deception* that natural hormones are so potent they can produce very dramatic changes in cell activity with very small amounts (parts per billion or parts per trillion)—a figure so minute that only extremely sensitive tests can measure them. Hormones like insulin are measured at the parts-per-trillion (ppt) level, the equivalent of putting one drop of water into a 6-mile-long train with 660 tank cars. This should place the introduction of large amounts of insulin into the body in proper perspective. Doctors have used insulin homeopathically (in very small amounts) in a variety of ways. It does seem to help, although I have not conducted a long-term study on homeopathic insulin use. I use homeopathic insulin because it works on the energetic level and signaling level. Insulin may be toxic at high levels such as in hyperinsulinemia. Insulin works on many levels with complex feedback loops. Each of insulin's chemical reactions depends on bioelectric signals arising from insulin growth factor regulator (IGF-1), hormonal control, human growth hormone (HGH), and enzymatic reactions. Signaling activity begins with the insulin receptor insulin interface on the outside surface of the cell membrane. IGF-1 or anything that activates insulin receptor substrates will activate glucose uptake. This can actually happen with homeopathic insulin or IGF-1. The insulin molecule targets specific muscle fibers, fat tissues, and brain regions. Glucose metabolism is facilitated into the cell by glucose transporters and does not necessarily require insulin. Every cell in the body takes in glucose to some degree, yet every cell does not possess an insulin receptor. The insulin receptor family regulates nutritional metabolic pathways. IGF-1 receptors are in every cell in the body and create signals similar to insulin. Insulin receptor substrates transport glucose and stimulate metabolism.

Homeopathic insulin can also activate liver function. The liver is the first target of insulin and serves to increase storage of glucose as glycogen. Insulin upgrades the liver to a full state of glycogen and also stimulates glyconeolysis, the breaking down of glycogen to sugar. Insulin also uses magnesium as a second messenger. Insulin helps to stabilize intracellular magnesium levels. Insulin also promotes triglyceride synthesis and mineral uptake of phosphates and potassium. So homeopathic insulin has the capacity to stimulate many functions through cell signaling. The important point here is that insulin is a hormone and affects the whole hormonal system as a signaling protein. Insulin, as pointed out before, inhibits the breakdown of muscle fibers. IGF-1 can stimulate protein synthesis in fatty tissue and is influenced by insulin uptake of free fatty acids.

This is an immensely complex system. Type-2 diabetes and insulin resistance seem to be affected hormonally. This gives us another insight into the physiology. Insulin is released in response to elevated serum glucose and hyperinsulinemia and an increased insulin response to glucose are the first measurable responses. It's possible that one of the underlying causal physiologies of insulin resistance is a defect in the utilization of glycogen within the cell. Some 80 percent of glucose is stored in the muscles, and 20 percent is stored in the liver. So this is a defect that could permanently affect glycogen utilization within the muscle and prevents the muscle from using glycogen stores. When you have increased glycogen storage buildup, there is a possible backup of the transport of glucose across the cell membrane for storage within the cell. There is no more room in the cell for glucose utilization and storage. This results in hyperglycemia as part of the response to the intracellular backup. Hyperglycemia then causes an increase in the release of insulin. In small doses, insulin is an anabolic steroid that optimizes lean body mass and energy utilization. In excess, however, insulin impairs cyclic adenosine monophosphate (cAMP) and inhibits the release of anabolic steroids. Therefore, it increases catabolic processes and decreases the energy available to the organism.

Advanced health professionals are looking now at a new way of understanding this process, and this understanding is still at a theoretical level. But as we know, endocrinologists successfully treat diseases of hormone insufficiency such as hypothyroidism and hypoadrenalism, both of which I have seen very consistently in diabetes, as well as hypogonadism and somatotrophic deficiency of growth hormone treated by supplementing with hormones. In diseases of hypersecretion, we try to block the excess hormones. Thus treating the hyperinsulinemia associated with insulin resistance with more insulin just isn't logical.

Hormone Disruption

Hormone disruptors may be another contributing factor in diabetes. For example, Vietnam veterans exposed to endocrine disruptors such as Agent Orange (a potent mixture of several hormone-disrupting pesticides such as dioxins) have a higher incidence of diabetes, as well as abnormal glucose and insulin levels.[100] Women are even more strongly affected. Dioxin is also known as Agent Orange, a powerful carcinogen and toxin in general. A follow-up study on a dioxin accident in Seveso, Italy, examined blood from 31,000 people within months of the accident and followed the exposed people for more than 20 years. They found an increased incidence of diabetes, but only in females.[101] Berkson suggests that women are more greatly affected by chemical exposures than men, probably because they have a higher ratio of body fat and different metabolic and elimination rates than men.

Arsenic in Tap Water

Arsenic is another commonly found hormone disruptor suspected of playing a role in diabetes. Arsenic interferes with the action of glucocorticoid hormones, which belong to the same family of steroid hormones as estrogen and progesterone. Glucocorticoids turn on many genes that help regulate blood sugar and even ward off cancer. Repeatedly drinking water containing certain amounts of arsenic has been linked to increased rates of cancer and diabetes. The underlying mechanism is now thought to be hormone disruption.[102]

Testosterone Changes

Another fascinating aspect of hormonal physiology is the role of testosterone in diabetes. In the 1960s, J. Moller and other European clinicians used testosterone to treat men who had diabetes.[103] Some research suggests that testosterone can actually bring the glycosylated hemoglobin back to normal and lower insulin levels in men. The logic goes like this: Sex hormone binding globule (SHBG) binds testosterone, dihydrotestosterone, and estradiol to the cell wall. Without SHBG, no gonadal hormone can enter into the cell and generate the release of messenger RNA (mRNA) to activate gene expression. Men tend to have a lot less SHBG than women because SHBG is actually an estrogen amplifier. Higher SHBG and estradiol are found in men with central obesity, gynecomastia, and Type-2 diabetes. That is a very important piece in this whole hormonal imbalance. Healthy men have more free testosterone than free estradiol only when there is adequate testosterone and SHBG is less than 15 picomoles.[104] An increase in SHBG preferentially binds testosterone over estradiol, shifting the ratio to more free estradiol over testosterone, which isn't really great for men. By adding testosterone to the system, it's possible to create the shift away from estradiol dominance, increasing testosterone levels and lowering SHBG. Low levels of testosterone are found in diabetic men.[105, 106] The absence of testosterone or low testosterone seems to be connected with an increase in insulin resistance, showing up as a diminished insulin sensitive glycogen synthase enzyme activity.[107, 108] It's possible that in men, a low secretion of testosterone might be a primary event precipitating insulin resistance. Preliminary research shows that building testosterone to normal values reduces insulin resistance.[109] When we add testosterone, it lowers SHBG, and that lowers insulin levels. Lower SHBG improves the testosterone and estrogen ratio. Testosterone also lowers insulin resistance, and therefore insulin, and decreases obesity. The subtle mechanisms are best seen by clinical results of an increased testosterone decreases insulin resistance, but a deeper explanation is not so clear. Perhaps this is telling us how little we know about the whole hyperinsulinism syndrome, but it gives us a clue. There is not much research about testosterone and women in this system, so there is little I can say about it. Low testosterone seems to have some correlation with Syndrome X.

Syndrome X results from the underlying physiology and symptoms of hyperinsulinemia, which includes impaired glucose tolerance, Type-2 diabetes, obesity, hypertension, dyslipidemia, heart disease, and the inability to lose weight. N. M. Kaplan has observed that hyperinsulinemia precedes these disease states, which is a very important thing to understand in this whole process.[110] Syndrome X is an intermediary form of CDDS. The risk of ischemic heart disease is 4.5 times greater with elevated insulin. Other researchers have found that a decrease in an endogenous testosterone is associated with an increase in triglycerides and a decrease in HDL cholesterol. So it could be that in men, it is a decreased testosterone that is associated with hyperinsulinemia and Syndrome X.[111, 112] We can reasonably hypothesize that in men with Type-2 diabetes there is often a state of relative hypogonadism, which leads us to hyperinsulinemia. Increasing the testosterone may be an appropriate gender-specific treatment. There does seem to be a significant correlation between insulin sensitivity and SHBG levels in men with Type-2 diabetes.[113] Research suggests that increased testosterone and DHEA seems to be associated with lowered insulin in men, which leaves us open to the idea that adding testosterone to men with Syndrome X or Type-2 diabetes or middle-aged men who are obese (which is a tip-off of Syndrome X) may improve insulin sensitivity.[114, 115]

Living Enzymes

> Enzymes are substances that make life possible. No mineral,
> vitamin, or hormone can do any work without enzymes. They
> are the manual workers that build the body from proteins,
> carbohydrates, and fats. The body may have the raw building
> materials, but without the workers, it cannot begin.
>
> **Edward Howell, MD**

Included in the Culture of Life antidiabetogenic diet is a significant
benefit we derive from the living enzymes present in uncooked foods.
In research at George Washington University Hospital and Hygienic
Laboratory, Dr. Rosenthal and Dr. Ziegler found that when 50 g of
raw starch was administered to patients, their blood sugar rose only 1
mg and then decreased, but when the starch was cooked, there was a
dramatic increase of 56 mg in a half hour, 51 mg in 1 hour, and 11 mg
in 2 hours after the meal. Researchers also gave raw starch to diabetics
to whom no insulin had been given for several days. Average increase
in blood sugar in these diabetics from eating the raw starch was just
6 mg in a half hour, then a decrease of 9 mg in 1 hour, and a decrease
of 14 mg in 2.5 hours after the raw starch meal.[116] This significant difference in raw versus cooked foods in terms of blood sugar regulation
implies that the enzymes in the raw starch might be important. Also,
heating activates the breakdown of complex carbohydrates to simple
sugars more rapidly, thus raising the GI of the food. My clinical experience over some 40 years has been that a plant-source-only, raw-food,
healthy-fat diet with the use of food enzymes and supplemental digestive enzymes has been supportive in the treatment of adult Type-2
diabetes. Cooking affects weight gain as well. Research has found that
if raw potatoes are fed to hogs, they won't gain weight, but when fed
cooked potatoes, they gain weight.

In his book *Food Enzymes for Health and Longevity*, Dr. Howell
describes a study at Tufts School of Medicine related to weight gain
and inadequate enzymes. They examined 11 overweight individuals

and found lipase deficiency (lipase is needed to digest fats) in their fatty tissues as well as fatty tumors.[117] The lipase content of the adipose tissues of obese individuals and in lipomas was below the population norm.[118] Generally speaking, the amount of amylase (needed to digest carbohydrates) in diabetics is about 50 percent of normal. It has been shown that the amylase content of liver and spleen was raised from 2 to 17 times over the original when digestive enzymes containing amylase were given.[119] There is some suggestion that the external excretion of the pancreas becomes deficient in enzymes in diabetes, and that oral administration of enzymes had a beneficial effect.[120] Dr. Bassler reported a deficiency in amylase in the duodenum in more than 86 percent of cases of diabetes he studied. Dr. Harrison and Dr. Laurent, in 29 cases of Type-2, reported 14 cases with a significantly lower blood amylase and 13 cases with values from the low to lowest limits of the normal range.[121, 122]

In the area of fat digestion enzymes such as lipase, it is important to distinguish between cooked, saturated, and animal fats and raw fats, with their naturally high lipase content, such as we see in the indigenous Eskimo diet. Cold-pressed unrefined olive oil, avocado, raw nuts and seeds soaked overnight, and even sprouted grains are healthy sources of fat. Even raw animal fat does not seem as strongly associated with the onset of chronic disease, but eating the same diet cooked and without enzymes because they were destroyed with cooking may easily be associated with the enzyme deficiency that cooking creates. This could also be explained by the transformation of fats from cis to trans. More likely it is both. A low lipase enzyme level in the body is also connected to increased obesity. Enzyme research summarized by Miehlke and colleagues showed that artery obstruction was successfully treated and improved through high enzyme intake between meals, and it didn't seem to matter whether it was through the enzymes in the food or taken exogenously through supplementation.[123] Dr. Edward Howell's work with the Eskimos showed that they lived a disease-free life with a high-enzyme diet, rich with raw flesh foods (particularly blubber). Diabetes and degenerative diseases only became common when

Eskimos began cooking their food and consuming depleted, refined carbohydrates and processed foods, with the encroachment of Western culture. Cooking destroys enzymes in the raw fat and in the raw meat. According to Dr. Howell in *Food Enzymes for Health and Longevity*, through the introduction of cooking, the Eskimos have become one of the unhealthiest cultures. According to one study,[124] as of the late eighties, these were the top 10 foods eaten by Alaskan natives, ranked by frequency of consumption:

1. Coffee and tea
2. Sugar
3. White bread, rolls, and crackers
4. Fish
5. Margarine
6. White rice
7. Tang and Kool-aid
8. Butter
9. Regular soft drinks
10. Milk (whole and evaporated)

Notice that the only native food in the top 10 is fish, and that it is outranked in consumption by coffee, tea, sugar, and white bread. According to one study[125] by the Alaska Area Native Health Service in Anchorage, comparisons with past data indicate that the prevalence of diabetes in Eskimos has increased from 1.7 percent in 1962 to 4.7 percent in 1992, a nearly threefold increase.

Proteolytic Enzymes

Our program uses proteolytic enzymes, lipases, and general combinations of proteolytic lipase and amylase. Sufficient enzymes seem to be associated with a decreased tendency for clotting, help decrease the inflammation effect of the disease process in Type-1 and Type-2, and help unclog arteries. Dr. William Wong (in a personal communication) reported two cases in which Type-1 diabetes was cured using only proteolytic enzymes. One involved an 86-year-old with 50 years of Type-1 diabetes. She had a below-knee amputation on the right and was about to lose her left foot. She had paresthesia in her fingers and forearm, scar tissue in her eyes, a gray pallor, and dry skin, and was on four injections of insulin a day. She was given the proteolytic enzymes over three months. As scar tissue in her eyes cleared, her vision became 20/10, and her left foot had a full correction. An ultrasound done after three months found no arterial blockage whatsoever. Her skin in general (especially in her extremities) became pink. Her glycosylated hemoglobin went from 9 to 6, and she stopped taking insulin.

Another Type-1 diabetic was from the Flathead tribe in Montana. He was in his mid 30s, had acquired Type-1 in his mid 20s, and was receiving three to four injections of insulin a day. Toes in both feet had been amputated. He was suffering neurological degeneration in the legs and paresthesia in arms and hands. He had received one kidney transplant, and the other one was beginning to fail. After he took high intensity proteolytic enzymes for six months, his circulation improved and the regimen saved his toes and foot from further amputation. His need for insulin dropped to none. His neuropathy disappeared, which I hypothesize was secondary to fibrosis in the nerve trunks, or poor circulation due to inflammation. His kidneys began to function again. I hypothesize that the inflammation and subsequent scarring in the kidneys decreased through use of the proteolytic enzymes as his only new supplement. His creatinine, an indicator of kidney function, went to normal from previously abnormal.

These two cases suggest an interesting, additional, theoretical way to understand the disease process in Type-1 and Type-2 diabetes. A first step in the degenerative process is inflammation, termed *insulinitis* in Type-1, either due to antibody attacks on the beta cells of the pancreas from cow's milk antibodies, vaccinations, or certain viruses. The inflammation progresses to scarring. In Type-2 there is a progression from hyperinsulinism and its inflammation, in which the beta cells are stressed through overproduction and free radical production. The inflammation leads to a chronic scarring, which either blocks the flow of insulin from the beta cells, inactivates the beta cells, or perhaps blocks the circulation to the beta cells. The recovery, in one case from more than 50 years of Type-1 diabetes, theoretically suggests that the beta cell function is not destroyed but is only blocked by the scarring (as will be discussed in Chapter 5, with a theory of why at least 21 percent of Type-1 diabetics are healed with this program and 31 percent become insulin free). This may lead to a new way to understand the intermediary degenerative process in diabetes, and it gives us a new way to supplement the treatment approach by using high-potency proteolytic enzymes both for opening up general capillary, arterial, and major artery circulation and reestablishing the channel for insulin secretion from the blocked, but not destroyed, excretory function of the beta cells of the pancreas.

A third case was a person who developed Type-1 diabetes in his teens, starting with a rapid onset of diabetes with possible insulinitis and then scarring. He was hospitalized with an FBS of 1,200 and diagnosed as Type-1. One way to explain his rapid response to my program is to claim he was misdiagnosed, but that ignores the typical rapid onset and acute transition to a potentially life-threatening blood sugar of 1,200. In a previously healthy person, Type-2 is classically known to have a slow, gradual onset. Since the onset in his teens, he had been on approximately 20 units of insulin per day. In four days on the Dr. Cousens's Diabetes Recovery Program—A Holistic Approach, he was off all insulin, and in two weeks, his blood sugar was in the 70s. All symptoms disappeared, and he was in perfect health and has been diabetes-free ever since (for more than eight years, at the time of this writing). Four years after attending the program, his HgbA1c was 6.0, which was down from his initial HgbA1c of 11.8.

These three Type-1 diabetics experienced what is considered medically impossible. With two of them, only proteolytic enzymes were used, and the third benefited from the full program, which included the use of proteolytic enzymes as well as the low-glycemic and low-insulin-index live-food diet that in itself has an anti-inflammatory effect. My present statistics show that 31 percent of Type-1 diabetics are off all insulin by 21 days; in general, there is a 67.5 percent drop in insulin usage and about 21 percent have an FBS of less than 100.

To summarize my preliminary theories on the importance of high-intensity proteolytic enzymes, Type-1 and late-stage Type-2 involve a chronic inflammation and scarring of the beta cells of the pancreas and their peri-ductal outlets. In early stage Type-2, there is a constant overstimulation of the beta cells of the pancreas, eventually moving to hyperinsulinemia, inflammation, and fibrosis. The fibrosis blocks the ducts of the pancreas, and the hyperglycemia and inflammation appear to kill the beta cells of the pancreas. There is also inflammation and fibrosis in the glomeruli of the kidneys and fibrin, causing atherosclerosis. The proteolytic enzymes create a lysis of the fibrin plugs in the microcirculation, in the matrix of the plaque. What we see is a significant opening of peripheral circulation and therefore a decrease in the secondary degenerative symptoms. This is a theoretical explanation for why I feel the proteolytic enzymes work to help reverse the diabetic degenerative process.

I have now explored most contributory causes to Type-2 diabetes, except the mineral deficiencies, vitamin deficiencies, and metabolic toxins, which are the subject in Chapter 4. Minerals play a very important role, and I see specific deficiencies of magnesium, manganese, zinc, chromium, vanadium, and potassium in diabetic patients. These deficiencies could be a result of the blood hyperosmolality and the minerals being lost with excessive urination, in an attempt to get the sugar out of the system. There may be other reasons as well.

A Preliminary Unifying Theoretical Approach to Healing Diabetes

In summary, I am proposing that a degenerative metabolic process arises from a low-fiber diet high in sugar, cooked animal fat and protein, trans-fatty acids, white sugar, white flour, and processed and junk foods, combined with a lifestyle of stress, lack of exercise, and general toxicity that interfaces with and activates the diabetes-producing genes in both Type-1 and Type-2. My theory includes these genetic realities. Genes play a more predominant role in Type-2. Diabetes affects the metabolism on many levels of fat metabolism, protein metabolism, and glucose carbohydrate metabolism. The theory must also include hormone balance and enzyme levels, as the degenerative metabolic process affects the hormone flow and is affected by it. In addition, our enzyme levels and function affect the hormone flow, as diabetics have significantly less lipase, amylase, and proteases. The theory needs to include the process of para-inflammation advancing to fibrosis, which seems to be somewhat reversed by proteolytic enzymes, fasting, and live, raw foods, which also minimize and reverse the degenerative, para-inflammatory process of heart disease, kidney disease, retinopathy, and neuropathy that are the long-term complications of diabetes.

I am looking for a comprehensive understanding that can cut through the complexity of diabetes. The unifying theory and healing approach of the Dr. Cousens's Diabetes Recovery Program—A Holistic Approach is strongly based on the underlying principle that what one eats and how one lives speaks to one's genes. By what one eats and how one lives, one can either degrade one's phenotypic diabetic expression and activate the diabetic process or improve one's phenotypic expression for the prevention and reversal of diabetes.

Genotype means the actual genes that were given genetically. In essence, genotype is analogous to a computer's hard drive. Phenotype is the way the genes express themselves, which can vary according to the signaling systems that we give them through our diet and lifestyle. Phenotypic expression is analogous to our software programs. Put a healthy program in and we get a healthy response.

Since 1922, when Frederick Banting and Charles H. Best discovered insulin, which was a great contribution and saved many lives, the allopathic community has taken a more medical or drug-based approach to the treatment of diabetes. The cross-cultural studies show that diabetes is not a natural occurrence or a disease one catches; it is something one earns. It is caused by a Crime Against Wisdom style of eating and living in a way that downgrades our phenotypic expression so that the diabetic process is activated. Genes are polymorphic (slightly variable), and they can have multiple activators. Diet is a primary activator and exercise and lifestyle are secondary activators. Our diabetes-creating diet is a Crime Against Wisdom that brings increasing amounts of death and misery through the disease of diabetes to millions of people. I have already said that the research shows that a high white sugar, white flour, processed, junk food diet with a high saturated animal and trans fat diet tends to shut down healthy gene expression. I have seen that high intakes of cooked animal flesh, trans fat, high omega-6 to omega-3 ratios, glucose from junk food, and refined carbohydrates are causally related to a genetic downgrade that deregulates our phenotypic expression to one that sets off the diabetic process, initially as CDDS and eventually becoming Type-2 diabetes. The Dr. Cousens's Diabetes Recovery Program—A Holistic Approach starts out as a diet with 100 percent live food and macronutrients, depending on one's individual constitution. It is composed of moderate to low complex carbohydrates (25–45 percent), with low glycemic and insulin indexes; plant-source fats (25–45 percent); and moderate protein (10–25 percent). (The Centers for Disease Control suggests that the optimum protein intake is between 10–35 percent with 15 percent being average. In other words, these percentages are well within the range of general estimations with slightly less carbohydrate and slightly more fat.) The diet contains approximately daily 2,000 calories and is specifically designed to upgrade the phenotypic gene expression. All foods are raw. This dietary approach results in turning off the phenotypic diabetic expression and turning on the antidiabetogenic phenotypic expression.

Calories with Purpose

A key piece of research that supports my holistic theory was published in 2001 by Dr. Stephen Spindler. He underfed rats by 40 percent. Within a month they had a 400 percent increase in the expression of the antiaging genes and an increase in the anti-inflammation genes, antioxidant genes, and anticancer genes. Why a live-food diet is so successful is that it turns on antiaging genes, anti-inflammatory genes, and theoretically the antidiabetic genes. There is a powerful crossover between the diabetic degenerative gene program and the aging genetic program. This is because a live-food diet is a natural form of calorie restriction. When you cook your food, according to the Max Planck Institute, you coagulate 50 percent of your protein and destroy 60–70 percent of your vitamins and minerals and up to 95–100 percent of your phytonutrients. One of the phytonutrients, for example, called *resveratrol*, plays a very important role in activating the antiaging genes as well as the anti-diabetes genes. It is gaining growing recognition in fighting age-related diseases ranging from dementia to diabetes. On a live-food diet that is properly eaten, we actually eat 50 percent fewer calories as compared to a standard American diet but maintain a very high level of nutrition. The reason for this is that we are consuming nutrient-dense foods, not just calorie-dense foods such as those offered in restaurants and fast-food dispensaries all over the Westernized world. We are becoming nations of overfed, undernourished individuals. Our bodies are rebelling through the metabolic degeneration process called diabetes. They are asking us for nutrients that are not provided through our cooked, processed diet, typically found in the Culture of Death.

When I say "calorie restriction," it is in the Culture of Life context, which is a plant-source-only, live, organic diet; it should not be misunderstood as denying ourselves the fuel we need. Nor are we in a cycle of deprivation. On the Dr. Cousens's Diabetes Recovery Program—A Holistic Approach, described in Chapter 7 of this book and in my book *Rainbow Green Live-Food Cuisine*, people are eating a delicious, satisfying, natural, appropriate amount of calories that are nutrient-dense enough to activate an aliesthetic taste change. The aliesthetic change is experienced as when we feel pleasurably satisfied from eating. It is also known as the "stop eating" signal we get from our body. This taste change most commonly happens when eating raw food. In other words, it is unusual to overeat a salad. This is in contrast to eating a processed, cooked, fast-food hamburger diet laden with excitotoxins (such as MSG) that provide the double insult of low nutrient density combined with the supersensory proprietary opioid stimuli of artificial flavorings, driving body and mind to continue to ask for food long after our calorie needs would have been satisfied by a tasty nutrient-dense meal. You would think that by eating a lower-calorie diet that a feeling of restriction or deprivation would result, but when your body receives all the minerals, phytonutrients, vitamins, enzymes, protein, essential fats, complex carbohydrates, and water it requires through a plant-source-only meal, a feeling of deep satisfaction is experienced right down to the cellular level. We are satiated by these foods, which are high on the satiety index. A completely new sense of abundance is realized as we begin to seek quality over quantity in our food. When you eat in such a way that everything you consume has purpose, you are choosing to live in the Culture of Life. Instead of accelerating the chronic disease/aging process, my program turns on the antiaging genes and removes the underlying causes of almost every preventable chronic disease process being witnessed in the Westernized world, including diabetes.

This is a key concept: A properly eaten live-food diet turns on the antiaging and antidiabetic genes. On a live-food, plant-source-only diet, people naturally tend to go to their optimal weight. Because of this, you automatically lose weight on my program if you are overweight. The people in the *Simply Raw* movie had an average weight loss (with the exception of the two Type-1 diabetics who were very thin to begin with) of 22 pounds in the first month. Often we see people who are obese lose over a hundred pounds in a year on a live-food diet without doing anything but eating live foods. Since up to 82 percent of diabetics are overweight, and diabetes is related to obesity, the natural weight loss down to optimal weight on a live-food, plant-source-only diet in this context is a powerful plus. A live-food diet creates just the opposite effect of the low-fiber diet high in refined sugar, white flour, junk foods, and processed, cooked animal fat that is creating the pandemic today. The pandemic gets worse as we go more into industrialized foods. A 100 percent live-food, moderate-low complex carbohydrate diet (initially with no fruit or grain) combined with green juice fasting is the most powerful way to upgrade the phenotypic expression and turn off the diabetic genes in Type-2 diabetics. An initial Phase 1.0 healing diet, as referred to previously, is described in *Rainbow Green Live-Food Cuisine* and in Chapter 7 of this book. This is the diet that a person stays on for at least the first three months until FBS has stabilized below 100 and the glycosylated hemoglobin (HgbA1c) reaches 5.7 or less. Once we have stabilized into a healthy nondiabetic physiology, then low-glycemic fruits can be added, as found in Phase 1.5. I give people the option of shifting to a diet of 80 percent live foods in Phase 1.5, which is the minimum definition of being on live foods, according to the 2006 International Summit on Live Foods.

On this diet, there are some variations, but a general constitutional pattern is needed to activate healing. The general pattern, according to Ayurvedic principles, is that diabetes is a kapha disorder, although it can happen in any of the three doshas (Ayurvedic constitutional types). A rebalancing diet for kapha is low sugar and bitter, pungent, and astringent foods. Kapha imbalances are made worse by a high amount of animal protein and fat, a high amount of sugar, and low exercise. Kaphas tend to have constipation, so they are made better by a high-fiber diet. This antikapha approach has been a mode of treatment for several thousand years. The treatment program in this book is based on not only current research but thousands of years of effective treatment and understanding. I have simply added a preliminary unified theory that enables a very rapid approach to healing and reversing diabetes naturally. The rapid moving to normal blood sugar levels without any medications encourages people to stay with the Dr. Cousens's Diabetes Recovery Program—A Holistic Approach because they get immediate tangible results. As long as one stays on this diet, one will be diabetes free.

This is an ongoing protective diet, no matter what your genetic predisposition is. This is the breakthrough. I am not talking about simply decreasing medication; I am talking about Type-2 people coming off all their insulin and oral medications in as rapidly as four days. I am talking about very rapid effects. The average person I see in my program comes in with an unregulated FBS of 300 while on insulin and/or oral hypoglycemics, and in an average of two to three weeks often has an FBS that is less than 100. If a person has Syndrome X, or what we call metabolic syndrome, then it may take several weeks or even longer to reset the phenotypic expression and move out of CDDS. The Dr. Cousens's Diabetes Recovery Program—A Holistic Approach seems to work at almost any age. The oldest participant so far has been a 93-year-old female with Type-2 diabetes, hypertension, and arthritis so severe she was confined to a wheelchair. She was on 11 different medications. By the end of the 21-day program she was off all medications, with an FBS of less than 100 and normal blood pressure, and she was out of her wheelchair and pain free.

The Seven Stages of Disease

The Seven Stages of Disease, formulated by Dr. John Tilden more than a hundred years ago, gives another perspective on how to understand the degenerative process of diabetes and how to reverse the process. "Health is what you consistently do," and the same can be said of ill health. Disease is an acquired state that is earned over the years with identifiable stages that lead to the manifestation of symptoms and even death if one is not prudent enough to reverse the disease process and go backward through the seven stages. Even an acute viral-based Type-1 onset requires a disturbed terrain that allowed a weakened immune state that produced susceptibility to a viral infection, resulting in insulinitis and a rapid onset of Type-1 diabetes. Diabetes is a disease process with stages that we can progressively degenerate along, advancing the disease condition and creating complications—or we can reverse the disease process. It depends on whether we are aware of what is required to live a healthy life. Herbert Shelton called this understanding the laws of life. If you understand and follow these laws you'll be healthy. If you break them you will get sick. This is the meaning of Crimes Against Wisdom. Shelton writes, "The laws of life are not something imposed upon the organization of man. They are imbedded in the very structure of our being, in our tissues, our nerve and muscle cells, our blood-stream, into the total organism. . . . Since these laws are fundamental parts of us, we cannot revolt against them without revolting against ourselves. . . . We cannot run away from the laws of being without running away from ourselves."[126]

In the Dr. Cousens Diabetes Recovery Program—A Holistic Approach, I teach what these natural ways are and empower you to live by them. Let's look now at the Seven Stages of Disease.

Stage 1: Enervation

Enervation is the reduction of nerve energy, by which the body's normal maintenance and eliminative functions are impaired, especially in terms of the elimination of endogenous and exogenous toxins—those created from within (through normal metabolic processes) and from without (in modern times, including the 65,000 human-made toxins in our environment and the excitotoxins, food additives, and toxins created by the cooking and processing of food). A person who is enervated is generally inactive, living in a toxic environment and consuming toxins that are not being released from the body in a timely manner.

Enervation is also created by stress, which uses up the vital energy in the body that would be applied to maintenance and elimination. Constipation occurs in the bowel, lymph, and tissues of the body. This is the diabetogenic diet and lifestyle we have been illustrating throughout this book.

Stage 2: Toxemia

The stagnation of Stage 1 leads to a buildup of toxins in the body, and these substances begin to saturate the blood, lymph, and cells. Stage 2 is typified by sluggish energy, and in the case of diabetes, we already have cells that are developing the preconditions for being insensitive to the signaling of insulin and leptin due to their toxic state. John Tilden writes in the chapter "Toxemia" in Herbert Shelton's *The History of Natural Hygiene*:

The toxin theory of the healing art is grounded on the truth that toxemia is the basic source of all diseases. So sure and certain is this truth that I do not hesitate to say that it is by far the most satisfactory theory that has been advanced in all the history of medicine. It is a scientific system that covers the whole field of cause and effect—a system that synthesizes with all knowledge, hence a true philosophy.

When this truth first began to force itself upon me, years ago, I was not sure but that there was something wrong with my reasoning. I saw that it would bring me very largely in opposition to every established medical treatment. I held back, and argued with myself. . . . I fought to suppress giving open utterance to a belief that would, in all probability, cause me to be hissed at—subject me to the jeers and gibes of the better class of people, both lay and professional.

Little by little I have proved the truth of my theory. I have tried it out daily for the past twenty years. I myself have personally stood the brunt of my experimenting, and have willingly suffered because of it. Every day this trying-out of the theory has convinced me more and more that toxemia is the universal cause of disease.

As has been stated continuously in my writings for the past dozen years, the habits of overeating, overclothing, and excesses of all kinds use up nerve energy. When the nerve supply is not equal to the demands of the body, organic functioning is impaired, resulting in the retention of waste products. This produces toxemia.[127]

Common sources of toxemia include various exogenous and endogenous toxins, which will now be recognizable as the diabetogenic preconditions for diabetes.

Endogenous toxins include the following:

- Metabolic waste, ongoing, toxic by-products on the cellular level
- Spent debris from cellular activity
- Dead cells
- Emotional and mental distress and excess
- Physical fatigue, distress, and excess

Exogenous toxins include the following:

- Unnatural food and drink
- Natural foods deranged by cooking, refining, and preserving
- Improper food combinations that result in endogenous toxins
- Medical, pharmaceutical, herbal, and supplemental drugging
- Tobacco, alcohol, and all forms of recreational drugging
- Environmental, commercial, and industrial pollutants
- Impure air and water

Stage 3: Irritation

The body becomes irritated by the toxic buildup in the blood, lymph, and tissues, and the interstitial space between the cells begins to resemble a toxic waste dump. The cells and tissues where buildup occurs are irritated by the toxic nature of the waste, resulting in inflammation. The waste products interfere with the proper oxygenation and feeding of the cells as well as causing the accumulation of excess water in the tissues. Pain signals coming from the tissues have at least three causes: lack of oxygen, lack of nutrition (cellular food), and pressure. The cells, subjected to the lack of oxygen, the lack of food, and the increased pressure from the retained water, begin to send out pain signals. The cells are hence irritated. The conventional answer is either to ignore the pain and discomfort or to take a "pain" pill, adding more to the toxic burden as the sufferer continues living in the same manner. The toxic sufferer can feel exhausted, queasy, irritable, itchy, and even irrational and hostile. This leads to the next stage of disease and body degeneration, inflammation.

Stage 4: Inflammation

The enervated body is now suffering the results of toxemia. The cells have initially become irritated. The next step of cellular changes and body degeneration is inflammation. The inflammation process produces the common "-itis." With the skin it is dermatitis. In the throat it may be tonsillitis and, further on, esophagitis. In the stomach, we find gastritis; in the small intestine, ileitis; in the colon, colitis; in the heart we have carditis; and in the liver, it is hepatitis. You may have an inflammation (an "-itis") anywhere in the body.

The medical community has named as many of the 20,000 distinctly different diseases that, in reality, are different manifestations of these seven stages. Allopathic practice tends to name a disease after the site where the toxins have accumulated and precipitated their symptoms. Once the set of symptoms is named, doctors usually prescribe pharmaceuticals at Stage 4, which do not remove the underlying causes that we are now familiar with. With diabetes and its complications, we see this stage of disease in the heart, kidneys, pancreas, liver, and nervous system. By allowing the accumulation of toxemia to advance, the body will continue to decline in energy and vitality. Further cellular changes will be found. Left unchecked and unheeded, the next stage of disease is ulceration.

Stage 5: Ulceration

An ulcer can be viewed as a consequence of body degeneration. Ulceration can occur with any body tissue, but the usual connotation of ulcers has to do with the skin. Tissues are destroyed. The body ulcerates, forming an outlet for the poisonous buildup. The toxic sufferer experiences a multiplication and worsening of symptoms while the pain intensifies.

The allopathic medical practice is usually to continue drugging and often commence with surgery and other forms of treatment at this stage. Remember, diabetic foot complications are the most common cause of nontrauma-based lower extremity amputations in the industrialized world. Neuropathy, a major etiologic component of most diabetic ulcerations, is present in more than 82 percent of diabetic patients with foot wounds.[128] The incidence of diabetes-associated gangrene is 20 times higher than in nondiabetics, and the risk of lower-extremity amputation is 15 to 46 times higher in diabetics than in people who do not have diabetes mellitus.[129, 130]

Stage 6: Induration

Induration means a hardening or scarring of tissues. Induration is the result of long-standing, chronic inflammation with bouts of acute inflammation interspersed. The chronic inflammation causes an impairment or sluggishness of circulation, and as some cells succumb, they are replaced with scar tissue. This is the way we lose good, normal-functioning cells—by chronic inflammation and death of cells.

We also see low oxygen in the cells coming from induration in the blood vessels as they are glycosylated. Atherosclerosis is a form of induration. With low or no circulation, toxic buildup, and low oxygen, we have the conditions for the seventh stage of disease: fungation, or cancer.

Stage 7: Fungation

When the internal conditions have deteriorated to the extent that normal aerobic, oxidative processes are no longer possible, the cells can revert to a more primordial means of surviving. Biochemical and morphological changes from the depositing of endogenous and exogenous toxins bring about degenerations and death at the cellular level. The cells can carry on their life processes by anaerobic processes—the same processes that many bacteria use. When the cells have changed in form and function to this extent, this is when an oncologist will tell you that you have cancer. Many diabetics also have candida.

Tracking Back through the Seven Stages to Health

The root causes of diabetes and its complications must be eliminated to be totally successful. In the language of the seven stages, the most important stages to address in reversing the diabetogenic process are toxemia, inflammation, and induration. This is another way to understand the CDDS process and how to reverse it. The means for reversal of toxemia and deficiency are topics we are going to investigate for the remainder of the book. When a person supplies the body with superior building materials, begins to lower the level of toxemia, and increases vitality, the body will begin to repair and rebuild. Previous complaints may surface once again as the body "retraces" and heals. The true test of any theory of disease is how well it can affect the chronic diseases such as diabetes.

Chapter 3 Summary

Diabetes is a complex, chronic, degenerative metabolic and hormonal dysregulation that emerges as a symptom of the Culture of Death. The lifestyle and diet of the Culture of Life is the antidote.

Although I have shared the fundamentals of a holistic theory to be discussed further in the summary chapter, results based on the application of this holistic theory are what are most important. The results in 120 participants are very positive, with 97 percent of Type-2 participants off all diabetic medications in 21 days and many having an FBS of 85 in a few weeks. The average FBS among the participants entering the program, as highlighted in Chapter 4, was around 260 on medications and ended at an average 86.6. LDL cholesterol dropped an average of 67 points, or 44 percent, with an ending average level of 82. The rapid reversal of the seven stages is accelerated by green juice fasting and natural supplements (discussed in Chapter 4) of herbs, minerals, high-protease enzymes, and digestive enzymes with our food to build up the amylase and liquid zeolite (natural cellular defense). This can help pull out heavy metals and 65,000 environmental toxins from our diet. With this integrated approach, the results of the Dr. Cousens's Diabetes Recovery Program—A Holistic Approach are rapid and consistent. The quicker the healing, the more encouragement people have to stay with the program and the happier they are.

This approach, based on my clinical experience over 40 years and guided by a unifying theory of turning on the antidiabetes genes and turning off the diabetes-producing genes with green juice fasting and live foods, has helped to break the four-minute mile of diabetes. It is supported by a lifestyle that creates life and not death. The program I describe in the next chapter is a complete holistic approach with the Culture of Life plant-source-only, live-food cuisine and lifestyle as its foundation.

Notes

1. Himsworth, H P. "The syndrome of diabetes mellitus and its causes." *Proc R Soc Med*, 1949, 42(3): 323.

2. Campbell, G D. *Congr Abstr, S Afr Med Ass*, East London, 45. Cape Town: South African Medical Association, 1959. Cited in Cleave, T L. *The Saccharine Disease*. Bristol, PA: John Wright & Sons, 1974.

3. Campbell, G D. *S Afr Med J*, 1960, 34: 332. Cited in Cleave, T L. *The Saccharine Disease*.

4. Albertson, V. *Diabetes*, 1953, 2: 1184. Cited in Cleave, T L. *The Saccharine Disease*.

5. Cohen, A M. *Israel Med J*, 1960, 19: 6137. Cited in Cleave, T L. *The Saccharine Disease*.

6. Cook, C E. Personal communication with Dr. Cleave, 1963.

7. Campbell, C H. Personal communication with Dr. Cleave, 1963.

8. Prior, J A M, and Davidson, F. *N Z Med J*, 1966, 65: 375.

9. Ascherio, A, and Willet, W C. "Health effects of trans-fatty acids." *Am J Clin Nutr*, October 1997, 66(suppl. 4): S1006–S1010.

10. Norris, S. "Trans fats: The health burden." http://www.parl.gc.ca /content/LOP/ResearchPublications/prb0521-e.htm.

11. Bluher, M, Kahn, B B, and Kahn, C R. "Extended longevity in mice lacking the insulin receptor in adipose tissue." *Science*, January 24, 2003, 299(5606): 572–74.

12. Lane, M A, Ingram, D K, and Roth, G S. "Calorie restriction in nonhuman primates: Effects on diabetes and cardiovascular risk." *Toxicol Sci*, December 1999, 52(2 suppl.): 41–48.

13. Kemnitz, J W, Roecker, E B, Weindruch, R, Elson, D F, Baum, S T, and Bergman, R N. "Dietary restriction increases insulin sensitivity and lowers blood glucose in rhesus monkeys." *Am J Physiol*, April 1994, 266(4, part 1): E540–E547.

14. Kent, S. "BioMarker pharmaceuticals develops anti-aging therapy." *Life Extension*, June 2003, 9(6): 56–67. Fort Lauderdale, FL: Life Extension Foundation.

15. Suh, Y, Lee, K A, Kim, W H, Han, B G, Vijg, J, and Park, S. "Aging alters the apoptotic response to genotoxic stress." *Nat Med*, January 2002, 8(1): 3–4.

16. Mukherjee, P, El-Abbadi, M M, Kasperzyk, J L, Ranes, M K, and Seyfried, T N. "Dietary restriction reduces angiogenesis and growth in an orthotopic mouse brain tumour model." *Br J Cancer*, May 20, 2002, 86(10): 1615–21.

17. Kritchevsky, D. "Caloric restriction and cancer." *J Nutr Sci Vitaminol*, February 2001, 47(1): 13–19.

18. Moreschi, C. "The connection between nutrition and tumor promotion." *Z Immunitaetsforsch*, 1909, 2: 651.

19. Spindler, S R. "Reversing aging rapidly with short-term calorie restriction." *Life Extension Magazine*, 2001, 7(12): 40–61. Fort Lauderdale, FL: Life Extension Foundation. http://www.lef.org/magazine/mag2001 /dec2001_cover_spindler_01.html?source=search&key=Spindler%20 S%20R%20Reversing%20aging%20rapidly%20with%20shortterm%20 calorie%20restriction.

20. Yoshida, K, Inoue, T, Hirabayashi, Y, Nojima, K, and Sado, T. "Calorie restriction and spontaneous hepatic tumors in C3H1He mice." *J Nutr Health Aging*, 1999, 3(2): 121–26.

21. Widmer, S, Mauriz, M, and Gottesmann, S. "Posttranslational quality control: Folding, refolding, and degrading proteins." *Science*, December 3, 1999, 286(5446): 1888–93.

22. Kritchevsky, D. "The effect of over- and undernutrition on cancer." *Eur J Cancer Prev*, December 1995, 4(6): 445–51.

23. Bjørnholt, J V, Erikssen, G, Aaser, E, Sandvik, L, Nitter-Hauge, S, Jervell, J, Erikssen, J, and Thaulow, E. "Fasting blood glucose: An underestimated risk factor for cardiovascular death. Results from a 22-year follow-up of healthy nondiabetic men." *Diabetes Care*, 1999, 22: 45–49.

24. Fauci, A S, Braunwald, E, Kasper, D L, Hauser, S L, Longo, D L, Jameson, J L, and Loscalzo J. *Principles of Internal Medicine*. 13th ed. New York: McGraw-Hill, 1994, p. 2001. "In one study in normal persons (arterialized venous samples), insulin secretion ceased at a 4.6 nmol/L glucose (83mg/dl)."

25. Ibid., p. 2004. "Plasma insulin concentration generally reaches background levels for the assay when plasma glucose falls below 4.6 nmol/L (83mg/dl)."

26. Ibid., table 328-4, "Mean plasma glucose and insulin during fasting." (Zero values obtained after overnight fast. Results are mean values for 20 normal men and 60 normal women.)

27. Walford, R L, Harris, S B, and Gunion, M W. "The calorically restricted low-fat nutrient-dense diet in Biosphere 2 significantly lowers blood glucose, total leukocyte count, cholesterol, and blood pressure in humans." *Proc Natl Acad Sci USA*, December 1, 1992, 89(23): 11533–37.

28. Heller, R F. "Hyperinsulinemic obesity and carbohydrate addiction: The missing link is the carbohydrate frequency factor." *Med Hypotheses*, May 1994, 42(5): 307–12.

29. Goodpaster, B H, Katsiaras, A, and Kelley, D E. "Enhanced fat oxidation through physical activity is associated with improvements in insulin sensitivity in obesity." *Diabetes*, September 2003, 52(9): 2191–97.

30. Holt, S H, Miller, J C, and Petocz, P. "An insulin index of foods: The insulin demand generated by 1000-kJ portions of common foods." *Am J Clin Nutr*, November 1997, 66(5): 1264–76.

31. Holt, S H A, et al. *European J Clin Nutr* 1995, 49: 675–90.

32. Furber, J D. "Extracellular glycation crosslinks: Prospects for removal." *Rejuvenation Res*, Summer 2006, 9(2): 274–78.

33. Peppa, M, Uribarri, J, and Vlassara, H. "Glucose, advanced glycation end products, and diabetes complications: What is new and what works." *Clinical Diabetes*, 2003, 21: 186–87.

34. Werman, M J, et al. "The chronic effect of dietary fructose on glycation and collagen cross-linking in rats." *Am J Clin Nutr*, 1997, 66: 219.

35. McCarty, M F. "The low AGE content of low-fat vegan diets could benefit diabetics, though concurrent taurine supplementation may be needed to minimize endogenous AGE production." *Med Hypotheses*, 2005, 64(2): 394–98.

36. Qian, P, Cheng, S, Guo, J, and Niu, Y. "Effects of vitamin E and vitamin C on nonenzymatic glycation and peroxidation in experimental diabetic rats." *Wei Sheng Yan Jiu*, July 2000, 29(4): 226–28.

37. Ceriello, A, Quatraro, A, and Giugliano, D. "New insights on nonenzymatic glycosylation may lead to therapeutic approaches for the prevention of diabetic complications." *Diabet Med*, 1992, 9: 297–99.

38. Davie, S J, Gould, B J, and Yudkin, J S. "Effect of vitamin C on glycosylation of proteins." *Diabetes*, 1992, 41: 167–73.

39. Ceriello, Quatraro, and Giugliano. "New insights on nonenzymatic glycosylation."

40. Davie, Gould, and Yudkin. "Effect of vitamin C on glycosylation of proteins."

41. Jain, S K, McVie, R, Jaramillo, J J, et al. "Effect of modest vitamin E supplementation on blood glycated hemoglobin and triglyceride levels and red cell indices in Type-1 diabetic patients." *J Am Coll Nutr*, 1996, 15: 458–61.

42. Fife, B. *The Healing Miracles of Coconut Oil.* Colorado Springs: Health Wise, 2003, p. 110.

43. Nicholson, A S, et al. "Toward improved management of NIDDM: A randomized, controlled, pilot intervention using a low-fat, vegetarian diet." *Preventive Medicine*, 1999, 29: 87–91.

44. Barnard, N D, et al. "The effects of a low-fat, plant-based dietary intervention on body weight, metabolism, and insulin sensitivity." *Amer J Medicine*, 2005, 118: 991–97.

45. Stratton, I M, Adler, A L, and Neil, H A. "Association of glycaemia with macrovascular and microvascular complications of type 2 diabetes (UKPDS 35): Prospective observational study." *BMJ*, 2000, 321: 405–12.

46. Ornish, D, et al. "Can lifestyle changes reverse coronary heart disease?" *The Lancet*, 1990, 336: 129–33.

47. Petersen, K F, et al. "Impaired mitochondrial activity in the insulin-resistant offspring of patients with type 2 diabetes." *New England J Med*, 2004, 350: 664–71.

48. Goff, L M, et al. "Veganism and its relationship with insulin resistance and intramyocellular lipid." *Eur J Clin Nutr*, 2005, 59: 291–98.

49. Keen, H, and Mattock, M D. "Complications of diabetes mellitus: Role of essential fatty acids." In *Omega-6 Essential Fatty Acids. Pathophysiology and Roles in Clinical Medicine*, edited by D F Horrobin, 447–55. New York: Wiley-Liss, 1990.

50. Storlien, L H, Jenkins, A B, Chisolm, D J, et al. "Influence of dietary fat composition on development of insulin resistance in rats." *Diabetes*, 1991, 40: 280–89.

51. Dutta-Roy, A K. "Insulin mediated processes in platelets, erythrocytes, and monocytes/macrophages: effects of essential fatty acid metabolism." *Prostaglandins Leukot Essent Fatty Acids*, 1994, 51: 385–99.

52. Ibid.

53. Hagve, T-A. "Effects of unsaturated fatty acids on cell membrane functions." *Scand J Clin Lab Inves*, 1988, 48: 381–88.

54. Anderson, R A. "Chromium, glucose tolerance, diabetes and lipid metabolism." *J Advan Med*, 1995, 8: 37–50.

55. Horrobin, D F. "Essential fatty acid (EFA) metabolism in patients with diabetic neuropathy." *Prostaglandins Leukot Essent Fatty Acids*, 1997, 57: 256(abstr.).

56. Enig, M G, Atal, S, Keeny, M, and Sampunga, J. "Isometric transfatty acids in the U.S. diet." *J Am Coll Nutr*, 1990, 5: 471–86.

57. Pan, D A, Lilliioja, S, Milner, M R, et al. "Skeletal muscle membrane lipid composition is related to adiposity and insulin action." *J Clin Invest*, 1995, 96: 2802–8.

58. Storlien, L H, Pan, D A, Kriketos, A D, et al. "Skeletal muscle membrane lipids and insulin resistance." *Lipids*, 1996, 31: S262–S265.

59. Eritsland, J, Delijeflot, I, Abdelnoor, M, et al. "Long-term effects of n-3 fatty acids on serum lipids and glycemic control." *Scand J Clin Lab Invest*, 1994, 54: 73–80.

60. Clandinin, M T, Cheema, S, Field, C H, and Baracos, V E. "Impact of dietary fatty acids on insulin responsiveness in adipose tissue, muscle, and liver." In *Essential Fatty Acids and Ecosanoids: Invited Papers from the Third International Conference*, edited by A Sinclair and R Gibson, 416–20. Champaign, IL: AOCS Press, 1993.

61. Storlien, Pan, Kriketos, et al. "Skeletal muscle membrane lipids and insulin resistance."

62. Eritsland, Delijeflot, Abdelnoor, et al. "Long-term effects of n-3 fatty acids."

63. Kissebah, A H, and Hennes, M M I. "Central obesity and free fatty acid metabolism." *Prostaglandins Leukot Essent Fatty Acids*, 1995, 52: 209–11.

64. Foster, D W. "Diabetes mellitus." In *Harrison's Principles of Internal Medicine*, 11th ed, edited by E Braunwald, K J Isselbacher, R G Petersdorf, et al, 1778–81. New York: McGraw-Hill, 1988.

65. Heller, B, Burkart, V, Lampeter, E, and Kolb, H. "Antioxidant therapy for the prevention of Type-1 diabetes." *Adv Pharm*, 1997, 38: 629–38.

66. Mijac, V, Arrieta, J, Mendt, C. et al. "Role of environmental factors in the development of insulin-dependent diabetes mellitus (IDDM) in insulin-dependent Venezuelan children." *Invest Clin*, 1995, 36: 73–82.

67. Ibid.

68. Schmernthaner, G. "Progress in the immunointervention of Type-1 diabetes mellitus." *Horm Metab Res*, 1995, 27: 547–54.

69. Ibid.

70. Mijac, Arrieta, Mendt, et al. "Role of environmental factors in the development of insulin-dependent diabetes mellitus."

71. Karjalainen, J, Martin, J, Knip, M, et al. "A bovine albumin peptide as a possible trigger of insulin-dependent diabetes." *N Eng J Med*, 1992, 327: 302–7.

72. Saukkonen, T, Savilahti, E, Madascsy, L, et al. "Increased frequency of IgM antibodies to cow's milk proteins in Hungarian children with newly diagnosed insulin-dependent diabetes mellitus." *Eur J Pediatr*, 1996, 155: 885–89.

73. Saukkonen, T, Savilahti, E, Landin-Olsson, M, and Dahlquist, G. "IgA bovine serum albumin antibodies are increased in newly diagnosed patients with insulin-dependent diabetes mellitus, but the increase is

not an independent risk factor for diabetes." *Acta Paediatr*, 1995, 84: 1258–61.

74. Vahasalo, P, Petays, T, Knip, M, et al. "Relation between antibodies to islet cell antigens, other autoantigens and cow's milk protein in diabetic children and unaffected siblings at the clinical manifestation of IDDM." *Autoimmunity*, 1996, 23: 165–74.

75. Leslie, R D G, and Elliott, R B. "Early environmental events as a cause of IDDM." *Diabetes*, 1994, 43: 843–50.

76. Kostraba, J N, Cruickshanks, K J, Lawler-Heavner, J, Jobim, L F, Rewers, M J, Gay, E C, Chase, H P, Klingensmith, G, and Hamman, R F. "Early exposure to cow's milk and solid foods in infancy, genetic predisposition, and risk of IDDM." *Diabetes*, 1993, 42: 288–95.

77. Karjalainen, Martin, Knip, et al. "A bovine albumin peptide."

78. Akerblom, H K, et al. "Dietary manipulation of beta cell autoimmunity in infants at increased risk of Type-1 diabetes: A pilot study." *Diabetologia*, 2005, 48: 829–37.

79. Clyne, P S, and Kulczycki Jr., A. "Human breast milk contains bovine IgG: Relationship to infant colic?" *Pediatrics*, 1997, 87: 439–44.

80. American Academy of Pediatrics Work Group on Cow's Milk Protein and Diabetes Mellitus. "Infant feeding practices and their possible relationship to the etiology of diabetes mellitus." *Pediatrics*, 1994, 94: 752–54.

81. Brownlee, M, Vlassara, H, and Cerami, A. "Nonenzymatic glycosylation and the pathogenesis of diabetic complications." *Ann Int Med*, 1984, 101: 527–37.

82. Whitaker, J. *Reversing Diabetes*. New York: Warner Books, 2001, p. 82.

83. Esselstyn, C B, Ellis, S G, Medendorp, S V, et al. "A strategy to arrest and reverse coronary artery disease: A 5-year longitudinal study of a single physician's practice." *J Fam Prac*, 1995, 41: 560–68.

84. Esselstyn, C B. "Prevent and reverse heart disease." http://www.heartattackproof.com.

85. World Health Organization. "World health statistics annual, 1994–1998." http://www.who.int/whosis. Food and Agriculture Organization of the United Nations. "Statistical database food balance sheets, 1961–1999." http://www.fao.org. National Institutes of Health. "Global cancer rates, cancer death rates among 50 countries, 1986–1999." http://www.nih.gov.

86. Fuhrman, J. *Eat to Live*. New York: Little, Brown, and Company, 2003, pp. 51–52.

87. American College of Cardiology. "Children of diabetics show signs of atherosclerosis." Accessed July 2007. http://medicineworld.org/cancer /lead/6-2006/children-of-diabetics.html.

88. Ross-Flanigan, N. "Diabetes and periodontal disease: A complex, two-way connection." http://www.umich.edu/~urecord/9899/Jan25_99 /gums.htm.

89. Wyngaarden, J B, Smith, L H, and Bennett, J C. *Cecil Textbook of Medicine*. Philadelphia: W B Saunders, 1992.

90. Cogan, D G, Kinoshita, J H, Kador, P F, et al. "Aldose reductase and complications of diabetes." *Ann Int Med*, 1984, 101: 82–91.

91. Crane, M G, and Sample, C. "Regression of diabetic neuropathy with total vegetarian (vegan) diet." *J Nutritional Med*, 1994, 4: 431–39.

92. Pecoraro, R E, Reiber, G E, and Burgess, E M. "Pathways to diabetic limb amputation: Basis for prevention." *Diabetes Care*, 1990, 13: 513–21.

93. Lavery, L A, Ashry, H R, van Houtum, W, Pugh, J A, Harkless, L B, and Basu, S. "Variation in the incidence and proportion of diabetes-related amputations in minorities." *Diabetes Care*, 1996, 19: 48–52.

94. Armstrong, D G, Lavery, L A, Quebedeaux, T L, and Walker, S C. "Surgical morbidity and the risk of amputation due to infected puncture wounds in diabetic versus nondiabetic adults." *South Med J*, 1997, 90: 384–89.

95. Whitaker. *Reversing Diabetes*. pp. 6 and 146.

96. Thomas, S H, Wisher, M, Brandenberg, D, and Sonksen, P H. "Insulin action on adipocytes, evidence that the antilipolytic and lipogenic effects of insulin are mediated by the same receptor." *Biochem J*, 1979, 184: 355–60.

97. Baskin, et al. "Insulin receptor substrate 1 (IRS-1) expression in rat brain." *Endocrin*, 1998, 134: 1952–55.

98. Zhao, W, Chen, H, Xu, H, Moore, E, Meiri, N, Quon, MJ, and Alkon, D. "Brain insulin receptors and spatial memory. Correlated changes in gene expression tyrosine phosphorylation and signaling molecules in the hippocampus of water maze trained rats." *J Biol Chem*, 1990, 274: 34893–902.

99. Sonksen, P H. "Insulin, growth hormone and sport." *J Endocrinol*, 2001, 170: 23–25.

100. Berkson, L. *Hormone Deception*. New York: Contemporary Books, 2000, p. 208.

101. Bertazzi, P A. "Long-term health effects of dioxin exposure in a residential population." Presented at the Keystone Symposium on Endocrine Disruptors (B5) in Tahoe City, CA (January 31–February 5, 1999).

102. Berkson. *Hormone Deception.* p. 312.

103. Moller, J, and Einfeldt, H. *Testosterone Treatment of Cardiovascular Diseases: Principles and Experiences.* Berlin: Springer-Verlag, 1984.

104. Anderson, D C. "Sex hormone binding globulin." *Clin Endocrin*, 1972, 3: 69–96.

105. Haffner, S M, Shaten, J, Stern, M P, Smith, G D, and Kuller, L. "Low levels of sex hormone binding globulin and testosterone predict the development of non-insulin-dependent diabetes in men." MRFIT Research Group. Multiple Risk Factor Intervention Trial. *Am J Epidemiol*, 1996, 143(9): 889–97.

106. Haffner, S M, Valdez, R A, Morales, P A, Hazuda, H P, and Stern, M O. "Decreased sex hormone binding globulin predicts non-insulin dependent diabetes mellitus in women but not in men." *J Clin Endocrin Metab*, 1993, 77: 56–60.

107. Haffner, Shaten, Stern, et al. "Low levels of sex hormone binding globulin."

108. Haffner, Valdez, Morales, et al. "Decreased sex hormone binding globulin."

109. Tibblin, G, Alderberth, A, Lindstedt, G, and Bjorntorp, P. "The pituitary gonadal axis and health in elderly men: A study of men born in 1913." *Diabetes*, 1996, 45(11): 1605–9.

110. Kaplan, N M. "The deadly quartet. Upper body obesity, glucose intolerance, hypertriglyceridemia, and hypertension." *Arch Int Med*, 1989, 149: 1514–20.

111. Depres, J B, Lamarche, B, Mauriege, P, Cantin, P, et al. "Hyperinsulinemia as an independent risk factor for ischemic heart disease." *N Eng J Med*, 1996, 334(15): 952–57.

112. Zmuda, J M, Cauley, J A, Kriska, A, Glynn, N W, et al. "Longitudinal relation between endogenous testosterone and cardiac disease risk factors in middle-aged men. A 13-year follow-up of former Multiple Risk Factor Intervention Trial participants." *Am J Epidemiol*, 1997, 146(8): 609–17.

113. Birkeland, K I, Hanssen, K F, Tojesen, P A, and Valler, S. "Level of sex hormone binding globulin is positively correlated with insulin sensitivity in men with Type-2 diabetes." *J Clin Endocrin Metab*, 1993, 76(2): 275–78.

114. Haffner, S M, Valdez, R A, Mykkanen, L, Stern, P, and Katz, M S. "Decreased testosterone and dehydroepiandrosterone sulfate concentrations are associated with increased insulin and glucose concentrations in nondiabetic men." *Metab Clin Experim*, 1994, 43(5): 599–603.

115. Haffner, S M. "Sex hormone binding globulin, hyperinsulinemia, insulin resistance and non-insulin dependent diabetes mellitus." *Hormone Res*, 1996, 45(3–5): 233–37.

116. Rosenthal, S M, and Ziegler, E E. "The effect of uncooked starches on the blood sugar of normal and of diabetic subjects." *Arch Intern Med*, 1929, 44: 344–50.

117. Howell, E. *Enzyme Nutrition*. New York: Penguin Putnam, 1985.

118. *Zeit Ges Exp Med*, 1930, 71: 245–50.

119. *Am J Dig Dis & Nutr*, 1936, 3: 159–61.

120. *Nederlands Tij v Geneesk*, 1934, 78: 1529–36.

121. *Am J Dig Dis & Nutr*, 1934–1935, vol 1.

122. *Br Med J*, 1923, 1: 317–19.

123. Lopez, D A, Williams, R M, and Miehlke, K. *Enzymes: The Fountain of Life*. Charleston, SC: Neville Press, 1994.

124. Nobmann, E D, Byers, T, Lanier, A P, Hankin, J H, and Jackson, M. "The diet of Alaska Native adults 1987–1988." *Am J Clin Nutr*, 1992, 55: 1024–32.

125. Murphy, N J, Schraer, C D, Bulkow, L R, Boyko, E J, and Lanier, A P. "Diabetes mellitus in Alaskan Yupik Eskimos and Athabascan Indians after 25 years." *Diabetes Care*, October 1992, 15(10): 1390–92.

126. Shelton, H. *Getting Well*. San Antonio, TX: Dr. Shelton's Health School, 1946, pp. 233–34.

127. Shelton, H. *The History of Natural Hygiene and the Principles of Natural Hygiene*. San Antonio, TX: Dr. Shelton's Health School, 1946, pp. 59–60.

128. Pecoraro, R E, Reiber, G E, and Burgess, E M. "Pathways to diabetic limb amputation. Basis for prevention." *Diabetes Care*, 1990, 13: 513–21.

129. Lavery, Ashry, van Houtum, et al. "Variation in the incidence and proportion of diabetes-related amputations."

130. Armstrong, Lavery, Quebedeaux, et al. "Surgical morbidity and the risk of amputation."

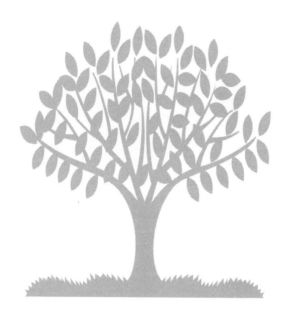

Dr. Cousens's Diabetes Recovery Program—A Holistic Approach

It is a part of the cure to wish to be cured.

Seneca, philosopher, legal scholar, and playwright

A truly good physician first finds out the cause of the illness, and having found that, first tries to cure it by food. Only when food fails does he prescribe medication.

Sun Ssu-mo, Tang dynasty Taoist physician, in *Precious Recipes*

Let nothing which can be treated by diet be treated by other means.

**Moshe Maimonides, MD (1135–1204 CE),
leading Jewish rabbi of his generation, philosopher,
and master holistic physician to the Egyptian sultan**

The first principle of the Dr. Cousens's Diabetes Recovery Program—A Holistic Approach is to heal diabetes naturally with a diet of organic, plant-source-only, live (raw) food, 25–45 percent moderate-low complex carbohydrates, 25–45 percent plant-based fats, moderate protein, low glycemic index, low insulin index, high minerals, no refined carbohydrates (especially white flour, white sugar, junk or processed foods), high fiber, and individualized moderate caloric intake, prepared with love.

This diet, updated with the concept of individualization as explained in detail in my book *Conscious Eating*, is also known as the Genesis 1:29 Garden of Eden diet. Some people need more protein (plant sourced), and others need a diet higher in complex carbohydrates, depending on one's constitution. Regardless of your constitution, however, this diet is high in vegetables, leafy greens, sprouts, high-fiber vegetables, and phytonutrients. A high-phytonutrient diet naturally includes a variety of antioxidants such as carotenes, vitamin E, vitamin C, phenol compounds, and resveratrol in the foods. You know you are getting these when there is a full rainbow of colors in your vegetables, and also fruits, beans, and grains (in the maintenance diet of Phase 1.5, including low glycemic fruits and grains), as colors are actually the pigments containing the phytonutrients, which turn on the antiaging, anticancer, antidiabetes, and anti-inflammatory genes. Most important, these phytonutrients turn off the diabetes-causing genes and turn on the antidiabetic genes. In *Genetic Nutritioneering*, Jeffrey Bland, PhD, explains how the hormone insulin indirectly speaks to the genes and alters gene expression. Insulin also influences the other hormones in the body. A healthy flow of insulin in the body not only helps us control blood sugar but is linked to a healthy balance of many other hormones, including insulin-like growth factor, human growth hormone, cortisol, somatostatin, serotonin, noradrenalin, and leptin.[1] Control of hormones is found through our diet, stress, exercise patterns, and of course the food we take into our body. Emerging research confirms that the type of carbohydrates one eats also influences the expression of one's genes through their effect on the secretion of insulin, glucagons, and other cell-signaling hormones. So when one eats, it is good to consciously consider that what is eaten speaks to our genes, and therefore positively or negatively affects gene expression.

Genes carry messages that describe how sensitive one is to insulin and blood sugar. In other words, there is free choice to modify the expression of these genetic messages, by what one eats, how one exercises, how one creates stress in one's life, and the toxins (such as drugs, alcohol, cigarettes, and heavy metals) that one brings into one's system. The point is that whether or not there is an onset of insulin resistance depends on our food and lifestyle. Insulin is a major regulator of the diabetic genes. When our insulin levels are not in homeostasis, our genes that favor the diabetic process are activated.

Studies have found that when individuals consume animal-protein-rich foods, their insulin output goes higher. This research done with the insulin index, as discussed in Chapter 2, shows that meat, dairy, and fish can create an excess release of insulin—that is, they have a high insulin index and therefore imbalance the system. Research by Gene Stiller, PhD, found that an animal-protein-enhanced diet often increases insulin resistance.[2] Research generally shows that diets containing whole and natural vegetable protein have a lower insulin response than refined high-fat foods. It has been found that the amino acid mix in vegetable protein, although complete, is slightly different than, and offers certain advantages over, animal protein. Specifically for diabetes, vegetable protein positively affects many aspects of our metabolism, including the improvement of insulin sensitivity and the reduction of toxic reactions.[3] Simply changing the excess of calories in the diet and improving the ratio of protein to carbohydrates and fat according to one's constitution can actually improve the regulation of blood sugar levels.[4]

Phytonutrients

One of the most potent components of food that affects gene expression on the molecular level is phytonutrients. Research on phytonutrients supports the general findings I've summarized; for example, 82 percent of 156 different published dietary studies found that fruit and vegetable consumption helped protect against cancer.[5] People who eat more fruits and vegetables have about one-half the risk of cancer mortality than those people who are not plant eaters. Plant-sourced diets are very high in phytonutrients, which include a variety of antioxidants, carotenes, vitamin E, vitamin C, phenolic compounds, and terpenoids. We get more than twice the phytonutrients from the same amount of calories on the nutrient-dense live-food diet, which is also a natural calorie-restricted diet. The Dr. Cousens's Diabetes Recovery Program—A Holistic Approach naturally stimulates and reactivates the antiaging, anti-inflammatory, anticancer, and antidiabetic genes and turns off the diabetes-causing genes with the aid of the rainbow menu of phytonutrients. These phytonutrients include the allyl sulfides in garlic and onions, potent stimulators of improved phenotypic expression for diabetes that aid in controlling blood sugar with their sulfur components important for insulin function; phytates in grains and legumes, with anticancer effects; glucarates in citrus, grains, and tomatoes, improving the gene expression of detoxification; lignans in flax, improving the metabolism of estrogen and testosterone; indoles, isothiocyanates, and hydroxybutene in cruciferous vegetables, improving detoxification against carcinogens; ellagic acid in grapes, raspberries, strawberries, and nuts, improving antioxidant function; and bioflavonoids, carotenoids, and terpenoids, reducing inflammation and improving immunity. Inflammation is definitely affected by our gene expression. My favorite anti-inflammatory food is ginger; it has active phytochemicals called gingerols, which have been shown to be quite effective in the treatment of arthritis and other inflammation problems. Used in conjunction with curcumin, these two have been shown to improve gene expression in regard to the anti-inflammatory response.[6] One popular flavonoid is quercetin. Found in apples, onions, and garlic, quercetin helps improve gene expression related to allergy and arthritis and helps maintain the integrity of vascular tissue for improved circulation. Bioflavonoids like quercetin are among the most important modifiers of gene expression, in addition to being antioxidants.

Once one understands this first principle about eating this diet, one starts to understand that what one takes into the body has very important healing effects. In an October 1997 article in *Science* by Dr. Caleb Finch, a professor at the Andrus Gerontology Center at the University of Southern California, Finch clearly makes the point that heredity plays a minor role in determining life-span.[7] After 40, genetics plays only about 25 percent of the longevity equation; lifestyle and diet play the other 75 percent of the outcome, including slowing the shortening of telomeres. If one does not activate the diabetes-producing genes with poor diet and lifestyle, then diabetes will not manifest.

Antiaging: Caloric Restriction and Resveratrol

To further make the point of the main principle of the Dr. Cousens's Diabetic Recovery Program—A Holistic Approach, *Life Extension*

(2004) reports that a phytonutrient, resveratrol, has been found by Harvard medical school researchers to activate a longevity gene in yeast that extends life by 70 percent. In an interview, leading resveratrol researcher Dr. Xi Zhao-Wilson told *Life Extension*, "There has been a great deal of attention focused on resveratrol in the past few years, following a study showing that resveratrol activates molecular pathways involved in life-span extension, now demonstrated in yeast, worms, flies, fish, and mice, and which possibly bear a relationship to mechanisms underlying caloric restriction."[8] The tremendous amount of scientific evidence on the effect of caloric restriction on upgrading our gene expression supports the link of caloric restriction to longevity. In humans, the preliminary evidence is very promising: Consuming a low-calorie, low-carbohydrate diet is associated with several possible markers of greater longevity, such as lower insulin levels and reduced body temperatures, along with less of the chromosomal damage that typically accompanies aging.[9] This research supports one of the main points of our program—that diabetes is an accelerated aging process and youthing through eating "restricted" but nutrient-dense foods reverses the accelerated aging associated with a diabetogenic diet and lifestyle.

Research History on Caloric Restriction

Research on caloric restriction goes back to the 1930s when Dr. Clive McKay of Cornell University found that the life-span of rats doubled when their food intake was halved. Not only did the calorie-restricted rats live longer, but they were more healthy and youthful, when compared to the control rats. He found that his control rats, allowed to eat as much as they wanted, became weak and feeble as they lived their normal life-span. Calorie-restricted rats, at the time when the control rats were dying out, were still alive, youthful, and vigorous. One of the rats lived to the equivalent of 150 human years. This research was repeated in the 1960s with calorie-restricted rats at the Morris H. Ross Institute, where the rats lived up to 1,800 days, or approximately 180 human years. In the 1970s breakthrough research was done by Dr.

Roy Walford and Dr. Richard Weindruch at the UCLA medical center, where they found that even gradual restriction of calorie intake in middle-age rats extended life-span as much as 60 percent. Research by Professor Huxley extended the life-span of worms by a factor of 19 times by periodically underfeeding them.[10] Research has also shown that undereating increases life-span in fruit flies, water fleas, and trout.[11] The research by Walford and Weindruch suggested that it doesn't matter what age you start—you can still turn on a healthy gene expression. That's good news for a lot of people.

The next breakthrough began in the 1990s with Dr. Richard Weindruch and Dr. Thomas Prolla at the University of Wisconsin. Using microchip technology, they measured the expression of thousands of genes in mice, rats, monkeys, and humans. Weindruch and Prolla studied gene profiles in the muscles in normal and calorie-restricted mice and found major differences in gene expression between the two groups. In this first study of gene expression, the scientists found that gene expression was significantly positively altered by caloric restriction in a way that seemed to show a slowing of the aging process.[12] Following this significant breakthrough was work done by Dr. Stephen Spindler, professor of biochemistry at the University of California-Riverside. Using gene technologies, Spindler studied the expression of 11,000 genes in the livers of young normally fed and calorie-restricted rats and found that 60 percent of the age-related changes in gene expression from calorie-restricted mice occurred within a few weeks after they started the calorie-restricted diet. The full effects of caloric restriction on the genetic profile for antiaging develop quickly. Spindler found that caloric restriction results in a specifically produced genetic antiaging profile and resulted in reversal of the majority of age-related degenerative changes that showed up in the gene expression. As diabetes is an age-related degenerative process, so it follows that a general antiaging effect should have an antidiabetogenic effect. Spindler found a 4-fold increase in the expression of the antiaging genes in short-term caloric restrictions and a 2.5-fold increase in the expression of youthing genes in long-term caloric restriction. He was able to reproduce this with a 95 percent success rate.

Spindler noted that caloric restriction not only prevented deterioration or genetic change gradually over the life-span of the animal, but actually reversed most of the aging changes in a short period of time. His research lasted only a month with the rats. In another study, he found that the most rapid change from a genetic aging profile to an antiaging profile occurred in older animals as well as young and middle-age ones, thus making the point that it doesn't matter at what age you begin. Caloric restriction does appear to turn on the expression of the antiaging genes and turn off the expression of the aging genes and most likely turns off the expression of diabetic genes. We have a full memory of all our gene expression in our chromosomes; all we have to do is push the right dietary button to get a healthy expression.

Cultural Evidence Supporting Caloric Restriction

Human cross-cultural studies reveal the same results. Dr. Kenneth Pelletier, in his research on longevity, found that cultures in which people lived the longest, healthiest lives—the natives of the Vilcabamba region of Ecuador, the Hunza of West Pakistan, the Tarahumara Indians of northern Mexico, and the Abkhasians of the Georgia region of Russia— ate low-protein, natural, primarily plant-fat and carbohydrate diets that contained approximately one-half the amount of protein Americans eat and only 50–60 percent of the total calories.[13] Paavo Airola makes the point in *How to Get Well* that one never sees an obese centenarian.

Returning to Spindler, an important part of his research is that the short-term caloric restriction can turn on the majority of the antiaging genes. He found that weight loss from caloric restriction improves insulin sensitivity, improves blood glucose values, decreases blood insulin levels, decreases heart rate, and improves blood pressure. In summary, Spindler's results, published in the proceedings of the National Academy of Sciences, showed the following:

- No matter what age you are, you still get an antiaging effect with calorie restriction

- Antiaging effects can happen quickly on a low-calorie diet
- Caloric restriction of only four weeks in rats seems to partially restore the liver's ability for metabolizing drugs and for detoxification
- Caloric restriction seems to quickly decrease the amount of inflammation and stress even in older animals.[14]

We see these same positive results in our one-week green juice-fasting retreats at the Tree of Life in the United States and Tree of Life Israel–Europe.

What we eat feeds our genes (as well as what we do not eat). It is our choice. This is the key to understanding the diet for reversing diabetes. We will take it one step further, so it is very clear. The Dr. Cousens's Diabetes Recovery Program—A Holistic Approach starts with green juice fasting for seven days, because that is the most powerful form of caloric restriction, and therefore has the most potential effect on balancing the insulin messages to our genes to turn off the diabetogenic process. We begin to see positive effects within four to seven days. This is one of the reasons we are able to get people off all their medications, including insulin, in such a short time. When there is a great deal of genetic upgrading needed, as with Syndrome X, it may take even a year or so, but considering that most people still believe diabetes is not reversible, even this is not very long.

This diet, besides its other qualities, is also high in enzymes, high in electron energy, and high in biophoton energy. These areas are all discussed in depth in my book *Spiritual Nutrition*. Organic, unrefined, plant-source-only, live food provides the highest-quality nutrient concentrates, phytonutrients, vitamins, minerals, and bioelectrical energy, which are quite important for healing and building the vital life force. It is not only activating and energizing for the total system but also repairing it on every level. When we cut through the metabolic complexities of diabetes and we simply see it as an accelerated form of aging, which it is, then we can apply an approach that gets to the core of reversing the diabetic process—turning on the antiaging genes and the antidiabetic genes through the Dr. Cousens's Diabetes Recovery Program—A Holistic Approach cuisine.

This is the essence and the breakthrough of our program. Is this a new idea? It most certainly isn't. Genesis 1:29 says very specifically, "Behold, I have given you every plant yielding seed that is upon the face of all the earth, and every tree with seed in its fruit; you shall have them for food." In other words, we have already been given the optimal maintenance diet for a healthy lifestyle. But that doesn't mean that everyone chooses to follow it. The pandemic of diabetes has given us a chance to reconsider that this Biblical advice is worth following. Choosing to heal oneself from diabetes is a major diet and lifestyle choice. As it says in Deuteronomy, one of the five books of the Torah, you can choose life or death. Which culture do you choose to live in?

Aside from pancreas problems with diabetes, there is usually significant weakness in the adrenals. In my clinical experience, there are almost 10 times more problems with adrenals when people are on a high-sugar diet. Hypothyroidism is also a common tendency. Hypogonadism, with its accompanying low testosterone, in men is not unusual, and there are also herbs to improve that condition. Additional herbal and nutritional support is given for these issues according to the individualized needs of the client. Increasing the testosterone in low-testosterone male Type-2 diabetics has been shown to decrease insulin resistance and improve blood sugar regulation.

Client Results

It is time to present the clinical data from the first 11 people for whom we formally collected data. These data are now supported by the results of the 120 people who have participated in the program. It is my long-term intent to make a study that is significantly larger than this "pilot study" in the future, with tighter controls and a more extensive spectrum of lab values.

It might have made sense to wait until this projected 200-person clinical study was completed, but because the results have been so dramatic, and because the lives of millions are so dear to me, and because the preservation of life possible through this approach is so important, I wanted to get this information out as soon as possible.

I would like to do this clinical trial of at least 200 people, and I hope to receive funding to do so. I feel the results you are about to see merit such attention, and I am actively working to receive the proper funding.

Explanation of the Data

Fasting Blood Sugar (FBS)

This blood glucose level is taken with a monitor each morning before food is eaten, as well as three other times during the day. A range of 70 to 85 is the optimal FBS. Borderline impaired fasting glucose tolerance is 86 to 99, an FBS of 100 and higher is considered prediabetes, and two FBSs above 126 is diagnosed as diabetes. Below is a summary of the FBS results that we achieved for our 11 participants, all off their oral hypoglycemics or insulin. The initial FBS results were achieved with all on oral hypoglycemics and insulin. Everyone was off these medications within four days of beginning the program.

Client	Initial FBS	Ending FBS	FBS Point Drop	% Change
Client 1	293	88	205	70%
Client 2	287	74	213	74%
Client 3	400	85	315	79%
Client 4	400	109	291	73%
Client 5	248	83	165	67%
Client 6	130	82	48	37%
Client 7	111	87	24	22%
Client 8	300	70	230	77%
Client 9	144	82	62	43%
Client 10	120	65	55	46%
Client 11	279	126	153	55%
Averages	247	86	161	65%

Glycosylated Protein (HgbA1c)

The HgbA1c test measures the percentage of hemoglobin that is non-enzymatically linked to glucose, also known as *glycosylated hemoglobin*. The life-span of red blood cells is about four months, so the HgbA1c test gives a three- to four-month view on blood glucose control. But contrary to this traditional teaching, I often see significant HgbA1c drops in three to four weeks. People with diabetes have high blood sugar levels; high blood sugar levels result in more glucose being unnaturally glycosylated to the hemoglobin. An HgbA1c test result above 5.7 is considered diabetic.

Research shows, as we saw with the Pima Indians data on retinopathy, that HgbA1c levels of 6.0 or less is where complications are minimized and eliminated most significantly. It is estimated that for every 1 percent drop in HgbA1c levels, the reduced risk of long-term diabetic complications is as much as 37 percent.

Fructosamine

While the HgbA1c test measures blood glucose over the last three or four months, the fructosamine test gives an indication of glucose control over the past month. Fructosamine is a term referring to the linking of blood sugar onto protein molecules in the bloodstream. This is a useful test to use when changing protocols in a specific person because changes in diabetic control can be detected earlier than with the HgbA1c test.

LDL/HDL Cholesterol

In our results, you will notice that the low-density lipoproteins (LDL) went close to normal range, with an average drop of 67 points, or 44 percent, to an average LDL of 82 over a period of 21–30 days. LDL is known as "bad" cholesterol because a high reading is believed to be associated with increased risk of heart disease. Many authorities are now encouraging LDL levels at less than 80 for those with diabetes because the number one cause of death among diabetics is heart disease. Although an LDL of less than 80 is relatively safe, in general, risk of heart problems drops as LDL decreases, until it reaches a level of approximately 40 mg/dl.[15] HDL (high-density lipoprotein) is called "good" cholesterol because it carries cholesterol out of the body. Optimum target levels for HDL are above 45 mg/dl for men and 55 mg/dl for women. HDL can also be interpreted in relation to total cholesterol. A favorable HDL would be at least one-third of total cholesterol, so if 150 is our goal, then a healthy HDL would be 50 and over. As I point out in Chapter 5, the association of high cholesterol levels with heart disease, according to the latest massive quantity and variety of epidemiological studies, is seriously questionable except for those with the familial hypercholesterolemia genes. A higher cholesterol for older women has actually been found to be associated with greater longevity and less cardiac morbidity.

Triglycerides

These are fat particles traveling in the bloodstream. Normal concentration is less than 150 mg/dl. A high triglyceride level has a questionable causal association with cardiac mortality but seems to be associated with increased high low-density lipoprotein levels of dense, small, easily oxidized particles, which are associated with increased atherosclerotic cardiovascular disease (ASCVD). Clients' triglyceride levels dropped to what is considered a safe zone of 69 in contrast to the 10-percent-fat vegan research of Esselstyne, which was a high of 144. My clients routinely see their triglycerides going to normal after one month on moderate-low carbohydrate live foods.

C-Reactive Protein (CRP)

CRP is a proinflammatory cytokine that is a cardiovascular disease risk factor. The CRP reading indicates the degree of inflammation; it is determined by measuring the amount of a specific protein in the blood. Recent research suggests that patients with elevated levels of CRP are at increased risk for diabetes,[16] hypertension, and cardiovascular disease.

A study of more than 700 nurses showed that those in the highest quartile of trans-fat consumption had blood levels of CRP that were 73 percent higher than those in the lowest quartile.[17]

As the reader now knows, inflammation is the fourth stage of disease, so one can use this test to first determine how far along someone is in the disease process and, even more important, to mark one's progression back through the seven stages to a healthy physiology. Inflammation contributes to complications that are further along than the fourth stage of disease, such as ulceration (Stage 5), so seeing this marker come down is a significant sign of improvement in health. I measured an average CRP decrease of 70 percent, after one month on the program.

Weight

The results summarized in the success stories that follow are occurring in people who are dramatically overweight. I am not operating a weight-loss clinic, but my observation is that 82 percent of people will come into a normal weight within two years of adopting the Dr. Cousens's Diabetes Recovery Program—A Holistic Approach cuisine and lifestyle. In all cases people felt stronger and healthier. At the end of the movie made at Tree of Life titled *Simply Raw*, the five people felt so much better by all their indicators that they were able to climb Red Mountain, a 1,000-foot plus climb over difficult terrain. For many diabetics, even those in a postdiabetes physiology, weight loss may need to continue to further reduce the risk of the complications of overweight, including increased insulin resistance and the temptation to return to a diabetogenic lifestyle. The average weight loss after one month was 22.9 pounds for those who were overweight at the beginning of the program. The average for the 120 people was 18 pounds in 3 weeks, with one person losing 46 pounds and others routinely hitting 25–30 pounds.

Eleven Success Stories

Client 1

This 59-year-old male had a health history of Type-2 diabetes for 10 years and an FBS near 300 before starting the program. Additional chronic conditions included heart disease with pacemaker, hypertension, obesity, and stroke.

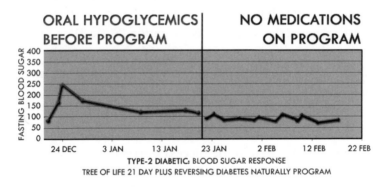

FIGURE 1. FBS for client 1

This client came to the Tree of Life with a history of blood sugar levels near 500, and at the start of the program, his blood sugar before lunch on January 14 was 330. Within a few days of officially beginning the program, on January 22, his FBS had already dropped to 123, and by January 27, just five days later, he reached an FBS of 88, close to a normal, nondiabetic FBS. When he began the program, his weight was 288; one month later he was down to 256. His fructosamine levels dropped into normal range, from 313 at the start to 262 after one month. CRP went from 8.8 to 3.8. Total cholesterol dropped from 147 to 107, and triglyceride levels held steady at 113.

Client 2

This 25-year-old male had a medical history of hospital-diagnosed Type-1 diabetes for more than 1.5 years. His medications included Lantis (15–20 units daily) and Glucophage (500 mg twice a day).

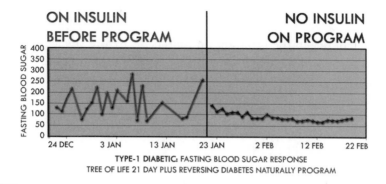

FIGURE 2. FBS for client 2

After just four days on the program, client 2 was off his insulin completely, with an FBS of 88. By two weeks, his FBS was consistently below 73 and remained there since. His fructosamine dropped from 480 to 340, within normal range, in three weeks. His glycosylated hemoglobin HgbA1c has returned to 6.0 from 11.8. Total cholesterol went from 216 to 150 and LDL cholesterol from 142 to 88. His triglyceride level fell from 65 to 53. Weight loss was not a serious need for this client, who was close to his optimal weight; he lost six pounds in 20 days and then gained back three pounds. To resolve the question of whether this patient was really Type-1, the patient (on his own) went to his local MD for further tests to determine whether he was Type-1 or Type-2. His beta cell antibody titers were significantly high at 8.9 (normal is 0–1.5), strongly suggesting that he is indeed a Type-1 diabetic. His clinical history, which was one of rapid and fulminating onset of diabetes, causing him to be hospitalized with a blood sugar of 1,200, is consistent with a medical history of Type-1 diabetes, as contrasted with Type-2, which is characterized by a slow onset of symptoms. It is interesting, and perhaps historic in the field of diabetes research, to note that in a one-year follow-up, his serum C-peptide, which is associated with a precursor protein to insulin, was originally less than 0.5 and is now 0.7. This suggests that the program is actually beginning to rebuild or reactivate the beta cells of his pancreas to produce insulin.

Client 3

This client began the program on March 27. Before she arrived, her blood sugar had hit levels as high as 465 just three weeks before the program.

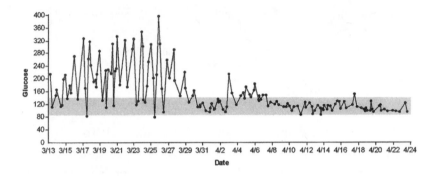

FIGURE 3. FBS for client 3

By her twenty-first day on the program, her FBS had reached 85, and weight loss was 25 pounds.

Client 4

This diabetic was 39 years old with Type-2 for five years and a medical history of hypertension and obesity—in my estimation, a classic example of Syndrome X. At the start of the program, her FBS was 400 and her weight was 352 pounds. After one month, her FBS dropped as low as 109 and her weight dropped to 329 pounds—a 23 pound loss. Her CRP dropped from 37.8 to 8.6. Her total cholesterol dropped from 237 to 171, and triglycerides dropped from 225 to 123 in one month.

Client 5

This client was a 55-year-old Type-2 diabetic for 10 years and had manifested a Syndrome X pattern. He started with an FBS of 248, and within 18 days on the program his FBS reached 83, off all medications.

Client 6

This Type-2 diabetic started with an FBS of 130 on oral diabetic medications. In one week while off all medications, her FBS dropped to 82. She also lost 13 pounds in three weeks. Her total cholesterol dropped from 217 to 140, and LDL went from 148 to 46.

Client 7

A 61-year-old female Type-2 diabetic for 10 years, this client had an average FBS of 111. By the end of the program her thinking, which had been noticeably slower, became clearer and more connected to the environment. By the end of the program her FBS was 87 and has remained in the 80s for more than a year, shown at our one-year follow-up, with an HgbA1c level of 5.5.

Client 8

Type-2 diabetes was diagnosed for this 55-year-old 35 years prior, two months after her last baby was born. She came to us with an average FBS of 300 and was using four doses of oral hypoglycemic medications each day. On day one, she eliminated her use of oral hypoglycemics and achieved an FBS of 105. Days two through four, her FBS was 50 and then rose to 77, 84, and 70 for days five, six, and seven, respectively. This is not an atypical pattern, as seen in my last 120 clients. Several weeks after her green juice fast, she continued to remain with an FBS of around 70, with one spike up to 170 when she got into sweets. This spike helped convince her not to succumb to the idea of "moderation" of the Culture of Death.

Client 9

This client had Type-2 diabetes for 10 years, with a history on Metformin and Gluco-Rite for the past three years. On day one, she stopped the use of medications. Her FBS was 144 on day one, 129 on day two, and by day seven was 102. On day eight, she achieved a nondiabetic FBS of 82.

Client 10

This Type-2 diabetic started the fasting program with an average FBS of 110–120. By day two, the FBS was 98, and by day seven, 65.

Client 11

This is an interesting Type-2 case because it shows that healing does not necessarily occur completely in three to four weeks. During her one-month program, she lost 26 pounds, went from using 35 units of insulin a day to 0 units, discontinued the use of the pharmaceuticals Lantis, Byetta, Neurontin, and Monopril within four days, saw a decrease in her CRP levels from 8.4 to 2.6, lowered her total cholesterol from 210 to 136 (with LDL dropping from 142 to 85 and HDL rising from 25 to 29), and lowered her FBS from 279 to 126, for a 55 percent drop without any medications. This particular client was well on her way to a healthy reversal when she returned home. Of the 86 percent of the insulin-dependent Type-2 diabetics who got off insulin in three weeks, there were 72 percent who did not get an FBS less than 100 in three weeks—many of those who stayed tightly on the program for the full year did go below an FBS of 100.

Foods, Juices, Herbs, Vitamins, and Minerals— An Eloquent Healing Message

The results summarized previously were achieved by a very conscious choice of foods, juices, herbs, vitamins, amino acids, minerals, and enzymes. The incredible transformation from a diabetic physiology to a nondiabetic physiology has as much to do with what we did include as what we removed from the diet and lifestyle. You are now aware that we have eliminated processed sugar, white flour, cooked vegetables (and all but leafy green, high-fiber vegetables and sprouts), all processed and junk foods, excitotoxins such as artificial flavorings and colorings, animal fats and protein, trans fats, cooked fats, smoking, and television. Before we discuss the nutritional and lifestyle elements that we do include in the program, it is important to mention that there are some plant-source foods that are typically eaten, and even recommended by medical professionals, as part of diabetes-amelioration programs that we do not use.

Wheat

Wheat, according to Ayurvedic principles, is kaphagenic (heavy and sweet) and therefore not recommended for diabetics. We do not include wheat, specifically white bread, also due to its alloxan content. Alloxan is the chemical that makes white flour look clean, white, and "beautiful." A remarkable discovery that a single injection of alloxan can produce diabetes mellitus in laboratory animals was made in 1942, in Glasgow, by John Shaw Dunn and Norman McLetchie.[18] Scientists and FDA officials have known about this connection for years. Alloxan causes diabetes by creating free radical damage to the DNA in the beta cells of the pancreas. The *Textbook of Natural Medicine* calls alloxan a "potent beta cell toxin." It is unfortunate that the FDA still allows companies to use it to process foods we eat. Research also shows that we are able to reverse the effects of alloxan with vitamin E. According to Dr. Gary Null's *Clinicians' Handbook of Natural Healing*, vitamin E effectively protected lab rats from the harmful effects of administered alloxan.

In support of that, researchers have found that among rats that are genetically susceptible to insulin-dependent diabetes mellitus (IDDM), feeding wheat gluten will cause 40 percent of the subjects to develop IDDM. Several other groups of rats with the same genetic inclination to develop IDDM were fed gluten-free diets, and only 10–15 percent developed IDDM. Further, the rate and severity of diabetes could be manipulated by varying the amount of gluten in the diet. Others have shown that delaying introduction of dietary gluten in animals delays or prevents diabetes. Most authorities in this specific area of diabetes research conclude that gluten is a major factor in causing the development of IDDM in genetically predisposed animals.[19]

Soy

Soy is also a diabetogenic and kaphagenic food. It is a low-mineral food that robs the body of minerals. About 92–96 percent of all soy is genetically modified (GMO). Soy is also one of the top seven allergens and is widely known to cause immediate hypersensitivity reactions. While in the last 40 years soy has occupied an important place in the transition from an unhealthy meat-based diet to vegetarian and vegan cuisine, it is time for us to upgrade our food choice to one having more benefits and fewer negative possibilities. In 1986, Stuart Berger, MD, placed soy among the seven top allergens—one of the "sinister seven."[20] At the time, most experts listed soy around tenth or eleventh: bad enough, but way behind peanuts, tree nuts, milk, eggs, shellfish, fin fish, and wheat.[21] Scientists are not completely certain which components of soy cause allergic reactions. They have found at least 16 allergenic proteins, and some researchers pinpoint as many as 30.[22] Kaayla T. Daniel writes in *The Whole Soy Story*:

> Allergic reactions occur not only when soy is eaten but when soybean flour or dust is inhaled. Among epidemiologists, soybean dust is known as an "epidemic asthma agent." From 1981 [to] 1987, soy dust from grain silo unloading in the harbor caused 26 epidemics of asthma in Barcelona, seriously affecting 687 people and leading to 1,155 hospitalizations. No further epidemics occurred after filters were installed, but a minor outbreak in 1994 established the need for monitoring of preventive measures. Reports of the epidemic in Barcelona led epidemiologists in New Orleans to investigate cases of epidemic asthma that occurred from 1957 [to] 1968, when more than 200 people sought treatment at a Charity Hospital. Investigations of weather patterns and cargo data from the New Orleans harbor identified soy dust from ships carrying soybeans as the probable cause. No association was found between asthma-epidemic days and the presence of wheat or corn in ships in the harbor. The researchers concluded: "The results of this analysis provide further evidence that ambient soy dust is very asthmogenic and that asthma morbidity in a community can be influenced by exposures in the ambient atmosphere."

Soy contains built-in insecticides called isoflavones (genistein and daidzein). Isoflavones are estrogen-like substances that have the same effect in the body as estrogen, and eating soy can make a person estrogenic, contributing to problems such as cancer, irritability and mood swings, fat gain from the waist down, fibrocystic breast disease, and uterine fibroids.[23, 24, 25] Isoflavones decrease thyroid hormone production. This can stunt children's growth. Hypothyroid is associated with raised serum cholesterol and tends to create fatigue and obesity.[26, 27, 28] This further encourages and enhances a diabetogenic reality. Isoflavones decrease the good cholesterol (HDL), thus contributing to heart disease, the number one killer of diabetics.[29, 30]

Soy may also be connected with Alzheimer's disease, which is also a complication of hyperglycemia and diabetes. In a major ongoing study involving 3,734 elderly Japanese American men, those who ate the most tofu during midlife had up to 2.4 times the risk of later developing Alzheimer's disease. As part of the three-decade-long Honolulu-Asia Aging Study, 27 foods and drinks were correlated with participants' health. In addition, men who consumed tofu at least twice weekly had more cognitive impairment than those who rarely or never ate the soybean curd.[31, 32] Going further, higher midlife tofu consumption was also associated with low brain weight, suggesting that soy consumption is associated with brain cell destruction and loss. Brain atrophy was assessed in 574 men using MRI results and in 290 men using autopsy information. Shrinkage occurs naturally with age, but for the men who had consumed more tofu, lead researcher Dr. Lon R. White from the Hawaii Center for Health Research said, "Their brains seemed to be showing an exaggeration of the usual patterns we see in aging."

In men, eating soy isoflavones can significantly reduce testicular function and lower luteinizing hormone (LH) production, which is what signals the testicles to work. A high soy intake and potentially lower level of LH increases the probability of estrogen dominance in men, contributing to hair loss, swollen and cancerous prostates,[33, 34] and insulin resistance. Dorris Rapp, MD, a leading pediatric allergist, asserts that environmental and food estrogens are responsible for the worldwide reduction in male fertility.[35] Soy intake has been associated with a 50 percent decrease in sperm fertility.

For women, female children fed the estrogens in soy formula and products hit puberty early, sometimes as young as ages six to eight.[36] Eating soy products during pregnancy may affect the sexual differentiation of the fetus toward feminization; studies even show malformations of the reproductive tract or offspring born with both male and female sexual organs.[37] Kaayla T. Daniel writes:

> Ingrid Malmheden Yman, PhD, of the Swedish National Food Administration, wrote to the Ministry of Health in New Zealand informing the agency that children with severe allergy to peanut should avoid intake of soy protein. To be on the safe side she further advised parents to make an effort to "avoid sensitization" by limiting both peanuts and soybeans during the third trimester of pregnancy, during breast feeding, and by avoiding the use of soy formula. Controversy has raged since the 1920s as to whether or not babies could be sensitized to allergens while still in utero. In 1976, researchers learned that the fetus is capable of producing IgE antibodies against soy protein during early gestation and newborns can be sensitized through the breast milk of the mother and later react to foods they've "never eaten." As Dr. Stefano Guandalini, Department of Pediatrics, University of Chicago, writes, "A significant number of children with cow's milk protein intolerance develop soy protein intolerance when soy milk is used in dietary management." Interestingly enough, researchers recently detected and identified a soy protein component that cross reacts with caseins from cow's milk. Cross reactions occur when foods are chemically related to each other.

Matthias Besler of Hamburg, Germany, and an international team of allergy specialists report on their website (www.allergens.de) that adverse reactions caused by soybean formulas occur in at least 14 to 35 percent of infants allergic to cow's milk. On another valuable allergy website (www.medicine.com), Dr. Guandalini reports the results of an unpublished study of 2,108 infants and toddlers in Italy, of which 53 percent of the babies under three-months old who had reacted poorly to dairy formula also reacted to soy formula.[38]

"The amount of phytoestrogens that are in a day's worth of soy infant formula equals 5 birth control pills," says Mike Fitzpatrick, a New Zealand toxicologist.[39] A study reported in *The Lancet*[40] found that the "daily exposure of infants to isoflavones in soy infant-formulas is 6–11-fold higher on a bodyweight basis than the dose that has hormonal effects in adults consuming soy foods." This dose, equivalent to two glasses of soy milk per day, was enough to change menstrual patterns in women.[41] In the blood of infants tested, who were on soy milk as a substitute for mother's milk, concentrations of isoflavones were 13,000 to 22,000 times higher than natural estrogen concentrations in early life.

Soy is a mineral-deficient food and, adding insult to injury, contains phytin, which chelates essential minerals such as iron, zinc, and magnesium out of the body before they can be absorbed.

In 2003, a study[42] was done comparing the bodily IGF-1 increase promoted by 40 grams of soy (the amount in one soy candy bar and a soy shake, or four soy patties) versus 40 grams of milk protein. Soy was found to be almost twice as powerful as milk protein in increasing IGF-1 levels (36 percent for milk versus 69 percent for soy). This new IGF-1 data potentially places soy in the category of a powerful cancer promoter of the breast, prostate, lung, and colon.[43] The implications are, first, that this further scientifically establishes soy as a very kaphagenic food, as IGF-1 is the end product of growth hormone stimulation. Although it is controversial, there are many in the medical world who feel that excessive IGF-1 could stimulate the aforementioned cancers if they are already present. This is why Canada does not allow rBGH milk from the United States: because it is so much higher in IGF-1. In essence, this is still at the level of theoretical speculation, but we feel it merits a preventive attention. Common sense, given the scientific data, is that one should have, at best, a minimum of soy in the diet if including any cooked food as part of an 80 percent live-, 20 percent cooked-food diet. The following chart shows how pervasive soy is in our so-called health foods. The 40 gram level of IGF-1-creating soy protein from the study, as you will see in the chart, is easy to achieve.

Eating Processed Soy Easily Adds 40 Grams of Harmful Protein Concentrate to Your Diet

Item	Serving	Grams of Protein
Desserts and Snacks		
Cliff® Builder's Bar	1 bar	20
Cliff® Bar (Oatmeal, Raisin Walnut)	1 bar	10
Revival Soy Bars®	1 bar	17
Atkins Nutrition Bars®	1 bar	21
ZonePerfect Nutrition Bars®	1 bar	15
Revival Soy Shakes® Splenda®	1 shake	20
Meats		
Morningstar Farms® Sausage Patties	1 patty	10
Boca© Breakfast Links	1 link	8
Gardenburger® Chik'n Grill	1 patty	13
Boca Burger® Original	1 burger	13
Boca® Ground Burger	2 ounces	13
Boca® Chicken Patties	1 patty	11
Smart Dogs®	1 dog	9
Boca® Chili	1 serving	20
Cheeses		
Veggie Shreds® (Cheese)	2 ounces	6
Boca® Pizza	1 slice	13
Tofu with Added Isolates		
Lite Tofu®	3 ounces	5
Flour		
Benesoy® High Protein Soy Flour	1 ounce	15

John McDougall, *The McDougall Newsletter,* April 2005, 4(4), www.drmcdougall.com.

Eliminating soy from your diet can be tough if you are just eating processed vegetarian or vegan food. Many prepackaged and prepared foods contain soy as an ingredient, but it may be listed as "textured vegetable protein" (TVP), "textured plant protein," "hydrolyzed vegetable protein" (HVP), "vegetable oil," or "MSG" (monosodium glutamate). You may also find "lecithin," "vegetable broth," "bouillon," "natural flavor," or "mono-diglyceride" ingredients that are often soy products. I suggest eating a live, plant-sourced diet that is not processed or cooked and avoiding restaurants that serve foods with soy products in them. The recipe section of this book will provide you with ample foods that are nutrient-dense, nonallergenic, delicious, and filling and will have you wondering why you ever ate processed, soy-containing meals.

Excitotoxins

Excitotoxins represent another health disaster associated with the better-living-through-chemistry paradigm of the Culture of Death. In an attempt to avoid dealing with the problems associated with the craving for the sweet taste of sugar, and instead of facing our sweet-taste issues (which are more of an acquired taste at the level of excess that is practiced in the world today), we have invented artificial sweeteners and excitotoxins. The negative health consequence of this has become more and more significant. Russell Blaylock, author of *Excitotoxins: The Taste That Kills*, writes: "There are a growing number of clinicians and basic scientists who are convinced that a group of compounds called excitotoxins play a critical role in the development of several neurological disorders including migraines, seizures, infections, abnormal neural development, certain endocrine disorders, neuropsychiatric disorders, learning disorders in children, AIDS, dementia, episodic violence, lyme borreliosis, hepatic encephalopathy, specific types of obesity, and especially the neurodegenerative diseases, such as ALS, Parkinson's disease, Alzheimer's disease, Huntington's disease, and olivopontocerebellar degeneration."[44, 45]

An enormous amount of both clinical and experimental evidence has accumulated over the past decade supporting this basic premise.[46] These excitotoxins are food additives such as MSG, hydrolyzed vegetable protein, and aspartame. This excitotoxins increase our cravings for the junk foods they are added to and thus make people more vulnerable to the problems associated with junk foods and diabetogenic foods because the excitotoxins stimulate the appetite rather than activating the satiety response. In this context, excitotoxins are great for building the wealth of the food companies and excellent for destroying the health of the population. For example, since 1948 the amount of MSG added to foods has doubled every decade. By 1972, 262,000 metric tons were being added to foods each year. More than 800 million pounds of aspartame have been consumed in various products since it was first approved. Ironically, these food additives have nothing to do with preserving food or protecting its integrity. They are used to alter or "enhance" the taste of food.

Monosodium Glutamate (MSG)

When one cooks soy, evidence suggests that MSG is a naturally created by-product. Many people in the live-food movement thought that the creators of Bragg's Liquid Aminos were adding MSG to the product, because people were having MSG reactions to it. They were not adding MSG. Patricia Bragg, a famous advocate for healthy living, would never do that. Instead, what was happening was that people were reacting to the normal MSG created by the heating of the soy.

Ingesting MSG creates an excess of glutamate, which the body has trouble converting. MSG causes a very large insulin response after it is ingested because there are glutamate receptors in the pancreas that are activated by the glutamate increased by the MSG and then cause a release of insulin. MSG also opens calcium channels, thus constricting blood vessels—this may put diabetics with high blood pressure at risk by negating calcium channel blocker medication.

Conventional wisdom has been that MSG does not result in a corresponding increase in blood levels of free glutamic acid, but according to research done in Canada, MSG does result in higher plasma concentrations of free glutamic acid and aspartate and higher insulin levels. In addition, plasma insulin concentration almost triples in response to MSG ingestion. This increase in plasma insulin can exacerbate hypoglycemia.[47] This is especially important in diabetics since prolonged elevation of the blood sugar produces a down-regulation of the glucose transporter and a concomitant "brain hypoglycemia" that is exacerbated by repeated spells of peripheral hypoglycemia common to Type-1 diabetics. A high insulin also contributes to increasing insulin resistance.

MSG has also been associated with damage to the hypothalamus and concomitant, resulting obesity. In 1968, John W. Olney, MD, a respected researcher at Washington University Medical School, St. Louis, Missouri, and member of the National Academy of Science, found that mice in his laboratory that had been administered MSG had resulting retinal damage and become grotesquely obese. Since 1969, many scientists have confirmed Dr. Olney's findings of damage to the hypothalamus from MSG with resulting obesity. There is abundant literature demonstrating that MSG and aspartic acid cause hypothalamic lesions, which, in turn, can cause gross obesity. Although there are a number of causes for obesity, there is no question that one of the contributing causes for the obesity epidemic is the ever increasing use of MSG and aspartame. The damage to the hypothalamus is even worse in the womb and the first two years of life, when the young child is developing. The use of MSG during this critical developmental time may create severe endocrine problems later in life including decreased thyroid function, increased tendency toward diabetes, and higher cortisone levels than normal. A child consuming a soup containing MSG plus a drink with NutraSweet will have a blood level of excitotoxins six times the blood level that destroys hypothalamus neurons in baby mice.

Aspartame

Aspartame, commonly thought to be a benefit to diabetics as a sweetener because it is low glycemic and low caloric, has actually been linked to the activation of diabetes. According to research conducted by Dr. H. J. Roberts, a diabetes specialist, a member of the American Diabetes Association, and an authority on artificial sweeteners, aspartame leads to the creation of clinical diabetes, causes poorer diabetic control in diabetics on insulin or oral drugs, causes convulsions, and leads to the aggravation of diabetic complications such as retinopathy, cataracts, neuropathy, and gastroparesis. Dr. Roberts found that "the loss of diabetic control, the intensification of hypoglycemia, the occurrence of presumed 'insulin reactions' (including convulsions) that proved to be aspartame reactions, and the precipitation, aggravation or simulation of diabetic complications (especially impaired vision and neuropathy) while using these products."[48] Russell Blaylock, MD, author of *Health and Nutrition Secrets*, writes, "Diabetics who drink large amounts of aspartame-sweetened drinks are more likely to go blind. Aspartame is composed of the excitotoxin aspartic acid; phenylalanine; and methanol, a known eye toxin."

General Antidiabetogenic Diet

The following charts show low-glycemic, low-insulin-score Rainbow Green food for Phases 1.0 and 1.5 of the Tree of Life cuisine program, as previously described.

Rainbow Green Cuisine, Phase 1.0 (The Therapeutic Antidiabetes, Anticandida, Anti-CDDS, Cancer-Prevention, and Antiaging Diet)

All vegetables except cooked carrots and cooked beets

All sea vegetables

Nonsweet fruits: tomatoes, avocados, cucumber, red pepper, lemons, limes

Fats and oils: flax oil, hemp oil, sesame oil, walnut, almond, sunflower, olive oil (only with fresh vegetables and salads), avocado, and coconut oil/butter

Nuts and seeds

Superfoods: Klamath Lake blue-green algaes (E-3Live is the most active), spirulina, chlorella, green superfood powder mixes

Sweeteners: stevia, cardamom, cinnamon, xylitol (from birch bark)

Salt: Transformational Salts, Himalayan salt, and other raw harvested salts

Fermented and cultured foods: apple cider vinegar, miso (nonsoy), sauerkraut, probiotic drinks

Rainbow Green Cuisine, Phase 1.5 (Additions to Phase 1.0)

All vegetables: carrots (raw), beets (raw), squash (raw)

Fruits: low-glycemic fruits—blueberries, raspberries, cherries, fresh and unsweetened cranberries, pomegranate, goji berries, grapefruits, lemons, limes

Condiments and sweeteners: mesquite, carob

Bee pollen granules

Grains: quinoa, buckwheat, millet, amaranth, spelt, brown rice

Notes:

Phase 1: no grains, no sweets

Phase 1.5: grains stored less than 90 days, low-sweet fruits, and fermented food

Phase 1.5: a small amount of Phase 2 fruits and veggies in a large salad

Diabetic Transition Chart
(Transitioning to a Low-Glycemic, Low Insulin Index Culture of Life Cuisine)

Old-World Flesh-Centered Cuisine	New-World Plant-Source-Only Cuisine
Meat	**High-Protein Plant Foods**
Beef, pork, lamb, chicken, turkey, tuna, and all fish	Nuts and seeds; nut and seed pâtés and cheezes; high-protein superfoods—spirulina, blue-green algae, green superfood mixes, hemp protein, maca; beans
Eggs	Flax with omega-3 fatty acids
Dairy Products	
Milk and cream	Nut and seed mylks
Butter, margarine, shortening, lard	Coconut oil, cold-pressed oils, cacao butter

Dairy Products (continued)

Cheeses	Nut and seed cheezes; fatty nuts–brazil, pine, macadamia, and pecan
Yogurt	Walnut nogurt; coconut cream (plain or fermented); cultured nut and seed mylks with probiotics
Sour cream	Sunflower and sesame sour cream
Ice cream	Nut-based ice creams; sorbets made in high-speed blender with frozen blueberries, raspberries
Whipped cream	Coconut cream
Milk chocolate bar	Raw chocolate bar made with cacao

Grains

White rice, whole wheat	Amaranth, millet, quinoa, spelt, buck wheat, and brown rice
Cakes and pastries	Live carrot cake
White or whole wheat bread	Flax crackers, nut and seed crackers and breads
Commercial cereals	Buckwheaties; live granola

Roasted/Salted Nuts and Seeds

Peanuts, cashews, almonds, macadamia nuts, and their butters	Raw nuts and seeds and their nut and seed butters–walnuts, flax seed, almonds, brazil nuts, sesame seed, chia seeds, pumpkin seeds, sunflower seeds

Vegetables–Cooked and Processed

Instant foods; frozen, canned, fried, boiled, salted, and baked vegetables	Fresh vegetables, salads, soups, green smoothies, dehydrated foods

Fruit–Canned and Sweetened, Dried and Sulphered, Frozen

	Fresh, low-glycemic fruits; dehydrated fruits

Beverages

Chlorinated, fluoridated tap water	Filtered, blessed, structured, distilled, or reverse-osmosis water
Fruit juices–pasteurized	Fresh juices, preferably low-glycemic green vegetable juice only

Beverages (continued)

Soda	Herbal noncaffeinated teas and fresh vegetable juices
Alcoholic beverages	Herbal noncaffeinated teas and fresh vegetable juices
Coffee	Noncoffee herbal substitutes (transitional)

Sweeteners

White sugar, brown sugar, molasses, corn syrup, dextrose, maple syrup, sucrose, fructose, aspartame, mannitol, saccharin, and sorbitol	Stevia, licorice root, and xylitol

Oils

Hydrogenated vegetable oils	Cold-pressed oils: coconut, flax, hemp, sesame, almond, sunflower, avocado, olive (accompanied by high antioxidant foods or supplements)

Salt

Iodized table salt	Transformational Salts, Himalayan crystal salt, Celtic sea salt

Particular Antidiabetogenic Foods

Cabbage

The protective action against the oxidative stress of red cabbage (*Brassica oleracea*) extract was investigated in diabetes-induced rats for 60 days.[49] Researchers found a significant increase in reduced glutathione and superoxide dismutase activity and a decrease in catalase activity and in the total antioxidant capacity of the kidneys. Daily oral ingestion of *B. oleracea* extract from cabbage for 60 days reversed the adverse effects of diabetes in rats. They found lowered blood glucose levels and restored renal function and body weight loss. In addition, the cabbage extract attenuated the adverse effect of diabetes on malondialdehyde, glutathione, and superoxide dismutase activity as well as catalase activity and total antioxidant capacity of diabetic kidneys. In conclusion, the antioxidant and antihyperglycemic properties of *B. oleracea* in cabbage may offer a potential therapeutic source for the treatment of diabetes.

Huckleberry

The huckleberry juice compounds may also offer significant protection against diabetic retinopathy and cataracts. Such huckleberry compound extracts are being widely used throughout Europe in the prevention of diabetic retinopathy. All this work with huckleberry in ophthalmology actually began back in World War II when some Royal Air Force pilots in Great Britain swore that eating huckleberry jam or drinking huckleberry cordials prior to flying night missions over Germany significantly improved their visual acuity in the darkness. Such reports generated a lot of interest in the medical community in Europe, which led to a number of studies being done with the berry.

Bitter Melon

Bitter melon, also known as *Momordica charantia* or balsam pear, is a tropical fruit known throughout Asia, Africa, and South America. Its green fruit looks like an ugly cucumber. Bitter melon is made of several compounds that have antidiabetic properties, including charantin, which has been shown to be more powerful than the hypoglycemic drug tolbutamide, and an insulin-like polypeptide called *polypeptide-P*, which lowers blood sugar when injected into Type-1 diabetics.[50] In one study, it decreased the glucose tolerance by 73 percent when people were given 2 ounces of the juice.[51] In another study, there was a 17 percent reduction in glycosylated hemoglobin in six people. Still another study found that 15 grams of the aqueous extract of this herb produced a 54 percent decrease in blood sugar after eating and a 17 percent reduction in the glycosylated hemoglobin in six patients.[52]

There are different preparations. The fresh juice is probably the strongest in terms of its effect. A variety of human clinical trials have established blood-sugar-lowering action of the fresh juice or abstract.[53, 54] More than a hundred studies have demonstrated bitter melon's ability to decrease the blood sugar, increase the uptake of glucose, and activate the pancreatic cells that manufacture insulin. The peptide it has acts like bovine insulin. So it has several effects: improved glucose tolerance without increasing insulin levels, stimulating the beta cells of the pancreas, suppressing the urge to eat sweets, and action similar to that of insulin.

Unripe bitter melon is available at Asian markets, and the fresh juice is probably the best, per the traditional use in the studies. Bitter melon is difficult to make palatable, as its name implies. The best way to use this effective plant is to juice 2 ounces and hold your nose as you drink it with celery-cucumber juice and some lemon.

Cucumber

Cucumber contains a hormone needed by the beta cells of the pancreas to produce insulin. The enzyme erepsin in cucumbers is targeted toward breaking down excessive protein in the kidneys. In our program, we use a lot of cucumber juice, for drinking as well as in salads.

Celery

Celery also has some general antidiabetogenic effects, as well as being helpful for people with high blood pressure such as we see with Syndrome X. Celery juice has a calming effect on the nervous system, due to its high concentration of organic alkaline minerals, especially sodium. The minerals contained in celery juice make the body's use of calcium more effective, balancing the blood's pH. Celery should be the center of your green vegetable juices and can be included in green soups and smoothies to alkalinize a system taxed by acidifying Culture of Death foods and lifestyle choices.

Nopal Cactus

Nopal is prickly pear cactus, widely used as a traditional food throughout Latin America. Researchers[55] gave eight fasting diabetics 500 grams of nopal. Five tests were performed on each subject, four with different cooked or raw preparations and one with water. After 180 minutes, fasting glucose was lowered 22–25 percent by nopal preparations, as compared to 6 percent by water. In a rabbit study, nopal improved tolerance of injected glucose by 33 percent (180-minute value for comparison) as compared to water.[56] Nopal researchers concur that although cooked and raw cactus are effective, preparations from commercially dehydrated nopal are not.

Garlic and Onion

Garlic and onions contain sulfur compounds that are believed to be responsible for their antidiabetic qualities. S-allyl cysteine sulphoxide in garlic is one of these. It has been reported to decrease fasting blood glucose and lower cholesterol levels in diabetic rats,[57] and in one human study, onion extract was shown to reduce hyperglycemia in a dose dependent manner.[58]

Grains and Beans

The following grains and beans are high-fiber complex carbohydrates that have been found to be useful for the prevention and part of a maintenance diet once diabetes is healed. They are part of the indigenous diets, especially of the Native Americans, that made diabetes a rarity before these cultures began to accept the Western diet in the 1940s (when their rate of diabetes began to soar):

- Millet
- Brown rice
- Oats
- Buckwheat
- Amaranth
- Mung beans
- Garbanzo beans
- Pinto beans
- White tepary beans
- Green beans
- String beans
- Papago beans

Nuts and Seeds

Recent research suggests that regular nut consumption is an important part of a healthy diet,[59] despite the fact that in the past, nuts were considered unhealthy because of their relatively high fat content at 14–19 grams/ounce. Most of the fats in nuts are the healthier monounsaturated and polyunsaturated fats.[60] Monounsaturated fats, such as those in olive oil, almonds, and avocados, improve insulin sensitivity.[61] A Harvard study in 2002 on the benefits of nuts concluded that high dietary nut consumption decreased the risk of sudden cardiac death, a leading cause of death among diabetics. Nuts and seeds are also high in plant sterols (phytosterols), which decrease cholesterol and improve heart health.[62, 63] In the intestinal lumen, phytosterols displace cholesterol and inhibit cholesterol absorption.[64]

Nuts and seeds are great for plain eating and for making pâtés, soups, salad dressings, and nut mylks. When you see the nut mylk recipes in Chapter 7, you will wonder what you were ever doing with cow, soy, and rice milk. The antidiabetogenic and nutritional benefits of nuts and seeds are worth knowing.

In a study presented to the American College of Cardiology March 14, 2000, Richard Vogel, MD, head of cardiology at the University of Maryland in Baltimore, suggested that olive oil may be nearly as dangerous as saturated trans fats in clogging arteries. He found that olive oil impaired vascular function to the same extent as a Big Mac, fries, or Sara Lee cheesecake—an arterial constriction of 34 percent. These vascular constrictions are significant because they injure the endothelium of the blood vessel and may contribute to heart disease because they predispose one to atherosclerotic cardiovascular disease. He also found that oils with high omega-3s, which olive oil does not have, did not impair blood vessel function. Dr. Vogel pointed out that it is not a question of whether it is monounsaturated or polyunsaturated but a question of the omega-3 levels. Olive oil is very high in omega-9. This raises a more serious question, which Dr. Vogel has answered: it was not the olive oil that was key in the Lyon Diet Heart Study of the Mediterranean cuisine, but rather, it may have been the fruits, vegetables, nuts, bread, and fish that were key, in conjunction with less meat in the diet. Actually, Vogel points out, the Lyon Diet did not use olive oil.

The research suggests that olive oil is not heart-healthy, although olive oil is clearly healthier than foods saturated with trans fats. However, being better than those foods is not saying much. When researchers at the University of Crete compared residents who had heart disease with those free of the disease, those with heart disease ate significantly higher quantities of olive oil and all fats in their diet. In essence, what Dr. Vogel has pointed out is that the protective elements in the Mediterranean diet are the antioxidants found in the plant sources of the cuisine. He felt that there was some protection against the direct impairment of endothelial function produced by high trans-fat foods, which also includes olive oil. In another study exploring the same issue, reported in the *American Journal of Cardiology*, they also found that the constriction was worse in 12 healthy and 12 high-cholesterol subjects after consuming olive oil.

Extra virgin olive oil does contain polyphenols that give some antioxidant protection. However, most plant foods are rich in polyphenols and provide more polyphenols per calorie than olive oil. For example, an 11-calorie serving of green leafy lettuce gives you the same amount of polyphenols (30 mg) as 120 calories of olive oil. Another group of researchers studied two hundred men using three different olive oils for three weeks; one of the oils was extra virgin, and the other two were not and low in polyphenols. The scientists found that the extra virgin had better heart health effects, including higher HDL cholesterol levels and less oxidative stress. The oxidative stress is what increases inflammation in the arteries, disrupting the endothelial cells and predisposing one to plaque rupture and heart attack.

Olive oil does not lower LDL cholesterol, a potential indicator for heart disease. However, the studies have produced some confusion, as people substitute olive oil for their intake of saturated fats and trans fats and see the LDL going downward. The point is that it may not be the addition of olive oil but the removal of harmful fats from the diet that has decreased harmful LDL cholesterol.

Given the preponderance of evidence from these studies, we cannot say that olive oil is heart healthy. In fact, the people with the longest life expectancy and fewest heart attacks have diets low in olive oil but high in plant foods.

Please keep in mind that there are very few studies on the topic at this moment, so I can only make a suggestive warning rather than a definitive statement about the adverse effect of olive oil on cardiovascular health. One study reported in the March 27 issue of the *Archives of Internal Medicine* showed that eating olive oil can lower high blood pressure. In a group of 23 patients, Italian researchers found that after eating olive oil for six months, blood pressure medications were lowered by 48 percent, and eight participants were able to discontinue their medications altogether. Sunflower oil had no effect on their blood pressure.

In the December 1999 issue of the *American Journal of Clinical Nutrition*, Danish researchers reported that olive oil worked better than canola oil at inhibiting blood clots after a fatty meal.

Even Dr. Vogel, who found the 34 percent endothelial constriction, suggested that when olive oil is combined with the eating of antioxidant-rich fruits and vegetables, the vessel-constricting effect disappears. Therefore, on a live-food diet rich in antioxidants, or with supplements such as vitamin E (400–600 IU), vitamin C (2,000 mg), L-arginine (2,000 mg), garlic, alpha-lipoic acid (300 mg/day), and flavonoids (there being 5,000 different flavonoids—potent antioxidants found in plant foods) all improved endothelial function and blood vessel tone. Therefore, if one is healthy, on a live-food diet high in antioxidants, and uses extra virgin olive oil on one's salad, the vascular constricting endothelial effect of olive oil should be mitigated.

I also would suggest that people with serious ASCVD eliminate olive oil but feel safe with walnuts, almonds, Brazil nuts (and other raw nuts and seeds), and avocados. Likewise, those people diagnosed with diabetes for more than a year have, with nearly 100 percent certainty, a degeneration of the endothelium of the arteries, and are most prudent to avoid or minimize the use of olive oil until the diabetic physiology has been reversed completely for two years. Even though the high-antioxidant, high-omega-3 oils are a good alternative, I do also recommend that one consider creating dressings from whole pulverized nuts and seeds rather than the oils of these high-quality nuts and seeds, which only contain the fat-soluble antioxidants. I recommend that one keep a fat intake of approximately 25–45 percent of total calories in the process of healing diabetes through a live-food diet. Taken in this context, because on a live-foods cuisine you can eat half as much with the same nutritional benefit, this is actually healthier and theoretically superior to having 10–15 percent of calories from fat in a cooked-food diet.

The best oils to use in salad dressings are those high in omega-3 such as walnuts, flax, and hemp, as well as sesame oil, which is very high in antioxidants. We recommend in our recipes that one can try substituting these oils for olive oil.

My clients put on a 100 percent living- and raw-foods diet with 25–45 percent raw plant fat, including raw nuts, seeds, and avocado, saw an average 44 percent drop in LDL with an average drop to an LDL of 82. They saw relief from all diabetic degenerative symptoms, including improved mental function. The improved mental function suggests an increase in blood flow to the brain. These results support the large studies cited about the beneficial use of whole raw nuts and seeds, such as walnuts and almonds.

Walnuts

Walnuts are exceptionally high in monounsaturated fat and the omega-3 fatty acid, alpha-linolenic acid. A study published in November 2004 by Kris-Etherton et al. showed that alpha-linolenic acid reduced cholesterol and fats in the blood and also C-reactive protein (CRP), an inflammatory marker associated with heart disease.[65] Additionally, walnuts combine these heart healthy fats with a hefty dose of the antioxidants, including at least 16 antioxidant phenols, vitamin E, and ellagic and gallic acid. In 1993, the *New England Journal of Medicine*[66] reported that eating six to eight walnuts per day decreased total and LDL cholesterol by 5–10 percent and reduced incidence of stroke and clogging of arteries up to 70 percent.[67] Additional research has confirmed that when walnuts are eaten as part of a healthy raw fat diet, the result is a more cardioprotective fat profile in diabetic patients than can be achieved by simply lowering the fat content of the diet. In a study published in the *Journal of the American Dietetic Association,* all 55 study participants with Type-2 diabetes were put on low-fat diets, but the only group to achieve a cardioprotective fat profile were those who ate walnuts (30 grams—about one ounce—per day).[68] Other studies have found similar results.[69, 70, 71, 72] Dr. Emilio Ros of Barcelona reported in the October 17, 2006, *Journal of the American College of Cardiology* that eating walnuts could reverse the impairment of endothelial function associated with eating a fatty meal, but olive oil did not show any measurable effect. He found that eating a handful of walnuts prevented the increase in inflammation in the arteries and of endothelial dysfunction, while olive oil did prevent the increase in inflammatory molecules but did not prevent the endothelial dysfunction associated with eating fatty foods. In a previous study reported by Dr. Ros, he showed that eating walnuts over four weeks helped repair endothelial dysfunction. Dr. Ros pointed out that walnuts have several components that help in this repair function, including polyunsaturated fats, alpha-linolenic acid, omega-3 fats, arginine, and many antioxidants. He recommends eating at least six to eight walnuts a day.

Almonds

Almonds may also play a role in controlling diabetes. In a study[73] involving 20 free-living individuals, researchers examined the effect of 100 grams (about 3.5 ounces) of almonds a day. Researchers found that LDL and total cholesterol levels decreased while glycemic control did not change. In the crossover arm of this study, total and LDL cholesterol decreased 21 and 23 percent, respectively, and glycemic control was unaffected. This study shows that almonds can be incorporated into a healthful diet without negatively affecting glycemic control while also lowering cholesterol. The *Journal of Nutrition* also reported that when walnuts and almonds were added to a meal, they gave glycemic control after eating a high-carbohydrate meal. A 160-calorie handful of almonds supplies vitamin E, magnesium, and fiber. All are important in protecting against diabetes. Almonds and walnuts are the two most studied nuts in regard to diabetes and heart disease.

Sea Vegetables

People all over the world have been eating sea vegetables (known generically as seaweed) for thousands of years. Four varieties of sea vegetables have been found preserved in Japanese burial grounds that were 10,000 years old. The Australian Aborigines use three different types of sea vegetables. The Native Americans include alaria (wakame-like), nori (laver), and kelp in their traditional diets. The Atlantic coastal people of Scandinavia, France, and the British Isles also have been eating sea vegetables for centuries.

Gram for gram, they are higher in minerals and vitamins than any other class of food. They are rich in vitamins A, B, C, and E. The minerals in sea vegetables are found in similar ratios to those in the blood. Sea vegetables produce substantial amounts of proteins, complex carbohydrates, carotenes, and chlorophyll. For example, dulse and nori have 21.5 and 28.4 grams of protein, respectively, per hundred grams of sea vegetable. They have approximately 2–4.5 percent fat, and 40–45 grams of carbohydrate per hundred grams of sea vegetable. Alaria (essentially identical to the Japanese wakame) and kelp are extremely high in calcium. All sea vegetables seem to be high in potassium, with kelp being the highest, followed by dulse and alaria. Alaria and kelp are high in magnesium, each having three times the recommended dietary allowance (RDA) per 100 grams. Kelp and alaria have very high amounts of iodine; 100 grams of kelp have approximately 10 times the estimated RDA of iodine. One hundred grams of alaria and nori have approximately 8,487 and 4,266 IU of vitamin A. One hundred grams of most of the sea vegetables have about one-third the RDA of the B vitamins, one-tenth the RDA of vitamin C, and about one-third the

RDA of vitamin E. As pointed out earlier, these sea vegetables also contain chelating agents that are effective for protection against the absorption of radioactive particles.

Kelp

Kelp absorbs from seawater almost all the nutrients, minerals, and trace elements that are essential to life. Kelp contains more than 60 minerals and elements, 21 amino acids, simple and complex carbohydrates, and several essential plant growth hormones. Being rich in amino acids, vitamins, minerals, and trace elements is one of the key reasons why kelp is known as a great promoter of glandular health, especially for the pituitary, adrenal, and thyroid glands. Kelp was first used medicinally to treat enlarged thyroid glands. Physicians didn't know why kelp was effective, until it was discovered that it was exceptionally rich in iodine and that enlarged thyroids were caused by iodine deficiency. Because iodine stimulates the thyroid gland, which controls the metabolism, it was noted that those who took iodine lost weight more easily. From these observations, kelp was then used to assist in weight loss. It has been suggested that kelp's positive effects in assisting metabolism may help in lowering cholesterol. This versatile sea-vegetable is also widely used to maintain healthy skin and hair. Kelp's most dramatic application is its ability to neutralize heavy-metal pollution and radiation in the body.

Algaes

Chlorella and Spirulina

Chlorella and spirulina are two of the most nutrient-dense foods known and easily qualify as whole, perfect superfoods. They have a balanced complement of protein (60 percent), carbohydrates (19 percent), fat (6 percent), bioavailable minerals (8 percent), and moisture (7 percent).

Chlorella gets its name from the high amount of chlorophyll in it—up to 10 times that of spirulina, which is itself very high in chlorophyll. Another hallmark of this superfood is chlorella growth factor

(CGF)—3 percent of the chlorella cell that is responsible for its ability to quadruple in quantity every 20 hours. CGF stimulates tissue repair, even if it has been ulcerated, as we see in advanced cases of diabetes. CGF has been proven effective against memory loss, depression, and other psychiatric diseases. It also helps boost the immune system, stimulating the production of interferon and the activity of macrophages (important defense cells in our immune system). Chlorella is the best algae for pulling heavy metals out of the system, particularly mercury, lead, cadmium, uranium, and arsenic—all known to be diabetogenic. The antiviral effects of chlorophyll and CGF have also been found beneficial in cases of blood sugar imbalances such as diabetes because chlorella's digestible protein smoothes blood sugar fluctuations. Chlorella helps diabetics by reducing advanced glycation end products (AGEs), the toxic metabolites resulting from consuming refined sugars.[74]

Spirulina is 60–70 percent protein and 95 percent assimilable. It contains gamma-linolenic acid (GLA), an essential fatty acid needed by diabetics. The Delta-6 desaturatase enzyme, which is necessary to convert linoleic acid to GLA, is inhibited in diabetes. And by giving GLA, an omega-6 fatty acid, researchers found that receivers of GLA did better in all 16 parameters evaluated in one study.[75]

GLA has been found to enhance nerve conduction and blood flow in diabetic rats. These essential fatty acids seem to improve circulation, improve nerve conduction, and increase prostaglandin PG-1, which has an anti-inflammatory effect and helps ameliorate neuropathy. Spirulina is also 95 percent digestible, higher than any food known. It contains more beta-carotene than any other whole food, as well as 92 trace minerals and other nutritional elements such as vitamins, chlorophyll, glycolipids, phycocyanin, carotenoids, and sulfolipids. It is also abundant in superoxide dismutase (SOD, an antioxidant), RNA, and DNA, which were identified in 1990 as essential nutrients. The high amounts of beta-carotene in spirulina have shown to be effective in fighting oral cancer in animals.[76] In India, the beta-carotene in spirulina was studied for its effectiveness and absorption in young children and found to be extremely effective.[77]

Spirulina and chlorella are excellent in juices, smoothies, on salads, and even in plain water. These are two superfoods you do not want to be without.

Sweeteners

Stevia is the primary sweetener I recommend. Having 15 times a sweeter taste than sugar, with no calories and a glycemic index of zero, the powdered leaf of *Stevia rebaudiana Bertoni* has recently become highly sought after as a supersweet, low-calorie addition to a low-glycemic diet. It gives a sweet taste and does not raise the blood sugar as all the other natural sweeteners do. Unlike nutrient-empty synthetic sugar substitutes, stevia is loaded with vitamins and minerals, including magnesium, niacin, riboflavin, zinc, chromium, and selenium. Stevia is also one of the oldest, safest, and most highly esteemed South American herbs known, with a centuries-long history of safe use. By 1921, stevia was being hailed by American trade commissioner George Brady as a "new sugar plant with great commercial possibilities." He was so convinced that it made "an ideal and safe sugar for diabetics" that he presented it to the United States Department of Agriculture.

Several modern clinical studies suggest that stevia may have the ability to lower and balance blood sugar levels, support the pancreas and digestive system, protect the liver, and combat infectious micro-organisms.[78, 79, 80, 81, 82] Xylitol is the only other sweetener I have tested that does not raise blood sugar in diabetics.

Xylitol is an alternative for sweetening your recipes. It has a fresh sweet taste. It can be used to transform any recipe that calls for sweetness. Some people experience diarrhea when they use too much of it. That is why is a good idea to use a little xylitol combined with stevia to get the best taste without getting the runs. Not all kinds of xylitol are the same, so make sure you buy non-GMO birch tree xylitol. You can purchase xylitol at the Tree of Life store (DrCousens.com).

Vitamins

Niacin (B-3)

As early as 1950, researchers had discovered that niacinamide could provide protection against the development of diabetes.[83] These studies, and some performed 30 years later, sparked several human-based studies that have again demonstrated niacin's ability to not only prevent Type-1 diabetes but, if given soon enough after diagnosis, to slow the progression of and sometimes even reverse the disease, restoring pancreatic function to the point that insulin is no longer required.[84]

Niacinamide has been shown to be effective in preventing the development of diabetes in high-risk children. Researchers divided a group of high-risk children into two groups; 14 were given niacinamide and eight were not. All eight of the untreated children eventually developed diabetes, compared to only one of the treated children.[85]

Researchers have now shown that niacinamide acts as a protective antioxidant. It also inhibits components of the immune system that target the pancreas.[86] Niacinamide also stimulates the pancreas to secrete more insulin and increases insulin sensitivity within cells.[87]

Enzymes that contain niacin play an important role in energy production and the metabolism of fat, cholesterol, and carbohydrates as a prehormone component in the sex and adrenal hormones, as well as a neurotransmitter precursor. Niacin is part of the glucose tolerance factor as well. Using niacinamide has had significant effects in Type-1 and Type-2 diabetes. There is some suggestion that niacinamide given within the first five years of the onset of Type-1 may help ameliorate the effect. It has also been shown to reduce total cholesterol and triglycerides and increase HDL levels. It may turn out to be an essential part of any diabetic program.

Niacinamide has the capacity in vitro of disrupting the pathogenic mechanisms of non-insulin-dependent diabetes mellitus (NIDDM). Animal studies have shown significant beta cell protection from niacinamide. Many of these studies have been done since 1987 and have played a role in helping prevent the destruction of pancreatic beta cells in patients newly diagnosed with Type-1 diabetes. Niacinamide prevents the depletion of intracellular NADH.[88, 89] Low intracellular NADH levels contribute to the death of islet cells of the pancreas. Niacinamide does seem to help prevent pancreatic beta cell death, but it does not seem to intervene in the inflammatory process, which is why the live-food diet and Culture of Life enzymes play an important role in reducing inflammation. B-3 is good for the functioning of glucose tolerance factor and it decreases lipid buildup.

Because of these interesting results, several pilot studies were designed to see if nicotinamide was a viable way to prevent Type-1 diabetes from manifesting, or after manifesting, to prevent the beta cells from further destruction or reduce the rate of destruction. In these studies, seven participants were given 3 grams of niacinamide a day. After six months, five patients in the niacinamide group and two in the placebo group no longer needed insulin. Their blood glucose levels and HgbA1c levels were normal. At 12 months, three patients in the niacinamide group and none in the placebo group remained diabetes-free.[90] Could niacinamide prevent diabetes from progressing? There have been at least 10 studies attempting to answer this question of the effectiveness of niacinamide treatment for recent onset of Type-1 or cases of less than five years duration. Of these 10 studies, 8 were double-blind, and of the 8, 4 showed a positive effect compared to placebo in terms of prolonged noninsulin need or lower insulin requirements, which, in essence, is better metabolic control. They also had increased beta cell functions as determined by C-peptide secretion.[91]

Because of these tentatively positive results, two large studies were conducted—the Deutsche Nicotinamide Intervention Study and the European Nicotinamide Diabetes Intervention Trial (ENDIT). Neither found significant benefit. However, in the face of some of these studies, if my child had Type-1 diabetes, I would certainly add niacinamide to the mix because of its minimal toxicity and the fact that it is inexpensive. A dosage of 2,000 mg a day would cost around $7.00 a month.

The typical dosage used is 500–1,000 mg three times a day, taken with food. Those at risk for developing Type-1 diabetes, or those who have already been diagnosed, are well advised to use niacinamide. The research has shown that it is most helpful either before or in the initial phases—that is, during the first five years of the disease. Dosage recommendations are approximately 25 mg of niacinamide for every 2.2 pounds of body weight, so a person weighing 150 pounds would need about 1.7 grams, or 1,700 milligrams a day. Studies have shown minimal side effects other than one case of diarrhea, and dosages up to 3 grams daily for six months have produced no problems. One study did show that in adult Type-1 diabetics treated with niacin for lipid value control, 16 percent suffered a bout of diabetic keto-acidosis.

If you are taking niacinamide, it is wise to use a B-complex supplement in conjunction with it, to ensure that the larger therapeutic doses create no other B-vitamin deficiencies. Food sources of niacin are spinach and hazelnuts.

Vitamin B-6

Vitamin B-6 is very helpful in reversing diabetic neuropathy and protects against peripheral nerve degeneration. Diabetics with neuropathy have been shown to be deficient in B-6 and benefit from supplementation.[92] It seems to also inhibit glycosylation of proteins.[93] It also helps with magnesium metabolism.

With regard to gestational diabetes, a study published in the *British Medical Journal* showed that women taking 100 mg of B-6 reversed the condition in 12 of the 14 women.[94]

Vitamin B-12

Thirty-nine percent of meat eaters are deficient in B-12 and up to 80 percent of vegans and live-food eaters are deficient in B-12 after six years. So it is absolutely essential that we supplement with this nutrient. Research has found that vitamin B-12 is also very helpful in maintaining proper function of the nervous system in individuals with Type-2 diabetes. Increased levels of B-12 were closely correlated with reduced oxidative stress in individuals with poor blood sugar control.[95] People's needs for B-12 are quite variable, and stress plays a big role in those needs. Vitamin B-12 deficiency can result in memory loss, depression, and numbness or burning feelings in the feet. We have used it along with the total program in helping to reverse diabetic neuropathy.

We recommend a form of B-12 that is plant-source-only, made from bacteria. It is called *Nano B complex*. Anyone on this diet is well advised to take it protectively. Adults need about 6 mcg twice a day as a minimum.

Biotin

Biotin is another vitamin that seems to be important for carbohydrate fat and protein metabolism. A plant-source-only diet seems to increase the intestinal bacteria in a way to enhance biotin synthesis and absorption. Biotin seems to increase insulin sensitivity, as well as activate glucokinase, which is involved in the utilization of glucose by the liver. This is important because in diabetics, glucokinase concentrations are low. Biotin also helps to decrease FBS. Biotin deficiency results in impaired utilization of glucose.[96] Blood biotin levels were significantly lower in 43 patients with NIDDM than in nondiabetic control subjects, and lower fasting blood glucose levels were associated with higher blood biotin levels. After one month of biotin supplementation (9 mg/day), fasting blood glucose levels decreased by an average of 45 percent.[97] Reductions in blood glucose levels were also found in seven insulin-dependent diabetics after one week of supplementation with 16 mg of biotin daily.[98] Biotin has also been found to stimulate the secretion of insulin in the pancreas of rats, having the effect of lowering blood glucose.[99] An effect on cellular glucose (GLUT-4) transporters is currently under investigation.

Biotin is appropriate for Type-1 and Type-2 diabetes. Type-2 diabetics were given 9 mg per day for one month and compared to a placebo group; the diabetics experienced an average drop of 45 percent in their blood glucose levels.[100] Similar improvements were noted in a study of Type-1 diabetics with a daily dose of 16 mg of biotin.[101] Biotin is very safe—no side effects have been reported. Food sources include avocados, raspberries, artichokes, and cauliflower.

Vitamin C

Vitamin C plays a very important role in the healing of diabetes and reversing complications. This antioxidant inhibits accumulation of sorbitol, reduces glycosylation of proteins, and preserves endothelial function. It inhibits aldose reductase, which creates a buildup of sorbitol, which is associated with many of the long-term complications of diabetes. One of the key gifts of vitamin C is its role in the function and manufacture of collagen, as well as maintaining the integrity of the connective tissue, which makes it important for two diabetic concerns: wound repair and maintaining healthy gums. Vitamin C seems to be important in the immune system and in the manufacture and metabolism of neurotransmitters and hormones. Insulin facilitates the transport of vitamin C into the cells, so when there is an insulin deficiency, what we actually get is a deficiency in intracellular vitamin C—thus the relative deficiency in vitamin C in many diabetics.[102] This leads to a subclinical scurvy problem, which creates an increased tendency to bleed, poor wound healing, microvascular disease, heart disease, elevation of cholesterol, and a depressed immune system.

Perhaps the most important effect of vitamin C (at doses of 2,000 mg/day) is its ability to reverse the glycosylation of proteins.[103, 104] The sorbitol accumulation and cross-linking, or glycosylation, are linked to many complications, especially eye and nervous system and circulatory disorders. Vitamin C may also be one of the best and safest nutrients for the inhibition of sorbitol accumulation in the cells. One study[105] showed that when researchers measured red blood cell sorbitol, then supplemented with either 100 mg or 600 mg vitamin C and measured participants again in 30 days for their red blood cell sorbitol, the controls had nearly double the sorbitol of those who received vitamin C supplementation. This normalization of the sorbitol seemed to be independent of changes in diabetic control. The researchers concluded that the vitamin C supplementation was distinctly effective in reducing the buildup of sorbitol in the red blood cells.

Even though the study was done with 100 or 600 milligrams of vitamin C, we suggest clinically that one should take 1,000 mg of food-sourced C three times a day because of the overall effects. Foods high in vitamin C include goji berries, grapefruit, lemons, broccoli, red peppers, brussels sprouts, camu camu berries, and acerola berries.

Vitamin D

Vitamin D is actually a hormone rather than, strictly speaking, a vitamin—one of the most powerful hormones in your body. It is active in quantities as small as one-trillionth of a gram.

Studies have shown vitamin D to have a protective effect against Type-1 diabetes. The results of a large pan-European trial, published in the journal *Diabetologica* in 1999, suggest that vitamin D supplements taken in infancy protect against, or arrest, the initiation of a process that can lead to insulin-dependent diabetes in later childhood. If this is the case, it seems reasonable to suggest that exposure to sunlight in early childhood may be important in preventing the onset of the disease.[106] For adults, studies have shown that the lower your vitamin D level, the higher your blood glucose.[107] One 20-minute full-body exposure to the summer sun will result in putting 20,000 IU into the body within 48 hours. However, if you are older, obese, or dark-skinned, you will get far less. In fact, using sunscreen of even a low SPF rating of 8 reduces vitamin D production by 95 percent.[108] Dr. Robert Heany of Creighton University, one of the top vitamin D researchers, has stated that as many as 75 percent of the women in the United States are deficient.[109]

Just in case you are wondering about vitamin D levels and a raw vegan diet, researchers led by Luigi Fontana, MD, PhD, of Washington University[110] looked at 18 men and women, ages 33 to 85, who had maintained a raw vegan lifestyle for an average of 3.6 years. They were compared with a matched group of 18 controls who ate a standard American diet containing animal fat and processed foods. The average vitamin D levels were higher in the raw vegan group than in the control group, despite an extremely low dietary intake of vitamin D—this may be indicative of the increased personal sun exposure.

If you live above 38 degrees north latitude (above Baltimore, St. Louis, Denver, and San Francisco), the sun is too weak from midfall through the following spring to stimulate significant vitamin D production. Other vitamin D absorption challenges are aging. As our skin becomes less efficient at producing vitamin D, excessive fat layers are found to inhibit production of vitamin D. The latter is a common concern for those of us who are healing obesity and diabetes.[111] Therefore, from a holistic perspective, I advise 5,000 to 10,000 IU daily.

The benefits of sunlight or supplementation for adequate vitamin D levels do not stop with Type-1 and Type-2 diabetes but significantly affect the complications associated with a diabetogenic history and a Westernized diet and lifestyle. Research shows that vitamin D has a variety of important benefits besides lowering blood sugar. It seems to protect against 18 different kinds of cancers, has a significant positive impact on the immune system in fighting colds and flus, viruses, and TB, and protects against rickets and osteoporosis.

Vitamin E

Diabetics seem to have an increased need for vitamin E. It reduces glycosylation, improves insulin sensitivity, and inhibits platelet clumping. It regulates intracellular calcium and magnesium in the blood vessels. It helps to protect against oxidation, helps improve the action of insulin, and helps prevent many of the long-term difficulties and complications of diabetes, including neuropathy.[112] A recent study found a biochemical marker of oxidative stress to be elevated in diabetic individuals.[113] Supplementation with 600 mg of synthetic alpha-tocopherol daily (equivalent to 300 mg of natural, RRR-alpha-tocopherol) for 14 days resulted in a reduction in the oxidative stress marker. One study reported improved control of blood glucose levels with supplementation of only 100 IU of synthetic alpha-tocopherol daily (equivalent to 45 mg of natural, RRR-alpha-tocopherol).[114]

In a human double-blind study, 24 hypertensive patients were given 600 mg of vitamin E per day. Those given vitamin E showed increased insulin sensitivity and improved concentrations of cellular magnesium. Magnesium is believed to protect against oxidative damage and normalize circulating glucose levels.[115] It can also play a role in preventing diabetes. One study followed 944 men, ages 42 to 60, who did not have diabetes at the beginning of the study. Forty-five men developed diabetes during the four-year follow-up. The study indicated that a low vitamin-E concentration was associated with 3.9 times greater risk of developing diabetes.[116]

It is important for optimal vitamin E effects that one use a natural vitamin E with all the tocopherols and tocotrienols factors.

Bioflavonoids

Recent research indicates that flavonoids may be useful in treating diabetes.[117, 118] Flavonoids include quercetin, which promotes insulin secretion and is a potent inhibitor of sorbitol accumulation. Quercetin has been found in vitro to inhibit sorbitol accumulation in human lenses[119] and has been found to slow the course of cataract formation.[120, 121] Other flavonoids include naringin and hespertin; both have been found to be aldose reductase inhibitors, therefore protecting against the accumulation of sorbitol.[122, 123]

The nutritional benefits of flavonoids include the increase of intracellular vitamin C levels, a decrease in the leakiness and breakage of small blood vessels, the prevention of easy bruising, and immune system support—all great benefit in diabetes.[124] Bilberry, grapeseed, and ginkgo are important plant sources of flavonoids.

Essential Fatty Acids

The essential fatty acids also play a very important role, which is why I am very hesitant to encourage dietary fat intake that is too low to get the benefits of EFAs.

In diabetes the essential fatty acid metabolism is impaired. The Delta-6 desaturatase enzyme, which is necessary to convert linoleic acid to gamma-linolenic acid (GLA), is inhibited in diabetes. By giving GLA, which is an omega-6 fatty acid, researchers found that in a study of 111 diabetics, those who received GLA supplements did better in all 16 parameters studied, compared to the placebo group.[125] GLA has been found to enhance nerve conduction and blood flow in diabetic rats. GLA and other essential fatty acids seem to improve circulation, improve nerve conduction, and increase prostaglandin PG-1, which has an anti-inflammatory effect and helps ameliorate neuropathy.

The omega-3 and omega-6 fatty acids are the biological precursors to a group of highly reactive, short-lived, molecular, hormone-like substances known as prostaglandins (PGAs). The PGAs play a role in regulating the second-by-second functioning of every part of the body. Each organ produces its own PGAs from the essential fatty acids stored in that organ. The PGAs are critical for cell membrane function because they become a part of the membrane construction themselves. PGAs help to balance and heal the immune system as well as reduce inflammatory reactions such as those seen in arthritis and allergic reactions. If there are dietary imbalances that lead to imbalances in the PGAs, then disease may arise. Although the research is not definitive, a ratio of omega-6 to omega-3 fatty acids of approximately 2:1 or 1:1 seems to be the best balance.

In the omega-6 series there is linoleic acid (LA), gamma-linolenic acid (GLA), dihomo-gamma-linolenic acid (DGLA), and arachidonic acid (AA). The omega-6 fatty acids are found in seed oils such as sunflower, safflower, corn, soy, and evening primrose. Peanut oil has some omega-6, as do olive, palm, and coconut oils. High amounts of GLA are found in mother's milk and primrose, borage, and black currant oils.

Fish are found to have high amounts of eicosapentaenoic acid (EPA) and some moderate amounts of the precursors of the omega-3 series. Fortunately, plant-source-only people do not have to worry about sources of omega-3 fatty acids because flax seed, hemp seed, purslane, chia seeds, walnuts, legumes, and sea vegetables have high concentrations. In the omega-3 series, there is alpha-linolenic acid. The long-chain omega-3s EPA and docosahexaenoic acid (DHA) are found in purslane, E3Live, and golden algae. As a high percentage of both meat eaters and plant-source-only people are low in long chain omega-3s, I recommend everyone take a DHA/EPA supplement.

Omega-3 Benefits

The omega-3 series should constitute approximately 10–20 percent of our fat intake. Some of the reported benefits of the omega-3s include protection against heart disease, strokes, and clots in the lungs; anti-carcinogenic activity against tumors; protection against diabetes; prevention and treatment of arthritis; and treatment for asthma, PMS, allergies, inflammatory diseases, water retention, rough or dry skin, and multiple sclerosis. The omega-3s are reported to increase vitality and contribute to smoother skin, shinier hair, softer hands, smoother muscle action, the normalization of blood sugar, increased cold weather resistance, and a generally improved immune system. Omega-3s are also important for visual function, development of the fetal brain, brain function in adults, adrenal function, sperm formation, and the amelioration of some psychiatric behavior disorders. It may take three to six months after starting high omega-3 foods or supplementation to see results. The conversion of short chain omega-3s to DHA and EPA is doubled when 1–3 tablespoons of coconut oil are taken with them. The importance of omega-3s will be discussed in more detail in Chapter 5.

Flax versus Fish Oil: Flax Wins

Flax seed contains 18–24 percent omega-3 (as do hemp and chia seeds in the approximately the same amounts, so in mentioning flax I am also including hemp and chia seeds), compared to the low content in fish of 0–2 percent. This is significant because many people mistakenly think that they need to eat fish in order to get the omega-3-derived EPA for heart and artery protection. Abundant research on the subject indicates that this is simply not true. The vegetarian flax seed has many major advantages over fish oil. The first is that the omega-3 is a basic building block in the human body for many functions, only one of which is to make EPA. The fish oil doesn't supply omega-3; it supplies the EPA and therefore limits the body's options to make what it needs from the omega-3. Thus the omega-3 is a better nutritional resource than the high-EPA fish oil.

Another major difference is the fiber that comes in the flax seed. Fish has no fiber and also is a highly concentrated food. Flax seed has a special fiber called lignin that our body converts to lignans, which help to build up the immune system and have specific anticancer, antifungal, and antiviral properties. High levels of lignans are associated with reduced rates of colon and breast cancer. Just 10 grams, or about 1–2 teaspoons of flax seed oil or 1–3 tablespoons of ground flax seed per day, raises levels of the lignans significantly.

The third advantage of flax seed oil over fish oil is the fact that fish are often high in toxic residues because they live in polluted waters, as well in possible radioactivity that is spread throughout the Earth's water bodies from Fukushima.

The fifth reason flax seed is more propitious is that high levels of fish oil are rich in vitamins A and D, which can be toxic in high doses. Please note that the provitamin carotene, which is converted by the body to utilizable vitamin A, cannot be toxic like animal-sourced vitamin A.

Alpha-Lipoic Acid

One of the most important antioxidants, although we need a variety of them, is alpha-lipoic acid. ALA helps with a variety of problems, one of which is the cardiovascular complications of diabetes having to do with small-vessel damage from inflammation. We also use a proteolytic enzyme called Culture of Life Intenzyme to neutralize and reverse this inflammatory process. Vitamin E also seems to play a role at 1,200 IU per day in creating a reduction in LDL oxidation.[126]

ALA is a physiological constituent of all cell membranes and is a very potent antioxidant in both lipid- and water-soluble areas of the body. It acts within the cell membrane, reacting with and neutralizing reactive oxygen species, including super oxide radical, singlet oxygen, hydrogen radicals, peroxide radicals, and hydrochloric acid.[127] It has been used successfully in Germany for the treatment of diabetic neuropathy.[128] Lipid peroxidation, which is free radical oxidation of the lipids, is increased in diabetic neuropathy and neutralized by ALA.

ALA also tends to prevent protein/lipid glycosylation oxidation, because it acts as an antioxidant and stimulates glucose uptake by the cells. ALA is actually approved for the treatment of diabetes in Germany for diabetic neuropathy. A high dose, about 600 mg per day, is needed to improve diabetic neuropathy.[129] ALA's primary effect is its antioxidant reaction. In summary, ALA improves blood sugar metabolism, reduces glycosylated protein/lipids, improves blood flow to peripheral nerves, and actually stimulates the regeneration of nerve fibers.[130, 131, 132, 133]

Research has shown that ALA increases insulin sensitivity. In one study, 74 patients with Type-2 diabetes were randomly assigned to receive either a placebo or 600; 1,200; or 1,800 mg a day of ALA.[134] After four weeks, those receiving ALA supplements had statistically improved insulin sensitivity, and all three dosages of ALA were effective. Other studies have supported these findings. There is some suggestion that lipoic acid reactivates vitamins C and E when they have performed their antioxidant function and works synergistically with niacin and thiamine, as well.

Gamma-Linolenic Acid (GLA)

GLA reportedly can reverse nerve damage to peripheral nerves in patients with diabetic neuropathy. GLA regulates insulin and seems to protect against diabetic heart, eye, and kidney damage. GLA has an insulin-sparing activity that allows insulin to be more effective. Diets that are relatively high in linoleic acid appear to decrease the progression of microangiopathy in diabetics.[135] Excellent sources are evening primrose oil and flax seed oil.

Amino Acids

Acetyl-Carnitine

Another nutrient, acetyl-carnitine, has been found to improve peripheral nerve function by normalizing nerve conduction. It seems to restore myoinositol levels that are depleted by sorbitol buildup.

L-Arginine

Arginine is another nutrient that seems to boost insulin sensitivity, as well as cardiovascular function. One study showed that insulin sensitivity was increased by 34 percent with the use of arginine, versus 4 percent for a control group. Supplementation of L-arginine can be beneficial for individuals who have increased AGEs and free-radical induced aging that accompanies poor control of blood sugar and insulin. In a clinical study done at the University of Vienna Department of Medicine, 1 gram of L-arginine was given twice daily to individuals who had oxidative stress as a consequence of poor blood sugar control. Results of the study revealed significant reduction in oxidative stress reactions, and L-arginine supplementation also reduced the amount of damage to DNA and other important cellular materials, thereby reducing the processes associated with accelerated aging.[136]

Arginine seems to increase the neurotransmitter nitric oxide. Nitric oxide also dilates the blood vessels and helps to decrease blood pressure and increase blood flow. The more blood flow there is, the more circulation and healthier your tissues can be.

Minerals

A highly mineralized body is a more disease-resistant and antiaging body. Minerals play an important role in the treatment of diabetes. Most diabetics suffer from mineral deficiencies beyond the depletion of minerals in the soil that affects everybody eating a nonsupplemented diet, due to mineral loss through polyuria (excessive urination). The key minerals that need to be replenished are vanadium, magnesium, chromium, calcium, zinc, manganese, and potassium. The beta cells of the pancreas are high in zinc, manganese, potassium, and chromium.

Planet Earth is made of minerals, and our bodies are made of minerals. Minerals are catalysts for enzymatic reactions in the body. They activate the vitamins and all the enzymes. They activate all the organ structures and, in fact, are the basis of all the organ and cellular structures of the body. Minerals are the builders of the system, and they act as the frequency rates in the system. They are not necessarily the energy makers, however. The human body is composed entirely of minerals and water. The water molecule is the one that acts as a powerful solvent in the human system, bringing in nutrients and washing out waste particles. Without the essential minerals and trace minerals, we could not survive.

Of a total of approximately 90 minerals, there are approximately 23 key minerals, including 16 major minerals and 7 minor, or trace, minerals. All key minerals are needed for the body to function at the highest level. They need to be replenished in the system through water-soluble ionic forms. As early as 1936, the U.S. Senate declared, "99 percent of the American people are deficient in minerals, and a marked deficiency in any one of the more important minerals actually results in disease." This is one of the most intelligent things that has ever come out of the U.S. Senate, and something that was beyond even the scope of medical school. Now, many years later, we are subjected to junk foods, foods that have been pesticided and herbicided, microwaved foods, and foods harvested from increasingly mineral-deficient soils. The situation has only gotten worse. This is why most everyone needs mineral supplementation, whether they are plant-source-only or meat eaters. Dr. Linus Pauling, winner of two Nobel prizes, said, "You can trace every sickness, every disease, and every ailment, ultimately, to a mineral deficiency." Research by Dr. Maynard Murray, author of *Sea Energy Agriculture*, shows that a highly mineralized body is a more disease-resistant and antiaging body.

For a mineral to be utilized at the intracellular level, it must be angstrom size (i.e., so infinitesimal it is measured in units of angstroms), and these particles must be completely water-soluble. Only the ionic form, on angstrom-size level, of minerals can enter the cells and activate the proper DNA structures to actuate the guiding frequencies for the function of the body. An angstrom (named after Johan Angstrom) is one-thousandth of a micron and one-millionth of a meter. The significance of this information is that almost all the mineral supplements on the market are larger than micron sizes. Now it can get a little confusing, but think about it this way: Particles that are micron in size and larger will be absorbed by the blood, but they are too large to be absorbed intracellularly and inside the nucleus. These larger forms stay in the bloodstream, and eventually become deposited in various tissue locations. Angstrom-size particles travel through the cells, and if the body doesn't need them, it will simply discharge them with no buildup of the minerals to create potential toxicity in the tissues.

We observe that the roots of the plants are designed to break down the soil and utilize and absorb mineral particles at angstrom size—that's what they do. With the help of fulvic acid in the humus material, plants are able to take in these minerals and break them down into angstrom-size particles, which they use. Once we understand that, we understand that the vegetables we eat transfer angstrom-size minerals from the soil to us via the plants. They do not absorb larger-size particles because they cannot assimilate them. Angstrom-size minerals are key to optimal mineral absorption. It takes about 12 years for farmland to become deficient of angstrom-size trace minerals. For this reason, traditionally, farmers would often move every 12 years.

Minerals of micron size or larger can cause a variety of problems. The paradox, which is hard to understand, is that while the tissues are full of minerals in a sense, the cell is lacking in the angstrom-size minerals. This is one reason it is important to use salt. High-energy salts include Transformational Salts and Himalayan salt. These are well absorbed intracellularly because they are in ionic angstrom-sizes. If salt isn't in the ionic form, one simply is not able to absorb it efficiently into one's body. Table salt (straight sodium chloride) is not available for use in the body and can cause a toxic buildup. This may also potentially apply to salts that are sun dried. The process of sun drying, like many other forms of heating, causes electrons not to be available and the ions to form more tight bonds that make them inaccessible for assimilation. If salt creates a savory and watery feeling in the mouth, then it is still ionic. If it dries the mouth, this suggests that it has converted to the less assimilable covalent form. Although larger mineral forms or covalently bonded salt may help us initially on one level, eventually they have the potential of building up to toxic overload.

Paradoxically, one of the most effective ways to pull out these accumulated minerals is to provide the same mineral in angstrom size. Angstrom-size minerals act as building blocks for the more than six thousand different enzymes needed for optimal function in our bodies. If we don't have the proper minerals for those enzymes to work in the particular organs where they are needed, we do not, in a sense, have the cellular building materials for repair and regeneration of our tissues. For example, in diabetes, because of all the refined foods we eat, we have created a deficiency of chromium because chromium is pulled out of our tissues to help metabolize the refined foods, which no longer have the chromium needed to metabolize them. The long-term result is a deficiency in chromium. So when we are taking in lots of refined carbohydrates and need chromium to help metabolize the sugar and to make the insulin work correctly, we become chromium deficient. When we eat junk foods, or food from depleted soils and synthetic fertilizers, we really aren't able to metabolize the sugars and carbohydrates properly. This adds to a diabetic condition.

In essence, minerals take us to the very formation of life. All qualities of positive or negative health can be traced back to a lack of minerals. To get adequate mineralization, as we said, the minerals need to be in angstrom-size form—0.001 micron. They need to be attached to covalent hydrogen in the water, which will pull them inside the cell. It is at the intracellular level where the action happens. When the minerals reach the nucleus and mitochondria of the cell, there's a transmutation on the cellular level that activates the DNA. The nucleus and the mitochondria are both the energy centers and the creative centers of the cell. Mitochondria also have a particular form of DNA, which is different than nuclear DNA. The minerals activate the primordial DNA. These minerals activate electromagnetic communications both intracellularly and extracellularly that organize the system and communicate about what activities must be done. Some of the DNA frequencies are received in the cell wall.

In essence, we can say that the soil in the United States, and in most of the world, is overworked and underfed—and getting worse. This soil exhaustion creates exhausted and diseased plants, exhausted and diseased animals, and exhausted and diseased human beings.

The Dr. Cousens's Diabetes Recovery Program—A Holistic Approach employs several routes to remineralization: fresh organic plant foods eaten, juiced, and blended (including sea vegetables); super-food powder blends; and bioavailable mineral supplementation. Our means for getting nutrient-dense plant foods will be fully discussed in the recipe section, but here let us investigate key minerals that can help support and heal the pancreatic beta cells, improve insulin sensitivity, regulate blood glucose levels, and prevent or reverse diabetic complications.

Vanadium

Vanadium is an important trace mineral in healing diabetes naturally. It seems to keep blood sugar from rising too high. It supports the absorption of blood sugar into the muscle system and protects against elevated cholesterol, particularly a buildup of cholesterol in the central nervous system. At the Tree of Life, we use vanadium frequently to help with insulin resistivity and Type-2 diabetes. Vanadium has been found to be helpful in protecting against diabetic cataracts and neuropathy.[137] It reduces gluconeogenesis and increases the development of glycogen deposits.[138] It seems to be associated with modest improvements in fasting glucose and hepatic insulin resistance. Clinical trials have found a significant decrease in insulin requirements in patients with insulin-dependent diabetes after vanadyl sulfate therapy. They have also noted a decrease in cholesterol levels for both IDDM and NIDDM. It has also been found to stimulate glucose uptake and metabolism that leads to glucose normalization. In some cases it helps to restore insulin production in diabetic rats.

Kelp and sea vegetables are good sources of vanadium.

Magnesium

Magnesium depletion is commonly associated with both IDDM and NIDDM and is one of the most important minerals to replace. Between 25 percent and 38 percent of diabetics have been found to have decreased serum levels of magnesium (hypomagnesemia),[139] and supplementation may prevent some of the complications of diabetes such as retinopathy and heart disease.[140] One cause of the depletion may be increased urinary loss of magnesium as a result of the increased excretion of glucose that accompanies poorly controlled diabetes. Magnesium deficiency has been associated with insulin resistance. Intracellular depletion of magnesium has been found to be a common feature of insulin resistance. Research has also shown that a decrease in insulin sensitivity occurs with a magnesium deficiency.[141] There seems to be a clear association between the lowest consumption of dietary magnesium and the highest amount of insulin resistance in nondiabetic subjects.[142] Other research has noted that magnesium deficiency resulted in impaired insulin secretion, and magnesium replacement restores insulin secretion. Dietary magnesium supplements (400 mg/day) were found to improve glucose tolerance in elderly individuals.[143]

In two new studies of both men and women, those who consumed the most magnesium in their diet were least likely to develop Type-2 diabetes, according to a report in the January 2006 issue of *Diabetes Care*.[144] Until now, very few large studies have directly examined the long-term effects of dietary magnesium on diabetes. Dr. Simin Liu of the Harvard Medical School and School of Public Health in Boston said, "Our studies provided some direct evidence that greater intake of dietary magnesium may have a long-term protective effect on lowering diabetes risk."[145]

Diabetics often have low magnesium levels in their cells and blood, and some researchers believe that they might even have a defect in the metabolism of magnesium that exacerbates the disease. Even if you're not a diabetic, you're likely to suffer from insulin resistance if you're low in magnesium. One recent study found that normal, healthy adults developed a 25 percent greater insulin resistance on a magnesium-deficient diet.[146]

Magnesium is also very alkalizing to the body and helps counter the tendency to acidity from a diabetogenic lifestyle and physiology. Its highest concentration is in leafy green vegetables, nuts, whole grains, unpolished rice, and wheat germ. Generally high-magnesium foods include apples, apricots, avocados, beet tops, berries, black walnuts, Brazil nuts, cabbage, coconuts, comfrey leaves, figs, dulse, endive, greens, spinach, rye, walnuts, watercress, and yellow corn.

The recommended dosage is 400 mg/day. Also, diabetics should take at least 50 mg of vitamin B-6 per day, as the level of intracellular magnesium is dependent on vitamin B-6 intake. Without B-6, it is difficult for magnesium to readily enter the cell.

Calcium

Calcium is an alkalinizing mineral that helps neutralize the acidity of diabetes. It has not been well studied in relation to diabetes, but following the use of calcium as a supplement, a patient of mine had decreased fasting plasma insulin levels and a significant increase in insulin sensitivity.

Zinc

Zinc seems to be important for preventing insulin resistance, as a low zinc level seems to be associated with increased insulin resistance. It seems to be involved in almost all aspects of insulin metabolism, including synthesis, secretion, and utilization. Lower levels may affect the ability of the islet cells of the pancreas to produce and secrete insulin, particularly in Type-2 diabetes.[147] Zinc seems to have a protective effect against beta cell destruction as well as antiviral effects. Increased urinary zinc excretion appears to contribute to the marginal zinc nutritional status that has been observed in diabetics,[148] and it needs supplementation for that reason. Zinc supplementation has been shown to improve insulin levels of both Type-1 and Type-2 diabetics.[149] Zinc also helps with wound healing, a phenomenon frequently observed in diabetics. Zinc deficiencies in diabetics are associated with excess free radical activity and the increased oxidation of fats.[150] When fats become oxidized, they become more reactive and damaging to the heart, arteries, and other integral parts of the vascular system.

Foods that contain zinc include legumes, nuts (especially almonds), and seeds (particularly pumpkin and sunflower seeds).

Potassium

Potassium helps reduce insulin resistance at postreceptor sites. It seems to improve insulin sensitivity and insulin secretion. For diabetics using insulin, the use of insulin therapy causes the loss of potassium. High potassium reduces the risk of heart disease and lowers high blood pressure. A number of studies indicate that groups with relatively high dietary potassium intakes have lower blood pressures than comparable groups with relatively low potassium intakes.[151] Data on more than 17,000 adults who participated in the Third National Health and Nutritional Examination Survey (NHANES III) indicated that higher dietary potassium intakes were associated with significantly lower blood pressures.[152] The results of the Dietary Approaches to Stop Hypertension (DASH) trial provided further support for the beneficial effects of a potassium-rich diet on blood pressure.[153] Compared to a control diet providing only 3.5 servings per day of fruits and vegetables and 1,700 mg per day of potassium, consumption of a diet that included 8.5 servings per day of fruits and vegetables and 4,100 mg per day of potassium lowered blood pressure by an average of 2.8/1.1 mm Hg (systolic blood pressure/diastolic blood pressure) in people with normal blood pressure and by an average of 7.2/2.8 mm Hg in people with hypertension.

There is some danger with potassium excess, especially with diabetes-associated kidney disease. If someone is receiving a high potassium supplementation, kidney function should be periodically evaluated. Potassium is also alkalinizing.

Good food sources of potassium are prunes, tomatoes, artichoke, spinach, sunflower seeds, and almonds.

Manganese

Manganese is an important cofactor in many enzyme systems that are associated with blood sugar control, energy metabolism, and thyroid hormone function.[154, 155] Guinea pig research showed that a deficiency of manganese resulted in diabetes and birth of offspring that developed pancreatic abnormalities. Most diabetics have about half the manganese levels of normal individuals, and a study revealed that urinary manganese excretion tended to be slightly higher in 185 diabetics compared to 185 nondiabetic controls.[156] A study of functional manganese status found the activity of the antioxidant enzyme, manganese superoxide dismutase (MnSOD), to be lower in the white blood cells of diabetics than in those of nondiabetic controls.[157]

The recommended dosage is up to (but no more than) 30 mg per day.

Chromium

Chromium is an essential nutrient for sugar and fat metabolism. Because chromium appears to enhance the action of insulin and chromium deficiency results in impaired glucose tolerance, chromium insufficiency has been hypothesized to be a contributing factor to the development of Type-2 diabetes.[158, 159] Individuals with Type-2 diabetes have been found to have higher rates of urinary chromium loss than healthy individuals, especially those with diabetes for more than two years.[160]

In 12 of 15 controlled studies of people with impaired glucose tolerance, chromium supplementation was found to improve some measure of glucose utilization or to have beneficial effects on blood lipid profiles.[161] Chromium used synergistically with biotin seems to work to improve beta cell function, enhance glucose uptake by both liver and muscle cells, and inhibit excessive glucose production in the liver. About 25–30 percent of individuals with impaired glucose tolerance eventually develop Type-2 diabetes.[162]

In 1997 the results of a placebo-controlled trial conducted in China indicated that chromium supplementation might be beneficial in the treatment of Type-2 diabetes.[163] In the study, 180 participants took either a placebo, 200 mcg/day of chromium, or 1,000 mcg/day of chromium (both of the latter groups in the form of chromium picolinate). At the end of four months, blood glucose levels were 15–19 percent lower in those who took 1,000 mcg/day compared with those who took a placebo. Blood glucose levels in those who took 200 mcg/day did not differ significantly from those who took a placebo. Insulin levels were lower in those who took either 200 mcg/day or 1,000 mcg/day. Glycosylated hemoglobin levels, a measure of long-term control of blood glucose, were also lower in both chromium-supplemented groups, but they were lowest in the group taking 1,000 mcg/day.

Women with gestational diabetes whose diets were supplemented with 4 mcg of chromium per kilogram of body weight daily as chromium picolinate for eight weeks had decreased fasting blood glucose and insulin levels, compared with those who took a placebo.[164, 165]

Niacin-bound chromium is more bioavailable than chromium picolinate. A recent study at the University of California found that chromium polynicotinate was absorbed and retained up to 311 percent better than chromium picolinate and 672 percent better than chromium chloride. Generally, chromium supplementation at doses of about 200 mcg/day, in a variety of forms for two to three months, has been found to be beneficial in various studies.

Herbal and Natural Teas

Caffeine elevates blood sugar by stimulating and aggravating the adrenal glucose axis, causing imbalanced and elevated blood sugars, and therefore hinders the attempts of the healing diabetic body to achieve a normal physiology. Caffeine is also a diuretic and creates dehydration, which is a tendency in diabetes because the body is trying to rid itself of excess blood sugar by urination (diuresis).

If you have prediabetes or diabetes, I suggest you not use caffeinated drinks such as black tea (containing 60 mg/cup caffeine), green tea (25–30 mg/cup), or even yerba maté (25 mg/cup). Do not drink coffees (100 mg/cup caffeine), even if they are decaffeinated. Instead, consider herbal teas and other teas made from natural plant sources.

String Bean Pod

According to Paavo Airola in *How to Get Well*, string bean pod tea is an excellent natural substitute for insulin and therefore extremely beneficial in diabetes. The skins of the pods of green beans are very rich in silica and certain hormone substances closely related to insulin. One cup of string bean skin tea is equal to at least one unit of insulin.[166] At the Tree of Life we juice the whole string bean in the juice aspect of the program.

A product called Beanpod Tea is an all-natural, mild, and pleasant-tasting tea that is very beneficial for diabetics. This tea is a natural detox tea, detoxifying the pancreas and related organs. Beanpod Tea is composed of the pods of kidney, white, navy, great northern, and baby lima beans. Beanpod Tea contains the amino acids tyrosine, tryptophan, and arginine, plus the B vitamin choline and the enzyme betaine. Patience is the key word in the usage of this tea. Most people will not experience instant relief with the usage of this tea. Diabetics must drink Beanpod Tea regularly for approximately three months in order to help normalize their blood sugar levels.

Kidney Bean

According to John Heinerman, kidney bean pods are effective in lowering elevated blood sugar levels. Since almost 16 pounds of pods would have to be consumed each day to have an effect, this works best as a tea. The pods should be picked before the beans inside ripen, and fresh pods are more effective than dried ones by 8 to 1.

Heinerman advises us to bring 3 quarts of water to a boil, toss in five handfuls of coarsely cut kidney bean pods, and simmer uncovered for three hours. Strain and drink three-quarters of a quart each day with meals.[167]

Dandelion

It has been said that dandelions are nature's way of giving dignity to weeds. Dandelion is well known for its beneficial effects on liver problems, including cirrhosis, jaundice, hepatitis, gallstone removal, and liver toxicity. Dr. David Peterson, a licensed, practicing medical herbalist in Great Britain, once wrote that the high insulin content of the root may be regarded as something "to prescribe for people with diabetes mellitus."

Heinerman suggests three capsules of dried root each day.[168]

Herbs

Gymnema Sylvestre

Gymnema sylvestre decreases glucose absorption from the intestines; it seems to regenerate the beta cells in the pancreas and improves insulin secretion. It also increases the permeability of cells so that they absorb more insulin. In the November 1999 *Journal of Endocrinology*, School of BioMedical Sciences, King's College, London, researchers S. J. Persaud and P. M. Jones reported, "Results confirming the stimulatory effects of gymnema sylvestre on insulin release indicate that this herb acts by increasing cell permeability."

Native to India, its Hindi name *gurmar* means "sugar destroyer," and it has been used for the treatment of diabetes for more than 2,000 years in that part of the world. Research on gymnema goes back to the 1930s. In one study, a water-soluble extract of gymnema leaf was administrated to 27 Type-1 diabetics at a dose of 400 mg/day for approximately a year. The subjects' insulin requirements decreased by half. Average blood glucose dropped from 230 to 152 mg per milliliter. The HgbA1c levels decreased in the first six to eight months but still remained above normal. Decreases in the amounts of glycosylated proteins, cholesterol, and triglycerides were also noted.[169] In another study, gymnema extract doubled the number of islets and beta cells in the pancreas, which supports the theory that it increases the insulin secretion by creating a regeneration of the pancreas.[170]

Considered one of the most powerful herbs for improving blood sugar status, gymnema has been shown to help normalize blood sugar and triglycerides, reduce sugar cravings, and decrease insulin needs. Other research has found that this herb causes a reduction in the activities of enzymes that are normally increased in diabetes such as glycogen phosphorylase, glyconeogenic enzymes, and sorbitol dehydrogenase. The researchers also found that the glycogen depletion in the liver and lipid accumulation in diabetic animals was reversed. In another study of Type-2 diabetics, 22 were given this herbal extract along with their own oral hypoglycemic drugs. These people all had an improved blood sugar control. Twenty-one of the subjects were able to reduce their drug dosage significantly. Five were able to discontinue their medication and maintained blood sugar control with this herb alone.[171]

The average dose per day in many of these studies was 400 mg.

Curcumin (Turmeric)

Curcumin is a strong antioxidant and has been associated with treating complications in diabetes. It inhibits oxidation—an internal rusting— because it protects against free radicals that are caused by the cross-linkages and high sugar. So curcumin prevents free radical damage, reduces oxidative stress associated with diabetes, and helps to clean up metabolic waste.

Curcumin is a very good herb for the liver, which is affected by diabetes.

Fenugreek

Fenugreek has been studied in India for the treatment of Type-1 and Type-2 diabetes.[172, 173, 174, 175] Administration of 5 g of powdered fenugreek seed (as a 2.5-g capsule twice daily) resulted in significant lowering of blood glucose (fasting and postprandial) in non-insulin-dependent diabetics with and without coronary artery disease (CAD). In the diabetic patients with CAD, fenugreek also significantly lowered total cholesterol and triglyceride levels.[176] In another study, defatted fenugreek seed powder was given to insulin-dependent diabetes patients at 100 g daily in two divided doses over 10 days. The treated group exhibited a 54 percent decrease in 24-hour urine excretion of glucose, as well as a reduction in total cholesterol.[177] Fenugreek seeds are also 55 percent fiber, so they slow down the rapid absorption of glucose. Fenugreek normalizes glucose after meals and improves insulin response in the body, and it lowers total cholesterol and triglycerides.

Cinnamon

Cinnamon is a powerful herb for blood sugar control. Dr. Richard Anderson, in a study with the U.S. Department of Agriculture's Beltsville Human Nutrition Research Center, found that cinnamon can improve glucose metabolism in fat cells by 20-fold.[178] Of the 49 herbs, spices, and medicinal plant extracts they studied on glucose utilization, they found that cinnamon was the most bioactive.[179] Cinnamon has a key substance called methyl hydroxy chalcone polymer (MHCP) that stimulates glucose uptake. Scientists at Iowa State University determined the polyphenols polymers in cinnamon are able to up-regulate the expression of genes involved in activating the cell membrane's insulin receptors, thus increasing glucose uptake and lowering blood glucose levels.[180] So cinnamon improves glucose intake by the cells, increases the effectiveness of insulin, and also increases the antibacterial, antiviral, and antifungal processes. In a study published in *Diabetes Care*, cinnamon was found to simultaneously reduce triglyceride levels, LDL cholesterol, and total cholesterol. Participants in three groups consumed 1, 3, or 6 grams of cinnamon daily. All three levels of cinnamon reduced mean fasting serum glucose levels by 18–29 percent. The 1 g dose also reduced triglyceride levels by 18 percent, LDL cholesterol by 7 percent, and total cholesterol by 12 percent. Higher doses of cinnamon produced even greater reductions in triglycerides, LDL, and total cholesterol.[181]

To achieve therapeutic effects similar to those in these studies, you will need to eat ¼ to 1 full teaspoon of powdered cinnamon a day. This is easy to do with smoothies, teas, and nut and seed mylks.

Cayenne

Also known as the common chili pepper, this herb contains the element capsaicin, which alleviates nerve pain (neuropathy) associated with diabetes.

Holy Basil

Holy basil, known as the herb of Vishnu, is considered in India to be an adaptogen, improving immunity and generally strengthening the body. A significant placebo-controlled study published in the *Journal of Clinical Pharmacy and Therapeutics* showed a 17.6-percent reduction in blood sugar. It also normalizes triglyceride levels in the blood, lowers cholesterol, and decreases blood pressure and inflammation in mild to moderate cases of diabetes.

Parsley

Parsley is excellent for kidney support in diabetics.

Banaba

Banaba leaf, known for its high concentration of corosolic acid, acts as a natural insulin agent. In animal studies, extracts of this herb created a significant decrease in blood glucose. It balances the blood sugar, transports blood sugar into our cells, and reduces the conversion of blood sugar into fats. It helps with weight loss and to decrease triglyceride levels. This herb helps transport blood sugar into our body cells. It also helps control carbohydrate cravings.

Aside from the banaba leaf, corosolic acid is found in queen's crepe myrtle. It is a promising blood sugar regulating herb. Studies in Japan have suggested that corosolic acid is an activator of glucose transport and decreases blood sugar. In one American study with 10 Type-2 diabetics, the blood sugar dropped 31.9 percent after two weeks of 480 mcg of corosolic acid per day. Nondiabetics had no change in their blood sugar. Repeated studies have found approximately the same results.

Shilajit

> There is hardly any curable disease which cannot be controlled
> or cured with the aid of Shilajit.
>
> **Vaid Charak (first century CE)**

Shilajit in Sanskrit means "conqueror of mountains and destroyer of weakness." The herb comes from the rocks in the lower Himalayas and is the most important natural remedy of Ayurvedic medicine. Shilajit is an ancient herbomineral extract from the Himalayas; it improves glycogen stores in the liver and has been shown to help reduce sugar in the urine, promote regeneration of the pancreatic beta cells, and reduce oxidative stress. It is not that well known, but we have used it for mineral replacement. The active principle of shilajit is fulvic acid, which improves the bioavailability of important trace minerals, and there is some feeling that it creates regeneration in the pancreatic cells. It is known as an adaptogen and should be taken mostly during the winter.

Coccinia Indica

Coccinia indica seems to have a blood glucose lowering effect that operates on the same mechanism as bitter melon.[182, 183]

Gingko Biloba

Gingko biloba has membrane-stabilizing flavones and anthocyanins, which seem to protect against retinopathy.[184]

American Ginseng

A team of researchers at the University of Toronto medical facility at St. Michael's Hospital in Toronto used American ginseng (*Panax quin-quefolius*) in the treatment of Type-2 diabetes.[185] The authors in an earlier study showed that 3 grams of American ginseng, either with or 40 minutes before a 25 g oral glucose challenge, significantly reduced the blood glucose levels in Type-2 diabetes.[186]

Another study was done with 10 Type-2 diabetics—6 men and 4 women who had diabetes from 2 to 12 years. Seven were on antidiabetic drugs and three were on diet alone. Their average age was 63. The American ginseng showed a clear benefit, reducing the total postprandial glucose by 15–20 percent over the two-hour trial. All three dose levels used seemed to come out the same. A 3 g dose of American ginseng taken two hours before the glucose challenge is just as effective as a much higher dose (25 g), so we just need 3 g three times a day. Also, American ginseng is a very good general adaptogen.

Goat's Rue

In medieval Europe, goat's rue (*Galega officinalis*) was traditionally used as a treatment for diabetes. Goat's rue contains guanidine, the herbal prototype for the pharmaceutical drug Metformin, which improves insulin sensitivity and is used to treat both Type-1 and Type-2 diabetes. Metformin has been claimed to be one of the best antiaging drugs currently available. Goat's rue causes a long-lasting reduction of blood sugar in rats and an increase in carbohydrate tolerance. In one study, goat's rue extract lowered the blood sugar of diabetic rats by 32 percent.[187] Goat's rue extracts have increased glycogen levels in the liver and myocardium of both healthy and diabetic rabbits. In addition, this potent herb lowers blood sugar in both normal and diabetic humans.[188]

Pterocarpus

Pterocarpus marsupium balances glucose and lowers cholesterol. It was able to reverse the damage to pancreatic beta cells in different studies. This is quite impressive. Even more so, it also helps to counter the effect of insulin resistance, maintains blood sugar levels, restores insulin release from the pancreas, and in some cases, resulted in almost complete restoration of normal insulin secretion.

Bilberry

Bilberry (*Vaccinium myrtillus*) has a long history of being used as a treatment for diabetes. Bilberry fruit contains flavonoids known as anthocyanidins, plant pigments that have excellent antioxidant properties. They scavenge damaging particles in the body known as free radicals, helping to prevent or reverse damage to cells. Antioxidants have been shown to help prevent a number of long-term illnesses such as heart disease, cancer, and the eye disorder called *macular degeneration*. Bilberry also contains vitamin C, another antioxidant.

Anthocyanidins found in bilberry fruit may also be useful for people with vision problems. During World War II, British fighter pilots reported improved nighttime vision after eating bilberry jam. Bilberry has also been suggested as a treatment for retinopathy (damage to the retina) in diabetics because anthocyanins appear to help protect the retina. Bilberry has also been suggested as treatment to prevent cataracts.

Bilberry was also able to lower glucose by 26 percent in diabetic rats and lowered triglycerides by 39 percent.[189] Bilberry has also been found to stabilize collagen[190] and decrease capillary permeability.[191] Increased capillary permeability, resulting in retinal hemorrhage with resultant abnormal collagen repair, is an underlying cause of diabetic retinopathy. Bilberry can decrease abnormal collagen formation and capillary permeability, thus helping prevent retinopathy.[192] In another study, 54 diabetic patients were treated with 500–600 mg per day of an extract for 8 to 33 months. Almost total normalization of collagen polymers was achieved, as well as a 30 percent decrease in structural glycoprotein.[193]

Prepare bilberry tea as an infusion, using one teaspoon of dried berries in 1 cup of water. Drink 1 cup per day. For blood glucose control, make a tea from ⅔ cup of leaves in 2 cups of water boiled for 25 minutes, and drink 2 cups daily.

Milk Thistle

Milk thistle has been found to be beneficial in a wide range of liver disorders. Eighty-percent silymarin extracts of milk thistle (e.g., a 200 mg capsule of milk thistle with 160 mg of silymarin) have been found to have antioxidant and glucose-regulating properties. In a study at Monfalcone Hospital in Groiza, Italy, 60 insulin-dependent diabetics took either 600 mg of silymarin or a placebo for 12 months. After the first month, in which fasting glucose levels were elevated, fasting glucose declined by 9.5 percent and average daily glucose dropped 14.9

percent among the treated group. In addition, glucosuria (sugar in the urine), glycosylated hemoglobin levels, and insulin requirements declined significantly.[194]

Additional Supplements from the Program

Culture of Life Intenzymes

There is some suggestion that Culture of Life Intenzymes, and other high-potency proteolytic enzymes, create a lysis, or loosening or dissolution, of the fibrin plugs in the vascular system and help reverse the general fibrosis scarring that goes on in the body for this reason, as well as diminishing the periductal scarring and B-cell scarring in the pancreas. It helps specifically to decrease the inflammation in diabetes, particularly Type-1 but also Type-2, where the organs are inflamed and stressed and begin to scar. Its very positive overall effect in diabetes is to improve insulin production and excretion from the pancreas and reverse diabetes-caused ASCVD, kidney degeneration, and neuropathy. I believe it also prevents cross-linking going to polymerization.

Chlorogenic Acid

Chlorogenic acid is a very effective extract from raw green coffee beans. It specifically inhibits the enzyme glucose-6-phosphatase, which causes increased production of endogenous glucose and increases with age. I discuss this in detail in Chapter 5. G-6-p, produced in excess amounts, causes a rise in both FBS and postprandial blood sugar spikes. Chlorogenic acid also suppresses postmeal glucose surges by inhibiting alpha-glucosidase. This enzyme breaks apart complex sugars in the intestines into simple sugars for faster absorption. Chlorogenic acid also increases the signal protein for insulin receptors in the liver cells, which increase insulin sensitivity, thereby lowering blood sugar. Researchers have found that the plant extract of chlorogenic acid has been able to reduce fasting blood glucose by up to 15 percent. In one study on reducing postprandial spikes, after a 30-minute period, there was up to a 14 percent decrease in the spike. There was up to a 22 percent reduction in the glucose spike after one hour. This is significant because with age many people are subject to an ever-increasing rise in FBS and post-prandial glucose spikes.

I recommend taking this extract to minimize FBS as well as post-prandial glucose spikes. Between 400 and 1600 mg of the coffee bean extract seems to be sufficient taken 30 minutes before meals or before bedtime. The 400 mg dose has been shown to reduce blood sugar by up to 28 percent after 1 hour. My clinical experience has found it to be especially helpful in people who begin the CDDS in their 50s, as the excess production of glucose-6-phosphatase is specifically age related and increases with age. Because of this, our endogenous blood sugar increases with age, which is a practical explanation of why 27 percent of people 65 years and older have Type-2 diabetes.

Digestive Enzymes

Digestive enzymes, according to my theory, help slowly overcome the general enzyme deficiencies that are documented in diabetics. They do this by helping the body use less of its own enzyme power for digesting the foods, so that these enzymes, by the law of adaptive secretion of enzymes theorized by Dr. Howell, will build up the depleted levels of amylase, lipase, and proteases in the system. Sometimes diabetics suffer from gastric paresis, which is a slowing of the emptying of the stomach associated with poor digestion. The general trend is that most people older than 45 or 50 have a progressive weakening digestion and are therefore not able to properly assimilate the nutrition in their food. This is why I also suggest the use of HCl supplementation to assist in the digestion of protein, assimilation of minerals, and B-12. In other words, digestive enzymes on many levels provide a tonic effect on the overall healing energy and capacity of the organism.

Natural Cellular Defense (NCD)

Another important component of our supplement program is the use of NCD (natural cellular defense), a liquid purified form of natural zeolite that safely chelates out heavy metals. Heavy metals, pesticides, herbicides, and a total of 70,000 chemicals are used commercially in the United States, according to the EPA. Sixty-five thousand of these chemicals are considered hazardous to our health. The Environmental Defense Council reports that more than four billion pounds of toxic chemicals are released into the environment each year. Although there is not a lot of data available, it does suggest that the heavy metals, especially arsenic, mercury, cadmium and lead, interfere with the specific function of insulin and the insulin receptors. Others, like fluorine in our water and a variety of pesticides and herbicides, are metabolic poisons that may further derange the already deranged metabolism of diabetics.

Since approximately 80 percent of Type-2 diabetics are overweight and most of these toxins are stored in the fat tissues, as people begin to lose weight, these toxins are released into the bloodstream and lymph in higher concentrations. In my preliminary clinical research at the Tree of Life, I have been able to measure the incidence of 26 toxins, including heavy metals, depleted uranium, and a variety of pesticides and herbicides. Usually people have all 26 that we check for. University research has shown that NCD is effective for removing heavy metals; when I combine it with our green juice fasting I have found a powerful synergy that greatly accelerates the removable of toxins and thus optimizes our ability to rapidly bring diabetics back to a healthy physiology. There have been some reports that the NCD also helps to decrease elevated blood sugar by directly absorbing it in its metallic structure and carrying it out of the system.

Lifestyle Habits

Exercise

In the case of insulin resistant or Type-2 diabetes, exercising regularly can mean the difference between pharmaceutical dependence and drug-free blood sugar control. Diabetics who exercise experience many levels of improvement, including enhanced insulin sensitivity, and therefore have less need for injecting insulin, improved glucose tolerance, reduced total cholesterol and triglycerides with increased HDL levels, and improved weight loss. The Diabetes Prevention Program (DPP) study, conducted in the United States from 1997 to 2001, showed that participants who lost 5–10 percent of their body weight, kept the pounds off if they did about half an hour a day of moderate exercise, cutting their risk of developing diabetes by 58 percent.[195] Some research suggests that exercise increases the number of insulin receptors in IDDM.[196] Exercise seems to activate the GLUT-4 receptors, which help to bring glucose into the muscle cells and consequently decrease blood glucose.

In Type-1 diabetics, there needs to be a little bit of attention when exercising because exercise may create an immediate release of lactic acid and glucagons, which may increase the blood sugar level, especially for those whose blood sugar levels are above 250 mg. Another danger of exercise is that if you have very low glucose while on your insulin, your body may switch to fat to get energy, and this could result in an increase in ketones. For this reason, your blood sugar level should be checked before intense exercise. Another risk could be aggravating a cardiovascular condition, as well as ocular complications. Exercise in Type-2 diabetes usually lowers the blood glucose. For this reason, before intense exercise, Type-1 and Type-2 diabetics should take less insulin or less oral hypoglycemics. If these precautions are met, we strongly recommend moderate exercise for all diabetics.

The best exercise in general is jumping on a high-quality rebounder for up to 16 minutes a day, four to five times a week. Other cardiovascular exercises would include moderately fast walking, jogging, swimming, and so on. There is no need to make exercise a complicated procedure—find exercise that is enjoyable and that finds you feeling positively stimulated rather than exhausted.

Rebounding

Jumping on a rebounder, or minitrampoline, is possibly the best and most fun cardiovascular and lymphatic stimulating exercise, requiring the least amount of time of any exercise system. It is my favorite aerobic and lymphatic-stimulating exercise. It can be effective for a minimum of 16 to 23 minutes.

Muscle Building

When you consider that muscle tissue is responsible for 80 percent of blood sugar uptake following a meal, it is easy to understand why every bit of extra muscle helps. Another important benefit of muscle tissue is that, unlike fat tissue, it constantly uses energy. The more muscle tissue you have, the higher your metabolic rate will be, because while you burn a certain amount of calories during exercise, your muscle tissue will continue to burn calories hours after you exercise.[197]

Meditation and Prayer

My program also includes training in meditation, as stress has been distinctly related to an increase in blood sugar secondary to an increase in epinephrine and corticosteroid secretion, which leads to an increase in insulin resistance. The value of meditation and yoga have been shown in such well-known programs as that of Dr. Dean Ornish, in which they were able to reverse atherosclerosis, as well as the large body of research linking meditation to general improvement in health, vitality, and longevity. It is interesting to note that researchers at the Medical University of South Carolina found that people with diabetes who regularly attend religious services had lower levels of C-reactive protein (CRP), an inflammatory risk factor for cardiovascular disease, which is the leading cause of death among diabetics.[198] On a deeper level, it has been my consistent observation that those who have some sort of spiritual connection increase their ability to heal. There is never enough food for the hungry soul, and meditation and prayer feed the hungry soul. Meditation and prayer create a quiet mind, which help you love yourself enough to want to heal yourself.

Yoga

In addition to meditation, we also teach Kali Ray TriYoga™, which is good for decreasing physical and mental stress. All forms of yoga in general are good and have more uses than just cardiovascular exercise. Yoga is a total system that creates a flow of energy through the body, helps to heal the body, and stimulates the pancreas and other internal organs. Although there are certain traditional poses specifically associated with the healing of diabetes, I prefer a total TriYoga flow: not only does it include these diabetes-healing poses, but the flowing system creates an energy that has a greater overall healing effect. In general, almost all forms of yoga provide a helpful tonic for the stimulation and healing of the internal organs such as the pancreas, liver, kidneys, and adrenals. Practiced regularly, yoga can help regulate blood glucose levels, reduce stress-hormone levels, and help with weight control. Find a knowledgeable and experienced yoga teacher in your local area who feels comfortable using yoga as a means for supporting the healing of your diabetes.

Skin Care

The most important thing about skin care is to be very observant of the skin condition of your feet, as that is one of the first places where the diabetic process manifests deterioration.

Alan Dattner, MD, a holistic dermatologist based in New York City, recommends lotions that are high in omega-6 fatty acids, essential fats that diabetics don't produce well. Jeanette Jacqui, MD, a holistic dermatologist in Phoenix, Arizona, suggests avoiding glycolic acid and other strong fruit acids, as they are too harsh for the skin. Also too strong are alcohol, iodine, mercurochrome, salicylic acid, and benzoyl peroxide.[199]

Zero Point Process

One of the most important parts of the program is the Zero Point course, a psycho-spiritual four-day training that helps people let go of their dysfunctional eating and lifestyle habits and let go of their paradoxical desire and resistance to heal from diabetes and the Culture of Death, to which many diabetics, like the rest of our society, are addicted. This course also helps the diabetic let go of the allopathic myth that Type-1 and even Type-2 diabetes are not curable and are both the equivalents of a slow and steady downhill death march. During the course participants open up the doors to loving themselves in a deeper way, which of course helps to facilitate healing.

This course takes place in the second week of the 21-Day+ Program. In the Zero Point process, clients receive two of the most important gifts one can receive in any healing program: first, learning the ability to clear negative thought forms usually associated with the shadow of the Culture of Death, which leads to the second, allowing you to love yourself enough to want to heal yourself and activating your belief in your power to heal yourself. The Zero Point course has the potential, if the participant is so inclined, to enhance the depth of their particular spiritual life.

Conscious Eating

Internationally acclaimed as one of the most holistic, comprehensive live-food training programs in the world, the Conscious Eating course offers an amazingly thorough exploration of the intricacies of a plant-based lifestyle. It illuminates the powerful role that live food has in the enhancement of all levels of being. Physically, a diet comprised of plant-based, live foods is associated with the amelioration of many diseases, including diabetes, depression, cancer, heart disease, osteoporosis, arthritis, and more, as well as being a foundation for optimal health. Emotionally, embracing compassionate food choices is a profoundly powerful practice in promoting peace with the self and with the ecology of the planet. Spiritually, a diet of live plant foods supports our bodies and energies as superconductors for the Divine. Optimal health, longevity, vitality, and spiritual attunement are hallmarks of a live-food lifestyle.

In this eye-opening journey, your relationship with food will be fundamentally altered. The aim of the program is not only to educate about the benefits of a live, plant-based lifestyle, but also to train participants in all elements of meal preparation. This includes lectures on detoxification and how to individualize the diet and food prep demonstration from Tree of Life café chefs. Another unique feature of the

Conscious Eating Intensive is that it is one of the few low-glycemic live-food preparation course in the world, making the recipes particularly useful for those with the CDDS, prediabetes, diabetes, hypoglycemia, insulin resistance, candida, and other blood-sugar related health challenges. I experience eating a live cuisine as an act of love, an opportunity for creative expression, and a potent portal opening to the divine.

Chapter 4 Summary

The use of herbs, nutrients, and supplements is one of the ways to support and accelerate the overall return to a normal physiology from the degenerative aging process of diabetes. With all these helpful additions to the healing process it is important to remember that a Phase 1.0 antidiabetogenic moderate-low carbohydrate organic live-food diet is the foundation for successful healing. The foundation for reversing diabetes is turning on the antiaging genes and turning off the expression of the diabetogenic genes. This profoundly and positively affects the protein, lipid, and carbohydrate metabolism in diabetes. As one turns off the diabetogenic CDDS process and activates the healthy genes with the use of the Dr. Cousens's Diabetes Recovery Program—A Holistic Approach, one creates the conditions for a rapid reversal of the diabetogenic process. This is the central focus of my program: reactivating one's healthy genetics. This has been the source of the success in my program for reversing diabetes naturally. By its very nature, my program also helps those who are overweight to naturally and easily lose weight because eating a live-food diet enables us to eat half as much as one does on a nutrient-poor standard American diet. This live-food, moderate-low carbohydrate diet is not one of deprivation but one that is satisfying, pleasurable, and nutritionally nurturing to our senses, as well as to our body and mind. It brings in a tremendous amount of live enzymes and electrical energy that improves the functioning of all cellular activities in the system. It brings in phytonutrients that further activate the antiaging and antidiabetic genetic effect. Generally, it improves all aspects of health. This is the key to the program, and everything else supports this foundation.

Once people have reached a certain level of repair and have returned to a normal healthy, nondiabetic physiology, they do not need to use all these herbs and supplements. One can move from a Phase 1.0 to a Phase 1.5 diet that includes a modest amount of low glycemic fruits, beans, and grains. I like them to sustain a nondiabetic physiology for at least three to six months before making the switch to Phase 1.5.

The delicious Dr. Cousens's Diabetes Recovery Program—A Holistic Approach antidiabetogenic cuisine at Phase 1.5 is, however, what we will always need to eat in order to maintain a healthy phenotypic expression and live a new whole way that prevents the onset of not only diabetes but chronic disease in general. This is a cuisine that inherently creates a healthy body, mind, and joyous spirit. The Culture of Life plant-source-only, 80-percent raw, moderate low-carbohydrate food diet is the primary foundation of the healing and maintenance program, and the herbs and supplements are secondary foundations that accelerate and support the healing.

A most important key to the success of the program is its sustainability. My clinical results with the use of live foods and green juice fasting leave no doubt that one can rapidly and safely take people off insulin and oral hypoglycemics with very rapid returns to a healthy FBS and a nondiabetic physiology. The key question that remains is the sustainability of living in the diet and lifestyle of the Culture of Life and not being swallowed again by the shadow of the Culture of Death, which is the predominant culture in the world today. It is this shadow of the Culture of Death in which diabetes is a pandemic symptom and our primary challenge here. The very life of the planet is at stake, but the world has been in denial. To a reasonable and scientific person it is apparent that a "moderate" solution takes us deeper into the shadow because it creates the feeling that we are doing something to significantly change what is happening, while in fact we are only dipping our toes in the water and calling it a bath.

One advantage of my program is its rapid results, which make the point clearly that something can be immediately done to reverse the diabetic physiology back to normal. The power of the immediate results is overwhelming. This is not a compromised or "moderate" approach that slows the march to diabetic death. My observation is that it takes about two years to become firmly rooted in this Dr. Cousens's Diabetes Recovery Program—A Holistic Approach lifestyle. Included in my program is a monthly follow-up with a variety of support systems including my monthly online diabetes support webinar. A key understanding is the teaching that what the Culture of Death euphemistically calls "moderation" actually kills. Moderation in this context kills because it reactivates the death sentence. There is an old Chinese saying that if you do not change the way you are going you will end up in the direction you are going. Moderation in this context does not change the way one is going. This is why the ADA and most doctors say that diabetes is not curable or reversible because they are prescribing moderation, which simply does not work by their own admission. In this context, it is actually a path of immoderation.

The approach I am offering is straightforward and one that brings immediate results. It succeeds in changing the way you are going and has the potential to save your life. That is true moderation: acknowledging the truth of a situation and doing what is appropriate to heal the situation. It is not living in the shadow of death and denial, which we euphemistically call "moderation," to give ourselves the illusionary warm, fuzzy feeling that we are acting reasonably.

I believe that the ultimate long-term success of the program depends on the support system created through the Zero Point course, the new dietary training, and the one-year follow-up, optional continuing support, and people loving themselves enough to heal themselves.

In the third week of the program, there is training in how to prepare Phase 1.0, plant-source-only, 80–100 percent live foods. This is a six-day course in which we like to include the family members. The focus is to empower people in the fundamentals of the Phase 1.0 and Phase 1.5 live-food plant-source-only cuisine. This will be covered in depth in the recipe section of this book.

For those who need ongoing work on losing weight, I recommend a 100 percent live-food program that can be continued at home until a client's weight returns to a normal healthy weight. The average weight loss is approximately 100 pounds yearly on a 100 percent live-food diet for people who are more than 100 pounds overweight.

In Chapter 6, I will cover in more detail the stabilizing and sustaining part of our program—helping people to fully integrate the Culture of Life into their personal lives at home. The happy continuation of this work goes on for one year with monthly check-ins to support people in staying in and celebrating this new lifestyle. It is during this time that we get HgbA1c readings every three months and create the time and space for people to stabilize their newfound healthy and joyous physiology. I do not really consider that a person is healed from the consciousness and physiology of diabetes until he or she has had two consecutive HgbA1c tests with results in the normal range of 5.7 or less and has a regular FBS less than 100 and optimally equal to or less than 85 regularly, without the use of any traditional diabetic medications.

Notes

1. Considine, R V, Sinha, M K, Heiman, M L, et al. "Serum immunoreactive-leptin concentrations in normal-weight and obese humans." *New Eng J Med*, 1996, 334: 292–95.

2. Spiller, G A, Jensen, C D, Pattison, T S, et al. "Effect of protein dose on serum glucose and insulin response to sugars." *Amer J Clin Nutr*, 1987, 46: 474–80.

3. Bland, J. *Genetic Nutritioneering*. Lincolnwood, IL: Keats, 1999.

4. Franz, M J. "Protein: Metabolism and effect on blood glucose levels." *Diabetes Education*, 1992, 18: 1–29.

5. Block, G. "Dietary guidelines and the results of food consumption surveys." *Amer J Clin Nutr*, 1991, 53: 56S–57S.

6. Xu, Y X, Pindolia, K R, Janakiraman, N, et. al. "Curcumin, a compound with anti inflammatory and antioxidant properties, down regulates chemokine expression in bone marrow stromal cells." *Exper Hematology*, 1997, 25: 413–22.

7. Finch, C E, and Tanzi, R E. "Genetics of aging." *Science*, October 17, 1997, 278(5337): 407–11.

8. Barclay, L. "Growing evidence links resveratrol to extended life span." *Life Extension*, Spring 2007, pp. 33–40.

9. Heilbronn, L K, de Jonge, L, Frisard, M I, et al. "Effect of 6 month calorie restriction on biomarkers of longevity, metabolic adaptation, and oxidative stress in overweight individuals: A randomized controlled trial." *JAMA*, April 5, 2006, 295(13): 1539–48.

10. Kulvinskas, V. *Survival into the 21st Century*. Woodstock Valley, CN: Twenty-First Century Publications, 1975.

11. Howell, E. *Food Enzymes for Health and Longevity*. Woodstock Valley, CN: Omangod Press, 1946.

12. Lee, C, Klopp, R, Weindruch, R, and Prolla, T. "Gene expression profile of aging and its retardation by caloric restriction." *Science*, 1999, 285(5432): 1390–93.

13. Kramer, P. "Health and longevity: What centenarians can teach us." *Yoga Journal*, September/October 1983, pp. 26–30.

14. Cao, S X, Dhahbi, J M, Mote, P L, and Spindler, S R. "Genomic profiling of short- and long-term caloric restriction effects in the liver of aging mice." *Proc Natl Academy of Sciences*, 98(19): 10630–35. Cited in Fahy, G, and Kent, S. "Reversing aging rapidly with short-term calorie restriction." *Life Extension*, May 2001.

15. Grundy, S M, et al. "Implications of recent clinical trials for the National Cholesterol Education Program Adult Treatment Panel III Guidelines." *Circulation*, 2004, 110: 227–39.

16. Pradhan A D. "C-reactive protein, interleukin 6, and risk of developing type 2 diabetes mellitus." *JAMA*, 2001, 286: 327–34.

17. Lopez-Garcia, E. "Consumption of trans fatty acids is related to plasma biomarkers of inflammation and endothelial dysfunction." *J Nutrition*, 2005, 135(3): 562–66.

18. Shaw Dunn, J, Sheehan, H L, and McLetchie, N G B. "Necrosis of the islets of Langerhans produced experimentally." *The Lancet*, 1943, 244: 484–87.

19. Braly, J, and Hoggan, R. *Dangerous Grains*. New York: Penguin Putnam, 2002, p. 126.

20. Berger, S. *Dr. Berger's Immune Power Diet*. New York: New American Library, 1986.

21. Daniel, K T. *The Whole Soy Story*. http://www.wholesoystory.com.

22. Ibid.

23. Casanova, M, et al. "Developmental effects of dietary phytoestrogens in Sprague: Dawley rats and interactions of genistein and daidzein with rat estrogen receptors alpha and beta in vitro." *Toxicol Sci*, October 1999, 51(2): 236–44.

24. Santell, L, et al. "Dietary genistein exerts estrogenic effects upon the uterus, mammary gland and the hypothalamic/pituitary axis in rats." *J Nutr*, February 1997, 127(2): 263–69.

25. Harrison, R M, et al. "Effect of genistein on steroid hormone production in the pregnant rhesus monkey." *Proc Soc Exp Biol Med*, October 1999, 222(1): 78–84.

26. Divi, R L, Chang, H C, and Doerge, D R. "Identification, characterization and mechanisms of anti-thyroid activity of isoflavones from soybeans." *Biochem Pharmacol*, 1997, 54: 1087–96.

27. Fort, P, Moses, N, Fasano, M, Goldberg, T, and Lifshitz, F. "Breast and soy formula feedings in early infancy and the prevalence of autoimmune disease in children." *J Am Coll Nutr*, 1990, 9: 164–65.

28. Setchell, K D R, Zimmer-Nechemias, L, Cai, J, and Heubi, J E. "Exposure of infants to phytoestrogens from soy based infant formula." *The Lancet*, 1997, 350: 23–27.

29. Ashton, E, and Ball, M. "Effects of soy as tofu vs. meat on lipoprotein concentrations." *Eur J Clin Nutr*, January 2000, 54(1): 14–19.

30. Madani, S, et al. "Dietary protein level and origin (casein and highly purified soybean protein) affect hepatic storage, plasma lipid transport, and antioxidative defense status in the rat." *Nutrition*, May 2000, 16(5): 368–75.

31. White, L R, Petrovich, H, Ross, G W, and Masaki, K H. "Association of mid-life consumption of tofu with late life cognitive impairment and dementia: The Honolulu-Asia Aging Study." Presented at the Fifth International Conference on Alzheimer's Disease, July 27, 1996 (Osaka, Japan).

32. White, L R, Petrovitch, H, Ross, G W, Masaki, K H, Hardman. J, Nelson. J, Davis. D, and Markesbery, W. "Brain aging and midlife tofu consumption." *J Am Coll Nutr*, April 2000, 19(2): 242–55.

33. Nagata, C, et al. "Inverse association of soy product intake with serum androgen and estrogen in Japanese men." *Nutr Cancer*, 2000, 36(1): 14–18.

34. Zhong, Ying, et al. "Effects of dietary supplement of soy protein isolate and low fat diet on prostate cancer." *FASEB J*, 2000, 14(4): a531.11.

35. Rapp, D J. *Is This Your Child's World?* New York: Bantam Books, 1996, p. 501.

36. Irvine, C H G, Fitzpatrick, M G, and Alexander, S L. "Phytoestrogens in soy based infant foods: Concentrations, daily intake and possible biological effects." *Proc Soc Exp Biol Med*, 1998, 217: 247–53.

37. Levy, J R, Faber, F A, Ayyash, L, and Hughes, C L. "The effect of prenatal exposure to phytoestrogens genistein on sexual differentiation in rats." *Proc Soc Exp Biol Med*, 1995, 208: 60–66.

38. Daniel. *The Whole Soy Story.*

39. "Soy infant formula could be harmful to infants: Groups want it pulled." *Nutrition Week*, December 10, 1999, 29(46).

40. Setchell, Zimmer-Nechemias, Cai, et al. "Exposure of infants to phytoestrogens."

41. Cassidy, A, Bingham, S, and Setchell, K D. "Biological effects of a diet of soy protein rich in isoflavones on the menstrual cycle of premenopausal women." *Am J Clin Nutr*, September 1994, 60(3): 333–40.

42. Arjmandi, B H, Khalil, D A, Smith, B J, Lucas, E A, Juma, S, Payton, M E, and Wild, R A. "Soy protein has a greater effect on bone in postmenopausal women not on hormone replacement therapy, as evidenced by reducing bone resorption and urinary calcium excretion." *J Clin Endocrinol Metab*, March 2003, 88(3): 1048–54.

43. Yu, H. "Role of the insulin-like growth factor family in cancer development and progression." *J Natl Cancer Inst*, September 20, 2000, 92(18): 1472–89.

44. Ikonomidou, C, and Turski, L. "Glutamate in neurode generative disorders." In *Neurotransmitters and Neuromodulators: Glutamate*, edited by T W Stone, 253–72. Boca Raton: CRC Press, 1995.

45. Blaylock, R. *Excitotoxins: The Taste That Kills*. Santa Fe, NM: Health Press, 1997.

46. Whetsell, W O, and Shapira, N A. "Biology of disease. Neuroexcitation, excitotoxicity, and human neurological disease." *Lab Invest*, 1993, 68: 372–87.

47. Kalaria, R N, and Harik, S I. "Reduced glucose transporter at the blood-brain barrier and in the cerebral cortex in Alzheimer's disease." *J Neurochem*, 1989, 53: 1083–88.

48. Gold, M D. "The bitter truth about artificial sweeteners." http://www.curezone.com/foods/aspartame.html.

49. Kataya, H A H, and Hamza, A A. "Red cabbage (*Brassica oleracea*) ameliorates diabetic nephropathy in rats." *Evidence Based Complementary and Alternative Medicine*. http://www.ncbi.nlm.nih.gov/pmc/articles/PMC2529380.

50. Welihinda, J, Arvidson, G, Gylfe, E, et al. "The insulin-releasing activity of the tropical plant Momordica charantia." *Acta Bio Med Germ*, 1982, 41: 1229–40.

51. Welihinda, J, Karunanaya, E H, Sheriff, M H R, and Jayasinghe, K S A. "Effect of Momordica charantia on the glucose tolerance in maturity onset diabetes." *J Ethnopharmacol*, 1986, 17: 277–82.

52. Srivastava, Y, Venkatakrishna-Bhatt, H, Verma, Y, et al. "Antidiabetic and adaptogenic properties of Momordica charantia extract: An experimental and clinical evaluation." *Phytotherapy Res*, 1993, 7: 285–89.

53. Welihinda, Karunanaya, Sheriff, et al. "Effect of Momordica charantia."

54. Srivastava, Venkatakrishna-Bhatt, Verma, et al. "Antidiabetic and adaptogenic properties of Momordica charantia."

55. Frati, A C, Jimenez, E, and Ariza, R C. "Hypogylcemic effect of *Opuntia ficus indica* in non insulin-dependent diabetes mellitus patients." *Phytother Res*, 1990, 4: 195–97.

56. Trejo-Gonzales, A, Gabriel Ortiz, G, Puebla-Perez, A M, et al. "A purified extract from prickly pear cactus (*Opuntia fulignosa*) controls experimentally induced diabetes in rats." *J Ethnopharm*, 1996, 55: 27–33.

57. Sheela, C G, and Augusti, K T. "Antidiabetic effects of S-allyl cysteine sulphoxide isolated from garlic Allium sativum Linn." *Ind J Exper Biol*, 1992, 30: 523–26.

58. Sharma, K K, et al. "Antihyperglycemic effect on onion: Effect on fasting blood sugar and induced hyperglycemia in man." *Ind J Med Res*, 1977, 65: 422–29.

59. Hu, F B, and Stampfer, M J. "Nut consumption and risk of coronary heart disease: A review of epidemiologic evidence." *Curr Atheroscler Rep*, 1999, 1(3): 204–9.

60. Kris-Etherton, P M, Yu-Poth, S, Sabate, J, Ratcliffe, H E, Zhao, G, and Etherton, T D. "Nuts and their bioactive constituents: Effects on serum lipids and other factors that affect disease risk." *Am J Clin Nutr*, 1999, 70(3 suppl.): 504S–511S.

61. Rivellese, A A, and Lilli, S. "Quality of dietary fatty acids, insulin sensitivity and Type-2 diabetes." *Biomed Pharmacother*, March 2003, 57(2): 84–87.

62. Berger, A, Jones, P J, and Abumweis, S S. "Plant sterols: Factors affecting their efficacy and safety as functional food ingredients." *Lipids Health Dis*, 2004, 3(1): 5.

63. Katan, M B, Grundy, S M, Jones, P, Law, M, Miettinen, T, and Paoletti, R. "Efficacy and safety of plant stanols and sterols in the management of blood cholesterol levels." *Mayo Clin Proc*, 2003, 78(8): 965–78.

64. Nissinen, M, Gylling, H, Vuoristo, M, and Miettinen, T A. "Micellar distribution of cholesterol and phytosterols after duodenal plant stanol ester infusion." *Am J Physiol Gastrointest Liver Physiol*, 2002, 282(6): G1009–15.

65. Guixiang, Z, Etherton, T D, Martin, K R, West, S G, Gillies, P J, and Kris-Etherton, P M. "Dietary-linolenic acid reduces inflammatory and lipid cardiovascular risk factors in hypercholesterolemic men and women." *Amer Soc for Nutr Sci J Nutr*, November 2004, 134: 2991–97.

66. Sabate, J, Fraser, G E, Burke, K, Knutsen, S, Bennett, H, and Lindsted, K D. "Effects of walnuts on serum lipid levels and blood pressure in normal men." *N Engl J Med*, 1993, 328: 603–7.

67. *Stroke*, 1993, 26: 778–82. These results were first published in *The Lancet* in 1994 (343: 1454–59) and then subsequently in other reputable journals, such as *Preventative Medicine* (28: 333–39), *American Journal of Clinical Nutrition* (74: 72–79), and *Annals of Internal Medicine* (132[7]: 538–46).

68. World's Healthiest Foods. "Walnuts." http://www.whfoods.com/genpage .php?tname=foodspice&dbid=99.

69. Ros, E, Nunez, I, Perez-Heras, A, Serra, M, Gilabert, R, Casals, E, and Deulofeu, R. "A walnut diet improves endothelial function in hypercholesterolemic subjects: A randomized crossover trial." *Circulation*, 2004 109: 1609–14.

70. Abbey, M, Noakes, M, Belling, G B, and Nestel, P J. "Partial replacement of saturated fatty acids with almonds or walnuts lowers total plasma cholesterol and low-density-lipoprotein cholesterol." *Am J Clin Nutr*, 1994, 59: 995–99.

71. Iwamoto, M, Sato, M, Kono, M, Hirooka, Y, Sakai, K, Takeshita, A, and Imaizumi, K. "Walnuts lower serum cholesterol in Japanese men and women." *J Nutr*, 2000, 130: 171–76.

72. Lavedrine, F, Zmirou, D, Ravel, A, Balducci, F, and Alary, J. "Blood cholesterol and walnut consumption: A cross-sectional survey in France." *Prev Med*, 1999, 28: 333–39.

73. Lovejoy, J C, Most, M M, Lefevre, M, Greenway, FL, and Rood, J C. "Effects of diets enriched in almonds on insulin action and serum lipids in adults with normal glucose tolerance in type 2 diabetes." *Am J Clin Nutr*, 2002, 76: 1000–1006.

74. *J Medical Hypothesis*, 2005, 65: 953.

75. Keen, H, Payan, J, Allawi, J, et al. "Treatment of diabetic neuropathy with gamma-linoleic acid." The Gamma Linoleic Acid Multicenter Trial Group. *Diabetes Care*, 1993, 16: 8–15.

76. Schwartz, et al. "Inhibition of experimental oral carcinogenesis by topical beta carotene." Harvard School of Dental Medicine. *Carcinogenesis*, 1986, 7(5): 711–15.

77. Annapurna, V, et al. "Bioavailability of Spirulina carotenes in preschool children." National Institute of Nutrition, Hyderabad, India. *J Clin Biochem Nutrition*, 1991, 10: 145–51.

78. Oviedo, et al. "Hypoglycaemic action of Stevia rebaudiana Bertoni (Kaa-he-e)." *Exerpta Medica* (International Congress Series), 1971, 208–92.

79. Suzuki, H, Kasai, T, Sumihara, M, and Suginawa, H. "Influence of the oral administration of stevioside on the levels of blood glucose and liver glycogen in intact rats." *Nogyo Kagaku Zasshi*, 1977, 51(3): 45.

80. Ishii, E L, Schwab, A J, and Bracht, A. "Inhibition of monosaccharide transport in the intact rat liver by stevioside." *Biochem Pharmacology*, 1987, 36(9): 1417–33.

81. Alvarez, et al. "Effect of aqueous extract of Stevia rebaudiana Bertone on biochemical parameters of normal adult persons." *Brazilian J Med Biol Res*, 1986, 19: 771–74.

82. Boeckh, E A. "Stevia rebaudiana (Bert.) Bertoni: Clinical evaluation of its acute action on cardio-circulatory, metabolic and electrolytic parameters in 60 healthy individuals." *Third Brazilian Seminar on Stevia Rebaudiana (Bert.)*, July 1986, pp. 22–23.

83. Lazarow, A, Liambies, J, and Tausch, A J. "Protection against diabetes with nicotinamide." *J Lab Clin Med*, 1950, 36: 249–58.

84. Mendola, G, Casamitjana, R, and Gomis, R. "Effect of nicotinamide therapy upon B-cell function in newly diagnosed type 1 (insulin-dependent) diabetic patients." *Diabetologia*, 1989, 32: 160–62.

85. Elliott, R B, and Chase, H P. "Prevention or delay of type 1 (insulin-dependent) diabetes mellitus in children using nicotinamide." *Diabetologia*, May 1991, 34(5): 362–65.

86. Andersen, H U, et al. "Nicotinamide prevents interleukin-1 effects on accumulated insulin release and nitric oxide production in rat islets of langerhans." *Diabetes*, 1994, 43: 770–77.

87. Bingley, P J, Caldas, G, Bonfanti, R, and Gale, E A. "Nicotinamide and insulin secretion in normal subjects." *Diabetologia*, July 1993, 36(7): 675–77.

88. Karjalainen, J, Martin, J, Knip, M, et al. "A bovine albumin peptide as a possible trigger of insulin-dependent diabetes." *N Eng J Med*, 1992, 327: 302–7.

89. Gale, E A. "Theory and practice of nicotinamide trials in pre-Type-1 diabetes." *J Pediatr Endocrinol Metab*, 1996, 9: 375–79.

90. Cleary, J P. "Vitamin B3 in the treatment of diabetes mellitus: Case reports and review of the literature." *J Nutr Med*, 1990, 1: 217–25.

91. Murray, M. *How to Prevent and Treat Diabetes with Natural Medicine.* New York: Riverhead Books, 2003, p. 176.

92. Jones, C L, and Gonzalez, V. "Pyridoxine deficiency: A new factor in diabetic neuropathy." *J Am Pod Assoc*, 1978, 68: 646–53.

93. Solomon, L R, and Cohen, K. "Erythrocyte O2 transport and metabolism and effects on vitamin B-6 therapy in type-2 diabetes mellitus." *Diabetes*, 1989, 38: 881–86.

94. Coelingh-Bennick, H J T, and Schreurs, W H P. "Improvement of oral glucose tolerance in gestational diabetes." *BMJ*, 1975, 3: 13–15.

95. Takahishi, Y, Takayama, S, Itou, T, Owada, K, and Omori, Y. "Effect of glycemic control on vitamin B12 metabolism in diabetes mellitus." *Diabetes Res and Clin Practice*, 1994, 25: 13–17.

96. Zhang, H, Osada, K, Sone, H, and Furukawa, Y. "Biotin administration improves the impaired glucose tolerance of streptozotocininduced diabetic Wistar rats." *J Nutr Sci Vitaminol* (Tokyo), 1997, 43(3): 271–80.

97. Maebashi, M, Makino, Y, Furukawa, Y, Ohinata, K, Kimura, S, and Sato, T. "Therapeutic evaluation of the effect of biotin on hyperglycemia in patients with non-insulin dependent diabetes mellitus." *J Clin Biochem Nutr*, 1993, 14: 211–18.

98. Coggeshall, J C, Heggers, J P, Robson, M C, and Baker, H. "Biotin status and plasma glucose levels in diabetics." *Ann NY Acad Sci*, 1985, 447: 389–92.

99. Romero-Navarro, G, Cabrera-Valladares, G, German, M S, et al. "Biotin regulation of pancreatic glucokinase and insulin in primary cultured rat islets and in biotin-deficient rats." *Endocrinology*, 1999, 140(10): 4595–600.

100. Murray, M, and Pizzorno, J. *Encyclopedia of Natural Medicine.* Rocklin, CA: Prima, 1998.

101. Coggeshall, Heggers, Robson, et al. "Biotin status and plasma glucose levels."

102. Cunningham, J. "Reduced mononuclear leukocyte ascorbic acid content in adults with insulin-dependent diabetes mellitus consuming adequate dietary vitamin C." *Metabolism*, 1991, 40: 146–49.

103. Davie, S J, Gould, B J, and Yudkin, J S. "Effect of vitamin C on glycosylation of proteins." *Diabetes*, 1992, 41: 167–73.

104. Vinson, J A, et al. "In vitro and in vivo reduction of erythrocyte sorbitol by ascorbic acid." *Diabetes*, 1989, 38: 1036–41.

105. Cunningham, J J, Mearkle, P L, and Brown, R G. "Vitamin C: An aldose reductase inhibitor that normalizes erythrocyte sorbitol in insulin-dependent diabetes mellitus." *J Am Coll Nutr*, 1994, 4: 344–50.

106. Hobday, R. *The Healing Sun*. Scotland: Findhorn Press, 1999, p. 78.

107. Need, A G, et al. "Relationship between fasting serum glucose, age, body mass index and serum 25 hydroxyvitamin D in postmenopausal women." *Clin Endocrinol*, 2005, 62(6): 738–41.

108. Feskanich, D, Ma, J, Fuchs, C S, Kirkner, G J, Hankinson, S E, Hollis, B W, and Giovannucci, E L. "Plasma vitamin D metabolites and risk of colorectal cancer in women." *Cancer Epidemiol Biomarkers Prev*, 2004, 13: 1502–8.

109. *Alternatives for the Health Conscious Individual*, April 2007, 169: 176.

110. Fontana, L, et al. "Low bone mass in subjects on a long-term raw vegetarian diet." *Arch Intern Med*, 2005, 165: 684–89.

111. *Alternatives for the Health Conscious Individual*, April 2007, 169: 172.

112. Paolisso, G, et al. "Daily vitamin E supplements improve metabolic control but not insulin secretion in elderly Type-2 diabetic patients." *Diabetes Care*, 1993, 16: 1433–37.

113. Davi, G, Ciabattoni, G, Consoli, A, et al. "In vivo formation of 8-iso-prostaglandin f2alpha and platelet activation in diabetes mellitus: Effects of improved metabolic control and vitamin E supplementation." *Circulation*, 1999, 99(2): 224–29.

114. Jain, S K, McVie, R, Jaramillo, J J, Palmer, M, and Smith, T. "Effect of modest vitamin E supplementation on blood glycated hemoglobin and triglyceride levels and red cell indices in type I diabetic patients." *J Am Coll Nutr*, 1996, 15(5): 458–61.

115. *Vitamin Research News*, April 2000, footnote 30.

116. Salonen, J T, et al. "Increased risk of non-insulin diabetes mellitus at low plasma vitamin E concentrations: A four-year follow-up study in men." *BMJ*, 1995, 311: 1124–27.

117. Cody, V, Middleton, E, and Harborne, J B. *Plant Flavonoids in Biology and Medicine—Biochemical, Pharmacological, and Structure-Activity Relationships*. New York: Alan R Liss, 1986.

118. Cody, V, Middleton, E, Harborne, J B, and Beretz, A. *Plant Flavonoids in Biology and Medicine—Biochemical, Pharmacological, and Structure-Activity Relationships. Volume II*. New York: Alan R Liss, 1988.

119. Chaudhry, P S, Cabera, J, Hector, R, et al. "Inhibition of human lens aldose reductase by flavonoids, sulindac, and indomethacin." *Biochem Pharmacol*, July 1, 1983, 32(13): 1995–98.

120. Varma, S D, Schocket, S S, and Richards, R D. "Implications of aldose reductase in cataracts in human diabetes." *Invest Ophthalmol Vis Sci*, 1979, 18: 237–41.

121. Varma, S D, Mizuno, A, and Kinoshita, J H. "Diabetic cataracts and flavonoids." *Science*, 1977, 195: 205–6.

122. Nakai, N, Fujii, Y, Kobashi, K, and Nomura, K. "Aldose reductase inhibitors: Flavonoids, alkaloids, acetophenones, benzophenones, and spirohydantoins of chroman." *Arch Biochem Biophys*, 1985, 239: 491–96.

123. Varma, D. "Inhibition of aldose reductase by flavonoids: Possible attenuation of diabetic complications." *Prog Clin Biol Res*, 1986, 213: 343–58.

124. Kuhnau, J. "The flavonoids: A class of semi-essential food components: Their role in human nutrition." *Wld Rev Nutr Diet*, 1976, 24: 117–91.

125. Keen, Payan, Allawi, et al. "Treatment of diabetic neuropathy with gamma-linoleic acid."

126. Fuller, C J, Chandalia, M, Garg, A, et al. "RRR-alpha-tocopheryl acetate supplementation at pharmacologic doses decreases low-density lipoprotein oxidative susceptibility but not protein glycation in patients with diabetes mellitus." *Am J Clin Nutr*, 1996, 63: 753–59.

127. Packer, L, Witt, E H, and Tritschler, H J. "Alpha-lipoic acid as a biological antioxidant." *Free Radic Biol Med*, 1995, 19: 227–50.

128. Estrada, D E, Ewart, H S, Tsakiridis, T, et al. "Stimulation of glucose uptake by the natural coenzyme alpha lipoic acid/thioctic acid: Participation of elements of the insulin signaling pathway." *Diabetes*, 1996, 45: 1798–1804.

129. Packer, L. "Antioxidant properties of lipoic acid and its therapeutic effects in prevention of diabetes complications and cataracts." *Ann N Y Acad Sci*, 1994, 738: 257–64.

130. Nagamatsu, M, et al. "Lipoic acid improves nerve blood flow, reduces oxidative stress, and improves distal nerve conduction in experimental diabetic neuropathy." *Diabetes Care*, 1995, 18: 1160–67.

131. Jacob, S, et al. "Enhancement of glucose disposal in patients with Type-2 diabetes by alpha-lipoic acid." *Arzneim Forsch*, 1995, 45: 872–74.

132. Kawabata, T, and Packer, L. "Alpha-lipoate can protect against glycation of serum albumin, but not low-density lipoprotein." *Biochem Biophys Res Commun*, 1994, 203: 99–104.

133. Suzuki, Y J, Tsuchiya, M, and Packer, L. "Lipoate prevents glucose induced protein modifications." *Free Rad Res Commun*, 1992, 17: 211–17.

134. Jacob, S, Ruus, P, Hermann, R, et al. "Oral administration of RACalpha lipoic acid modulates insulin sensitivity in patients with Type-2 diabetes mellitus: A placebo controlled pilot trial." *Free Radic Biol Med*, August 1999, 27(3–4): 309–14.

135. Houtsmuller, A J, van Hal-Ferwerba, J, Zahn, K J, and Henkes, H E. "Favorable influences of linoleic acid on the progression of diabetic micro and macroangiopathy." *Nutr Metab*, 1980, 24: S105–S118.

136. Lubec, B, Hayn, M, Kitzmuller, I, Vierhapper, H, and Lubec, G. "L-arginine reduces lipid peroxidation in patients with diabetes mellitus." *Free Radical Biol & Med*, 1997, 22: 355–57.

137. Bosia, S, Burdino, E, Grignola, F, and Ugazio, G. "Protective effect on nephropathy and on cataract in the streptozotocin-diabetic rat of the vanadium-lazaroid combination." *G Ital Med Lav*, 1995, 17: 71–75.

138. Shamberger, R J. "The insulin-like effects of vanadium." *J Adv Med*, 1996, 9: 121–31.

139. Tosiello, L. "Hypomagnesemia and diabetes mellitus. A review of clinical implications." *Arch Intern Med*, 1996, 156(11): 1143–48.

140. White, J R, and Campbell, R K. "Magnesium and diabetes: A review." *Ann Pharmacother*, 1993, 27: 775–80.

141. Nadler, J L, Buchanan, T, Natarajan, R, et al. "Magnesium deficiency produces insulin resistance and increased thromboxane synthesis." *Hypertension*, 1993, 21: 1024–29.

142. Humphries, S, Kushner, H, and Falkner, B. "Low dietary magnesium is associated with insulin resistance in a sample of young, nondiabetic Black Americans." *Am J Hypertens*, 1999, 12: 747–56.

143. Paolisso, G, Sgambato, S, Gambardella, A, et al. "Daily magnesium supplements improve glucose handling in elderly subjects." *Am J Clin Nutr*, 1992, 55(6): 1161–67.

144. Van Dam, R M, et al. "Dietary calcium and magnesium, major food sources, and risk of Type 2 diabetes in U.S. black women." *Diabetes Care*, 2006, 29: 2238–43.

145. Song, Y, Ridker, P M, Manson, J E, Cook, N R, Buring, J E, and Liu, S. "Magnesium intake, C-reactive protein, and the prevalence of metabolic syndrome in middle-aged and older U.S. women." *Diabetes Care*, 2005, 28: 1438–44.

146. Klatz, R, and Goldman, R. *Stopping the Clock*. New Canaan, CN: Keats Publishing, 1996, p. 129.

147. Chausmer, A B. "Zinc, insulin and diabetes." *J Am Coll Nutr*, April 1998, 17(2): 109–15.

148. Blostein-Fujii, A, DiSilvestro, R A, Frid, D, Katz, C, and Malarkey, W. "Short-term zinc supplementation in women with non-insulindependent diabetes mellitus: Effects on plasma 5'-nucleotidase activities, insulin-like growth factor I concentrations, and lipoprotein oxidation rates in vitro." *Am J Clin Nutr*, 1997, 66(3): 639–42.

149. Hegazi, S M, et al. "Effect of zinc supplementation on serum glucose, insulin, glucagon, glucose-6-phosphatase, and mineral levels in diabetics." *J Clin Biochem Nutr*, 1992, 12: 209–15.

150. DiSilvestro, R A. "Zinc in relation to diabetes and oxidative disease." *J Nutr*, May 2000, 130(5S suppl.): 1509S–1511S.

151. Barri, Y M, and Wingo, C S. "The effects of potassium depletion and supplementation on blood pressure: A clinical review." *Am J Med Sci*, 1997, 314(1): 37–40.

152. Hajjar, I M, Grim, C E, George, V, and Kotchen, T A. "Impact of diet on blood pressure and age-related changes in blood pressure in the U.S. population: Analysis of NHANES III." *Arch Intern Med*, 2001, 161(4): 589–93.

153. Appel, L J, Moore, T J, Obarzanek, E, et al. "A clinical trial of the effects of dietary patterns on blood pressure." DASH Collaborative Research Group. *N Engl J Med*, 1997, 336(16): 1117–24.

154. Wimhurst, J M, and Manchester, K L. "Comparison of ability of Mg and Mn to activate the key enzymes of glycolysis." *FEBS Letters*, 1972, 27: 321–26.

155. "Manganese and glucose tolerance." *Nutr Rev*, 1968, 26: 207–10.

156. el-Yazigi, A, Hannan, N, and Raines, D A. "Urinary excretion of chromium, copper, and manganese in diabetes mellitus and associated disorders." *Diabetes Res*, 1991, 18(3): 129–34.

157. Nath, N, Chari, S N, and Rathi, A B. "Superoxide dismutase in diabetic polymorphonuclear leukocytes." *Diabetes*, 1984, 33(6): 586–89.

158. Food and Nutrition Board, Institute of Medicine. *Chromium: Dietary Reference Intakes for Vitamin A, Vitamin K, Boron, Chromium, Copper, Iodine, Iron, Manganese, Molybdenum, Nickel, Silicon, Vanadium, and Zinc.* Washington, DC: National Academy Press, 2001: 197–223.

159. Jeejeebhoy, K N. "The role of chromium in nutrition and therapeutics and as a potential toxin." *Nutr Rev*, 1999, 57(11): 329–35.

160. Morris, B W, MacNeil, S, Hardisty, C A, Heller, S, Burgin, C, and Gray, T A. "Chromium homeostasis in patients with type II (NIDDM) diabetes." *J Trace Elem Med Biol*, 1999, 13(1–2): 57–61.

161. Kobla, H V, and Volpe, S L. "Chromium, exercise, and body composition." *Crit Rev Food Sci Nutr*, 2000, 40(4): 291–308.

162. Goldman, L, and Bennett, J C. *Cecil Textbook of Medicine*. 21st ed. Philadelphia: W. B. Saunders, 2000.

163. Anderson, R A, Cheng, N, Bryden, N A, Polansky, M M, Chi, J, and Feng, J. "Elevated intakes of supplemental chromium improve glucose and insulin variables in individuals with type 2 diabetes." *Diabetes*, 1997, 46(11): 1786–91.

164. Lukaski, H C. "Chromium as a supplement." *Ann Rev Nutr*, 1999, 19: 279–302.

165. Jovanovic-Peterson, L, and Peterson, C M. "Vitamin and mineral deficiencies which may predispose to glucose intolerance of pregnancy." *J Am Coll Nutr*, 1996, 15(1): 14–20.

166. Airola, P. *How to Get Well*. Phoenix: Health Plus, 1984, p. 72.

167. Heinerman, J. *Heinerman's Encyclopedia of Healing Herbs and Spices*. New York: Penguin Putnam, 1996, pp. 52–53.

168. Ibid., p. 200.

169. Shanmugasundarum, E R, Rajeswari, G, Baskaran, K, et al. "Use of Gymnema sylvestre leaf in the control of blood glucose in insulin dependent diabetes mellitus." *J Ethnopharmacol*, 1990, 30: 281–94.

170. Prakash, A O, Mathur, S, and Mathur, R. "Effect of feeding Gymnema sylvestre leaves on blood glucose in beryllium nitrate treated rats." *J Ethnopharmacol*, 1986, 18: 143–46.

171. Baskaran, K, Ahamath, BK, Shanmugasundaram, K R, and Shanmugasundaram, E R B. "Antidiabetic effect of a leaf extract from Gymnema sylvestre in non-insulin dependent diabetes mellitus patients." *J Ethnopharmacol*, 1990, 30: 295–305.

172. Bordia, A, et al. "Effect of ginger (*Zingibwe officinale Rosc.*) and fenugreek (*Trigonella foenum graecum L.*) on blood lipids, blood sugar, and platelet aggregation in patients with coronary artery disease." *Prost Leuko EFA*, 1997, 56: 379–84.

173. Sharma, R D, Raghumram, T C, and Rao, N S. "Effect of fenugreek seeds on blood glucose and serum lipids in type-1 diabetes." *Eur J Clin Nutr*, 1990, 44: 301–6.

174. Sharma, R D. "Effect of fenugreek seeds and leaves on blood glucose and serum insulin responses in human subjects." *Nutr Res*, 1986, 6: 1353–64.

175. Madar, Z, et al. "Glucose-lowering effect of fenugreek in non-insulin dependent diabetes." *Eur J Clin Nutr*, 1988, 42: 51–54.

176. Bordia, et al. "Effect of ginger."

177. Sharma, Raghumram, and Rao. "Effect of fenugreek seeds."

178. Anderson, R A, Broadhurst, C L, Polansky, M M, et al. "Isolation and characterization of polyphenol type-A polymers from cinnamon with insulin-like biological activity." *J Agric Food Chem*, January 2004, 52(1): 65–70.

179. Broadhurst, C L, Polansky, M M, and Anderson, R A. "Insulin-like biological activity of culinary and medicinal plant aqueous extracts in vitro." *J Agric Food Chem*, March 2000, 48(3): 183–88.

180. Imparl-Radosevich, J, Deas, S, Polansky, M M, et al. "Regulation of PTP-1 and insulin receptor kinase by fractions from cinnamon: Implications for cinnamon regulation of insulin signaling." *Horm Res*, September 1998, 50(3): 177–82.

181. Khan, A, Safdar, M, Muzaffar Ali Khan, M, Nawak Khattak, K, and Anderson, R A. "Cinnamon improves glucose and lipids of people with Type-2 diabetes." *Diabetes Care*, December 2003, 26(12): 3215–18.

182. Shibib, B A, Khan, L A, and Rahman, R. "Hypoglycemic activity of Coccinia indica and Momordica charantia in diabetic rats: Depression of the hepatic gluconeogenic enzymes glucose-6-phosphatase and fructose-1,6 bisphosphatase and elevation of both liver and red-cell shunt enzyme glucose-6-phosphate dehydrogenase." *Biochem J*, 1993, 292: 267–70.

183. Day, C, Cartwright, T, Provost, J, and Bailey, C J. "Hypoglycemic effect of Momordica charantia extracts." *Planta Med*, 1990, 56: 426–29.

184. Droy-Lefaix, M T, Vennat, J C, Besse, G, and Doly, M. "Effect of Ginkgo biloba extract (EGb 761) on chloroquine induced retinal alterations." *Lens Eye Toxic Res*, 1992, 9: 521–28.

185. Vuksan, V, Stavro, M P, Sievenpiper, J L, Beljan-Zdravkovic, U, Leiter, L A, Josse, R G, and Xu, Z. "Similar postprandial glycemic reductions with escalation of dose and administration time of American ginseng in type-2 diabetes." *Diabetes Care*, September 2000, 23(9): 1221–26.

186. Vuksan, V, Sievenpiper, J L, Koo, V Y Y, Francis, T, Beljan- Zdravkovic, U, Xu, Z, and Vidgen, E. "American ginseng (*Panax quinquefolius L*) reduces postprandial glycemia in nondiabetic and diabetic individuals with type-2 diabetes mellitus." *Arch Int Med*, 2000, 160: 1009–13.

187. Petricic, J, and Kalodera, Z. "Galegin in the goat's rue herb: Its toxicity, antidiabetic activity, and content determination." *Ata Pharm Jugosl*, 1982, 32(3): 219–23.

188. Muller, H, and Reinwein, H. "Pharmacology of galegin." *Arch Expll Path Pharm*, 1927, 125: 212–28.

189. Cignarella, A, Nastasi, M, Cavalli, E, and Puglisi, L. "Novel lipid-lowering properties of Vaccinium myrtillus L. leaves, a traditional anti-diabetic treatment, in several models of rat dyslipidaemia: A comparison with ciprofibrate." *Thromb Res*, 1996, 84: 311–22.

190. Boniface, R, and Robert, A M. "Effect of anthocyanins on human connective tissue metabolism in the human." *Klin Monatsbl Augenheilkd*, 1996, 209: 368–72.

191. Detre, Z, Jellinek, H, Miskulin, M, and Robert, A M. "Studies on vascular permeability in hypertension: Action of anthocyanosides." *Clin Physiol Biochem*, 1986, 4(2): 143–49.

192. Boniface and Robert. "Effect of anthocyanins on human connective tissue."

193. Lagrue, G, Robert, A M, Miskulin, M, et al. "Pathology of the microcirculation in diabetes and alterations of the biosynthesis of intracellular matrix molecules." *Front Matrix Bio*, 1970, 7: 324–35.

194. Challem, J, et al. *Syndrome X*. New York: John Wiley and Sons, 2002, p. 220.

195. Knowler, W C, Barrett-Connor, E, Fowler, S E, Hamman, R F, Lachin, J M, Walker, E A, and Nathan, D M. Diabetes Prevention Program Research Group. "Reduction in the incidence of Type 2 diabetes with lifestyle intervention or metformin." *New Eng J Med*, February 7, 2002, 346: 393–403.

196. Pederson, O, Beck-Nielsen, H, and Heding, L. "Increased insulin receptors after exercise in patients with insulin-dependent diabetes mellitus." *N Eng J Med*, 1980, 302: 886–92.

197. Williams, D G. "The world's first diabetes cure." *Alternatives for the Health-Conscious Individual*, 2005, p. 4. http://www.drdavidwilliams.com.

198. King, D E, Mainous, II, A G, and Pearson, W S. "C-reactive protein, diabetes, and attendance at religious services." *Diabetes Care*, 2002, 25: 1172–76.

199. Pollack, A. "Skincare." *Alternative Medicine*, February 2007, p. 63.

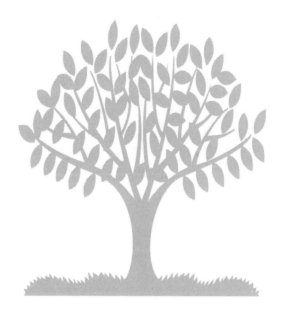

Dr. Cousens's Diabetes Recovery Program—A Holistic Approach: New Results from the Last 120 Diabetic Participants

In reviewing the last 120 diabetics that have come to the Tree of Life Rejuvenation Center to participate in Dr. Cousens's Diabetes Recovery Program—A Holistic Approach, I have found that 61 percent of cases of Type-2 non-insulin-dependent diabetes mellitus (NIDDM) and 24 percent of cases of Type-2 insulin-dependent diabetes mellitus (IDDM) were healed in three weeks. A collective percentage of 39 percent of all Type-2 diabetics were healed in three weeks. "Healed" is defined as fasting blood sugar (FBS) less than 100, with no need for any diabetes related medications. Eighty-six percent of IDDM Type-2 diabetics and 97 percent of all Type-2 diabetics were medication-free after three weeks. Also, 21 percent of the Type-1 diabetics, properly diagnosed with Type-1 diabetes with a positive GAD beta cell antibody test and a medical history of Type-1 diabetes, seem to have healed (which was initially shocking until I developed a theoretical explanation). Again, *healing* is defined as no insulin or oral hypoglycemic medications and an FBS less than 100. Thirty-one-point-four percent of all Type-1 diabetics were off all forms of insulin in three weeks but did not fully drop to an FBS of less than 100. There also seems to be a third category of these Type-1 diabetics, who were able to come off their insulin over a period of a few months to a year and slowly decrease their FBS to less than 100. They were more associated with the bulk of the 31.4 percent who came off all insulin in three weeks but had an FBS greater than 100 after three weeks. Additionally, the remaining 69 percent of the Type-1 diabetics, who remained on insulin, on average, had approximately a 70 percent drop in their insulin requirements—all of which was maintained for most of the people followed for one year after the 21-day cycle. Although I have no definitive explanation for these extraordinary results, I will offer my own theoretical explanations later in this chapter.

CDDS—A Broader Definition of Diabetes

In an effort to explain these results for all levels of Type-2 diabetics, I am offering an explanation that is, of course, also a guide for treatment. I have formulated a basic theory of understanding diabetes. This theory creates a new definition of the diabetes disease, which I call the chronic diabetes degenerative syndrome (CDDS). In this context, diabetes is an accelerated chronic degenerative aging process that is primarily a genetic and epigenetic toxic downgrade, resulting in leptin, insulin, and other hormonal and metabolic dysregulations, including protein, lipid, and carbohydrate imbalances. CDDS also involves a chronic inflammatory, accelerated aging process. This degenerative process arises from a diet primarily high in sugar (including both simple and complex carbohydrates), trans-fatty acids, processed and junk foods, and cooked animal fat and protein. It is made worse from a diet low in fiber combined with a lifestyle of stress; obesity; lack of exercise; lack of sleep; and general toxic exposure including pesticides, herbicides, heavy metals, and environmental toxins such as, and especially, Agent Orange. It is a diet with vitamin, mineral, and antioxidant deficiencies. The degeneration syndrome is often associated with insulin and sometimes leptin resistance. The tendency for developing CDDS increases with age. It is driven by a toxic degenerative epigenetic memory program associated with a change in histone and histone methyl-transferences in addition to the toxic metabolic memory. This toxic metabolic memory must be turned off to stop an ongoing cardiovascular and overall degeneration and proinflammatory cytokine release. This inflammatory program involves cytokine released from adipose tissues and other causes of inflammation, including ingestion of trans-fatty acids; advanced glycation end products (AGEs) from diets high in sugar (glucose and fructose); and AGEs from heated foods, burnt foods, boiled foods, and even infant formula,[1] as well as from stress and environmental toxins in the form of pesticides, herbicides, and radiation. Some preliminary research suggests that high electromagnetic frequencies (EMFs) in some cases may also be associated with temporary inflammation and diabetic hyperglycemic patterns.

Blood Glucose Spikes in Those with Normal FBS

My full definition of CDDS includes two additional categories of blood sugar dysregulation. The first is the prediabetes category, which is defined by an FBS of 100–125. According to the U.S. Centers for Disease Control (CDC), greater than one third of the general U.S. population is prediabetic, and 27 percent of Americans 65 and older have a diabetes diagnosis.[2] The other category includes those with an FBS of less than 100 but who have postprandial spikes of 125–140 mg of glucose in the blood. Research shows these people with blood sugar regulation problems have a significant increase in all the degenerative diseases associated with CDDS, although they are not officially diabetic in traditional terms. CDDS includes increased rate of cardiovascular disease,[3, 4, 5, 6, 7, 8, 9, 10, 11] Alzheimer's,[12] diabetic neuropathy,[13, 14] pancreas dysfunction,[15] kidney dysfunction,[16, 17] and cancer.[18, 19, 20, 21, 22, 23, 24] As expected, the risk of developing Type-2 diabetes increased sevenfold in individuals with an FBS of 105–109, as compared to those with an FBS of 85 or less.[25]

Because of this highly relevant research, I am defining CDDS in the broader context of not only all types of diabetes and prediabetes (FBS of 100–125), but also those with FBS of less than 100 (previously considered normal) who have blood sugar spikes of 125–140, or any postprandial spike of 40 points no matter what the blood sugar. CDDS includes all forms of blood sugar dysregulation that results in all levels of blood sugar imbalance, which activate and increase CDDS and its associated chronic degenerative conditions.

A complete treatment and ultimate healing of the diabetic degenerative syndrome requires addressing and reversing and turning off the full degenerative syndrome on all these levels. It is my hypothesis that the significance, efficacy, and power of the results in this clinical program, as previously discussed in the rest of this book, comes directly from creating a program that does indeed treat all these levels of CDDS and therefore turns off the toxic degenerative epigenetic and genetic memory and programs, thus allowing for a return to the normal, healthy, nondiabetic physiology.

As I look at the deeper causes of this toxic metabolic program, it would be best to start with research on its genetic and epigenetic aspects. As is generally known, 70–90 percent of Type-2 diabetics have a member in their immediate or extended family with Type-2 diabetes, and 45–85 percent share the disease with an immediate family member. This makes a strong case that there exists a genetic tendency toward Type-2 diabetes. This does not mean that one will get diabetes if there is a genetic tendency but that one may be predisposed to CDDS. A genetic predisposition toward diabetes loads the gun, but the Culture of Death lifestyle, with a diet high in sugar (simple and complex carbohydrate) trans-fatty acid, cooked animal fat and protein, junk food, with processed foods, white sugar and white flour, and genetically modified food (GMOs), in addition to inadequate exercise and inadequate sleep, pulls the trigger. There are other additional causes for diabetes, such as gestational diabetes, and now even electromagnetically caused diabetes, which is a newer syndrome that seems to be evolving related to electromagnetic fields. Electromagnetically caused diabetes results in an increased fasting glucose while in the EMF field, which then disappears when one is removed from electromagnetic fields. Chronic EMF hyperglycemia fulfills the conditions of CDDS. These glucose dysregulations may be brought forth by exposure to a variety of environmental toxins.

That being said, the research on the epigenetic causes of diabetes brings us some very interesting information. One of the leaders in the epigenetics research is the Baker Heart Institute in Melbourne, Australia. They essentially found that the epigenetic program remembers an exposure to sugar for up to two weeks, which results in prolonged poor eating habits and cravings for sugar after one single helping of sugar.[26] When extended, this epigenetic memory is capable of semipermanently altering DNA.[27] Research showed that on human heart tissue and in mice, DNA responded to one sugar exposure for approximately two weeks by switching off genetic controls designed to protect the body against diabetes and heart disease.[28] This is obviously significant in that once a person indulges in a high concentration of sugar, the results go far beyond the actual meal itself and literally alter the natural metabolic responses to our diet. Actually, it has the potential to pass on this epigenetic information for up to three generations.[29] This of course gives us an additional insight as to why diabetes tends to run in families. The research shows that the embryo within the mother who has the sugar input goes through the same epigenetic changes and begins craving sugar in utero. If it is a female embryo, that program enters into its ovocyte cells as well, making an extensive impact for three generations. This information is carried in the epigenetic field, which means there is no significant change in DNA but rather in the histoproteins, the epigenetic proteins associated with, and surrounding, the DNA genetic material, described as histone code changes. This has a particularly interesting effect on metabolic memory. Diabetic patients, despite what appears to be having controlled blood sugar levels, continue to develop aggressive, inflammatory complications, especially in terms of heart disease and other aspects of the degenerative syndrome. They found that diabetics continued developing ongoing organ injuries from previous periods of poor glycemic control.[30] This inflammation occurs in the realm of metabolic memory as a major determinant to continuing vascular complications. In order to change this metabolic memory, all aspects of the diabetic syndrome need to be addressed. The most important tool in reversing these negative aspects (which I have also discovered in my research), is maintaining a moderate low-glycemic diet consisting of completely whole, natural, live-food, plant-source-only, non-trans-fat, modest-calorie cuisine. This is not a "calorie restricted" diet, because as previously described, a live-food diet is natural and, without attending to restriction, contains about half the calories of a cooked-food diet, while containing more than an equal amount of nutrients. It therefore naturally turns on the antiaging and by association the antidiabetogenic genes.

Current research is unable to explain the mechanism for epigenetic memory leading to chronic diabetic vascular complications. One such complication is that a proinflammatory cytokine program from obesity will continue to express until obesity is ameliorated. The significance of this single understanding of reversing the vascular complications is that 75 percent of diabetics will die of heart disease if this para-inflammatory pattern is not reversed. (A para-inflammatory pattern is defined as a chronic metabolic inflammatory condition as opposed to an acute inflammatory condition.) Of particular interest is that even transient high levels of glucose, as a blood sugar of 140 after a meal, can actually activate persistent epigenetic changes and maintain an altered genetic expression during subsequent normal glycemic values. That is particularly significant and again speaks to the importance of how to turn off this epigenetic program. It is my experience that 90 percent of the nondiabetic people with hypertension I see during our spiritual fasting program at the Tree of Life Rejuvenation Center will have a permanent lowering of their blood pressure and are able to go off all blood pressure medications after as short as a 7-day fast (but some-times requiring a 14-day fast). Over the years, I began to theorize that indeed there is an epigenetic shift in this process that resets the blood pressure genetics back to normal. A key insight into this was gained from my research stimulated by the book *Genetic Nutritioneering* by Jeffrey Bland.[31]

This principle, which has been known for at least 30 years, is that your diet can actually shift the genetic program and the epigenetic program in either direction. Because of this, I have added to the treat-ment protocol for all Type-2 diabetics to do a one-week 50 percent water-diluted green juice fast, which seems to create a rapid shift of a decrease in the need for insulin and/or 100 percent discontinuance of any oral hypoglycemics. And so I hypothesized by observation that a one-week fast is a primary factor for rapidly upgrading the genetic and epigenetic program back to normal, which then is further strengthened and enforced with my Phase 1.0 dietary protocol following this.

Observations are now showing that repeated hyperglycemia, as previously explained, may actually cause persistent pathogenic effects, even when the blood sugars return to normal. This leads to an expla-nation on a molecular level of the variations and risks for diabetic complications. This gives us an ominous warning of the importance for maintaining a stable blood sugar in our diets. Even binge eating can have negative long-term effects. This new awareness of the importance of blood sugar spikes is different than the A1C results, which are a marker for chronic high blood sugar.[32]

The complication of this is that hyperglycemia that has not become diabetes has near the rates of chronic pathology as full diabetes. For example, one study showed, in an analysis of 1,800 older individuals on the coronary artery disease rate over a period of 10 years, that the rates of those considered prediabetic were nearly identical to those with full blown diabetes.[33] A summary analysis found that in 33,230 men, glucose levels of 86 and greater ("normal range") were associated with a 38 percent increase in deaths from digestive track cancers.[34] Other research showed that when the after-meal blood sugar was increased, even 21 percent in people with a normal glucose between 86–99, there was a 58 percent increase in heart attack risk,[35] and in the same framework they found a 26 percent increase in risk of cardiac failure and 27 percent increased risk of dying from stroke for every 18 mg greater than 83 mg of blood sugar. To give some perspective on this, if you have an FBS of 119, you have a 54 percent risk of death by stroke compared with someone with an FBS of 83.

Neuropathy damage in people who had "normal" blood sugar between 86 and 99 showed damage to their small nerve fibers. With any blood sugar range, the higher the glucose, the greater the involvement of large nerve fiber degeneration.[36] As previously mentioned, people with an FBS of 86–99 have a 40 percent higher rate of heart attacks.[37] In another study they found that when postprandial spikes were diminished, heart attack rates dropped 91 percent.[38] Another study showed that even with a heart attack, the amount of damage was reduced with decreased postprandial surges.[39, 40, 41] Another study showed the incidence of coronary artery disease was twice as high in patients with postprandial glucose levels between 157 and 189, as compared to those with surges below 144.[42] When postprandial glucose levels reached 225 or higher the incidence of sudden death was doubled. The Whitehall Study showed that if one had a blood glucose level two hours postprandial (after eating) of 96 or higher, they had a twofold increase in mortality from heart disease.[43] Another study showed that major coronary heart disease was 17 percent higher with people who had a postprandial glucose level of 140–199, as compared to 9 percent when people had a normal glucose tolerance.[44] An interesting study showed that for many nondiabetics, when their glucose became 140 or higher after a glucose tolerance test they suffered a significant increase in signs and symptoms of diabetic neuropathy,[45] though in some cases this was transitory. Two studies showed that 56 percent of neuropathy patients who had glucose tolerance levels falling in the prediabetic range suffered from damage to small nerve fibers.[46] Anecdotes suggested that foot pain in patients became worse when glucose levels were above 140 and diminished when levels dropped below.[47, 48] Retinopathy was discovered in people whose glucose rose above 200 and one large population study showed that 1 out of 12 people who had signs of prediabetes showed signs of retinopathy changes—these were individuals with an FBS of 100–125 as prediabetics or two-hour glucose tolerance test (GTT) ratings between 150 and 199. What they found was that postprandial glucose spikes over 150 were associated with tiny blood vessel changes leading to diabetic neuropathy.[49] As previously mentioned, diabetics have a higher rate of cancer. In diabetics with abnormal glucose regulation, when glucose was elevated the pancreas would secrete higher levels of insulin. This excess insulin was associated with increased cancer cell production, and in a study of 10,000 people over 10 years, they found that those with an FBS over 110 or a two-hour postprandial level over 160 had a significant increase in rates of cancer.[50] Other research showed, as I previously theorized, that not only do glucose spikes damage the tissue but also alter gene expression in a way that accelerates the aging process.[51, 52] People with an FBS of 100 to 104 have a 283 percent increased risk of developing Type-2 diabetes.[53] People with an FBS of 95–105 have a 100 percent increased risk of developing stomach cancer.[54] If the FBS is above 88, you have a 247 percent increase of a first-time heart attack over people with FBS of 85 and less.[55] If one has an FBS above 95, there is a 73 percent increased risk for need of coronary bypass or stent procedure.[56]

Excess high blood glucose seems to be related directly to destruction of beta cells in the pancreas, which produce insulin. This of course creates a diabetic situation. Beta cells are quite sensitive to slight increases in blood sugar and now there is evidence that these cells move into dysfunction when glucose levels stay over 100 mg per deciliter for more than few hours.[57] Research suggests that even incremental increases of glucose over the course of two hours can result in detectable beta cell failure. More beta cells will fail when a person's blood sugar rises above 86.[58] One study showed that beta cells start to die off when FBS is over 110.[59] Frankly this means that eating too many carbohydrates at one time will begin to kill off pancreatic beta cells and break down the pancreas and over time with age; this is why 26.9 percent of people 65 and older have IDDM. The good news is that studies in the lab have found that when the beta cells are removed from solutions that have high sugar, they can recover if this is done before a certain amount of time passes.[60, 61]

Research suggests that postprandial hyperglycemia results in the activation of protein kinase-C in the endothelium, which increases the production of adhesion molecules, bringing more leukocytes into the blood vessels, thus creating more congestion and disrupting endothelial function.[62] Also, high blood sugar has been found to increase platelet aggregation.[63] All these mechanisms accelerate atherosclerosis. Another effect of elevated postprandial glucose is increased hypercoagulability, which comes from increased thrombin production and decreased fibrogen breakdown. All this results in increased blood clotting or hypercoagulability. Hypercoagulability facilitates atherosclerotic plaque. It appears that the control of postprandial hyperglycemia has been associated with some reversal of the hypercoagulable state. High glucose in the blood results in increased glycosylation of vascular proteins and also lipids in the arteries and endothelium. This results in glycated LDL particles, which are easily oxidized and taken up by the macrophages. This, as I described, leads to higher foam cell production, which one gets with higher insulin levels. With higher foam cell production, there is more atherosclerotic plaque.[64] The other mechanism by which glycation contributes to atherosclerosis is that the AGEs form in the collagen of the vessel wall and accelerate the atherosclerotic process.[65]

King Solomon once said that the wise person knows the consequences of their actions. Knowing this information helps us to think more clearly about our choices to eat a high carbohydrate diet versus a moderate-low carbohydrate diet.

It is my experience that a significant portion of the "normal" public indeed has blood sugars above 110, and this creates glycemic conditions, which weaken or kill beta cells. I have used the term "burn-out" for Type-2 IDDM; this is a second and well-documented mechanism for the loss of beta cells and the consequential adult onset diabetes progressing to Type-2 IDDM.

My advice to people in this context: It is best if blood sugar doesn't rise above 120 two hours postprandially, although I previously mention that 125–140 is marginal. This is best achieved on the Phase 1.0 or 1.5 diets. Practically speaking, it is my feeling, with this limited information, that a blood sugar two hours postmeal of 140 for most is sufficient to consider beginning treatments and a diet to suppress these postprandial glucose spike levels. Without creating paranoia, it certainly makes a point that one should organize their food (particularly those 50 and older) in a pattern that minimizes carbohydrates and their glycemic spikes. As the data suggests, a high-carb diet may be seen as a threat to overall health and longevity when we remember that 80 percent of 46,000 in a previously mentioned study had an FBS greater than 85.

CDDS doesn't begin when one is diagnosed with diabetes, but rather approximately when one's FBS is greater than 85, and/or postprandial blood sugars spike higher than as little as 18 points above one's FBS. A spiking blood sugar above 125, in general, after two hours of a glucose tolerance test, or after eating a sweet meal, should be considered as the first stages of postprandial (postmeal) glucose spiking. It is part of an aging process where people who are taking in excess sugar undergo chronic cellular damage associated with high blood sugar. A moderate-low glycemic diet is the primary approach in minimizing this effect. The optimum range for an FBS is 70–85. As the new data points out, the postprandial (postmeal blood sugar spike at two hours) becomes equally, if not more, important. These surges of blood sugar seem to damage the blood vessels in the brain, heart, kidneys, and eyes and accelerate the general aging process in all our cells. Some of the research suggests that the postprandial spikes may be even more damaging than higher FBS.[66, 67, 68]

With age, there is a tendency for our FBS and our postprandial spikes to go higher. This comes from two sources—one is a process called *glycogenolysis*, which is the breaking down of glycogen that is stored in the liver for making sugar. The other source is gluconeogenesis, which is the new creation of glucose from protein and fat. With age, the glycogenolysis tends to not be suppressed appropriately. And the key enzyme for this glucose-6-phosphatase begins to express excessively with age, thus creating the increased release of glycogen from the liver. Glucose-6-phosphatase stimulates gluconeogenesis from protein and, to a lesser extent, from fat. This includes creating glucose from the protein in one's muscles while one sleeps. So with age it appears that people begin to make too much glucose in their bodies. These increases in internal (endogenous) sugar production is part of the reason 26.9 percent of people 65 or older have developed Type-2 diabetes.

The key enzyme responsible for these two problems, as I mentioned, is glucose-6-phosphatase (g-6-p), the control of which becomes impaired with age. The normal function of g-6-p is to increase the release of stored glucose from the liver and to create new glucose from protein. With age this enzyme gets more activated and moves out of harmony with the body physiology and produces more endogenous glucose than is healthy, which tends to raise the FBS, as well as the incidence of postprandial spikes. It is my clinical experience that fasting tends to reset this activation. There are also substances such as chlorogenic acid that can neutralize the dysregulation and excess of g-6-p. Besides stroke, high FBS and postprandial spikes also increase the risk of other cardiovascular emergencies.[69, 70, 71, 72, 73] In one study, they found that the lower the glucose the lower the cardiovascular risk. As I pointed out earlier, one study showed that there was a 40 percent increase in cardiovascular risk if FBS was 86 or higher. Another study showed that coronary heart disease risk was twice as high in patients with a postprandial blood sugar between 157 and 189, as compared to those with a postprandial spike below 144.[74] The rising of blood sugar is that for every 18 points beyond an FBS of 83, there is a 27 percent increase in risk of dying from stroke.[75] High blood sugars are also associated with an increase in certain cancers. There was a study in the *Oncologist*, which included almost half of Type-2 diabetics in Sweden,[76] that concluded that the risk of cancer escalated in direct correlation with blood sugar levels, even among people without diabetes. There were particular increases in the endometrial,[77] pancreatic,[78] colon,[79, 80] and colorectal tumors.[81] As pointed out earlier, the increase in insulin is associated with an increased cancer cell production. When blood sugar rises, insulin rises, and one is more likely to get cancer.

Another area of disease associated with high blood sugar is cognitive disruption. Research shows that as blood sugar rises, either within normal or diabetic ranges, there is a higher the risk for mild cognitive impairment and dementia.[82, 83] Surges in blood sugar were also associated with a greater production of fibrous kidney disease, and the surges seemed to be more significant than a higher blood sugar that was constant.[84] The research suggested that the fluctuations in glucose may be even more of a problem than a high FBS. As pointed out previously, high glucose levels also disorganize pancreatic function. High glucose levels also activated retinopathy and were associated with diabetic retinopathy syndrome, even if people never had diabetes. The same association is with neuropathy, where research is suggesting that the higher the glucose, even in prediabetic ranges, the greater the amount of damage on the large nerve fibers.[85, 86]

In summary, I am reporting a new perspective for looking at the blood sugar question, which examines not only the FBS but also the postprandial blood sugar spikes. These spikes affect many people and activate and accelerate the degenerative process even before the situation reaches diabetic proportions. This appears to be associated with an increasing lack of regulation of glucose-6-phosphatase with age. It is believed that the g-6-p enzyme regulation system creates a more excessive production and/or loses its signaling mechanism accuracy with age. This results in rising after-meal surges of blood sugar, especially if one is eating too much sugar in the meal. The safest and optimal ranges for people who are not diabetic are fasting glucose between 70 and 85 and postprandial glucose of less than 120–125. This is some of the more subtle rationale behind why I have chosen to emphasis a live-food, plant-source-only, moderate-low carbohydrate diet for both the treatment of diabetes and general well-being. I suggest Phase 1.0 for the treatment of diabetes and the readjusting of our enzymatic processes, beginning with 25–45 percent carbohydrates until one comes into a 70–85 FBS with postprandial spikes of 120–125 or less. Then I suggest moving into 30–50 percent carbohydrate intake in Phase 1.5, including some low glycemic fruit and a little grain if one chooses.

Para-Inflammation and Obesity

Chronic para-inflammation is another powerful degenerative force in Type-2 diabetes. Para-inflammation seems to be triggered by a variety of external causes. These include leptin and insulin resistance and para-inflammation from glycosylation (as discussed previously), especially from fructose, which has an AGE effect that is 10 times higher than glucose. Inflammation from obesity, trans-fatty acids, smoking, pesticides, herbicides, radiation, EMFs, and dental infections are some of the activating factors that are both endogenous and exogenous to the process of para-inflammation.

It is useful to take an evolutionary perspective on this to get a deeper understanding. There are two types of inflammation: one is acute inflammation and the other is para-inflammation, according to *Reumatologia*.[87] This para-inflammation is most likely responsible for the chronic inflammatory conditions associated with chronic degenerative diseases, including diabetes. These chronic inflammatory states do not seem to be caused by classic causes of acute inflammation, such as infection or injury, but seem more clearly associated with a dysfunction in the tissue that is both the cause and result of a homeostatic imbalance. This homeostatic imbalance is perhaps activated and mediated in a variety of ways reported in the literature, including inflammatory mediators, resident macrophages, and mass cells, and other mediators, including cytokines, adipose tissues, chemokines, eicosanoids, and some by-products of proteolitic cascades.[88, 89, 90] My focus in this discussion is more on the endogenous type of para-inflammation, although all the exogenous causes do contribute to CDDS. Primary forces are AGEs or glycosylation reactions that create free radicals and para-inflammation. This para-inflammation is caused by the glycosylation of proteins and lipids. It leads to gradual and increasing dysfunction of the proteins and lipids as biologically active complexes. Some of this para-inflammation pathology is connected to reactive oxygen species (free radicals). Reactive oxygen species are produced by phagocytes. They have a role in converting high-density and low-density lipoproteins into inflammatory signals by oxidizing their lipid and protein components.

For overview purposes, it helps to understand there are a variety of inflammatory mediators in general that can be cross-divided into seven groups according to their properties. In summary, there are meso-active amines, meso-active peptides, fragments or compliment components, lipid mediator cytokines, chemokines, and proteolytic enzymes. Another important group of inflammatory components are lipid mediators, eicosanoids, and platelet activating factors that come from phospholipids (which are in the inner layers of cell membranes, particularly in the mitochondrial level). An additional inflammatory set is the inflammatory cytokines, including tumor necrosis factor alpha, interleukin 1, and interleukin 6, particularly produced in adipose tissues by fat cells. These multilevels of para-inflammatory mediators also have important impacts on endocrine and metabolic function and on the maintenance of tissue homeostasis. My point is that the para-inflammation process is a complex interrelated biopathological degenerative inflammatory process that has many triggers, many of which are set off by a dysfunctional diet and lifestyle.

The interface (how metabolic and inflammatory processes overlap) gives us a potential insight for how obesity is linked with Type-2 diabetes and its concomitant para-inflammation. The long-term consequences of chronic para-inflammation, which, contrary to the healing effect of acute inflammation, has a degenerative effect, seems to be an important part of the ongoing program of degenerative disease, including CDDS. On some level, however, it helps to think about the para-inflammatory response as an attempt to heal a situation, which is ultimately to restore homeostasis to tissue. But in the case of chronic para-inflammation associated with obesity and diabetes, instead of healing, it causes an ongoing destructive pattern, which is particularly potent in its pathogenic interface with the cardiovascular system. The research is also becoming increasingly clear that this chronic para-inflammation creates an increase in insulin resistance.

From an acute point of view, insulin resistance increases during acute inflammation as a healthy response because a flow of glucose is needed to be moved from the general cellular function to the leukocytes to fight the cause of the acute situation and to other cells that need this increased for energy for an immune response. However, a sustained insulin resistance as part of the response to para-inflammation can lead to Type-2 diabetes. Obesity is now an aberration when viewed in light of early evolution in humans, when they did not have a continuous availability of high-calorie nutrients, low levels of physical activity, exposure to toxic compounds, or general inflammation, as is in the accelerated pathological process called aging. In examining the pattern of these chronic para-inflammatory conditions, including obesity, Type-2 diabetes, atherosclerosis, asthma, and a variety of neurodegenerative diseases,[91] increased sucrose intake is associated with an increase in C-reactive proteins (an inflammatory marker). Consumption of trans-fatty acids is also related to biomarkers of inflammation and endothelial destruction.[92] Ultimately, this para-inflammation leads to higher risk of cardiovascular disease.

In formulating an evolutionary overview of the interplay between obesity and diabetes, the World Health Organization reports that there are one billion overweight adults and three-hundred million who are clinically obese. According to the International Diabetes Federation, there are (as of 2011) as many as 366 million diabetics worldwide.[93] It is not unreasonable to theorize an association then between these metabolic and inflammatory responses and a high-caloric dietary intake. Epidemic obesity is a recent phenomenon. In the past, human beings' survival was dependent upon withstanding starvation cycles rather than enduring overeating. To avoid starvation, our genetics select for energy accumulation and storage of excess calories to be stored and accessed as food in lean times. Today, throughout the world, even though many are starving to death, there is a very different scenario because there is a continuous availability of calories for a majority of the population. At one point fat storage was good for survival, but a year-round excess creates adiposity and its concomitant chronic para-inflammatory diseases, which may lead to CDDS with insulin resistance and/or Type-2 diabetes, fatty liver disease, atherosclerosis, hypertension, and neuro-degeneration. It is pretty clear from the literature that obesity leads to para-inflammation and is also implicated in a variety of causes and effects with Type-2 diabetes. By constructing a theoretical model to understand this, I have been able to create a plan to reverse the chronic para-inflammatory process. This approach is guided by a comprehension of the interplay between the immune system, obesity, and the metabolic degenerative process I call CDDS.

There are some potential benefits of para-inflammation, at least in stress response, in blocking metabolic signaling pathways such as those of insulin and insulin growth factors. From a survival perspective, blocking insulin signaling diverts energy sources from building pathways into repair and management of the chronic disease process. In this context, it is no accident that stress and para-inflammatory signals, in preliminary research findings, are connected to disrupting insulin receptor signaling.[94] For this reason, the activated stress immune response pathways are associated with activating increased insulin resistance as a coping mechanism. The stress immune inflammatory response, in this context, is in essence a failed coping mechanism to a high caloric, continuous sugar and junk food excess from the Culture of Death diet. Generally, chronic metabolic disturbance in this inflammatory cascade are due to overnutrition. Most of the world population lives in a worldwide Culture of Death lifestyle that both creates a metabolic overload and is also associated with decreased physical activity and other toxic inflammatory behaviors and exposure. As pointed out before, obesity, insulin resistance, and Type-2 diabetes are closely associated with chronic para-inflammation. All these processes are characterized by excessive cytokine production and activation of a network of inflammatory signaling pathways.[95] There is, at this point in the scientific literature, a causal link between para-inflammation and the development of metabolic diseases and ultimately the complications of chronic degeneration emerging from this.[96, 97, 98]

One of the key players in this process is tumor necrosis factor alpha (TNF-alpha), which is hyperexcreted in the adipose tissue and is definitely a major inflammatory cytokine. TNF-alpha, the major proinflammatory cytokine, activates signal transduction cascades that result in critical inhibitors of insulin receptor site function. Inhibiting insulin receptor site function increases insulin resistance. In survival mode, when there is an excess of nutrients, there is a tendency to have excess insulin secretions to cope with the excess nutrients, particularly if it is an excess of carbohydrates, which it often is. This creates a situation where the tissues, particularly the liver, muscle, and then fat tissues, become insulin resistant in a progressive manner. The associated para-inflammation increases the insulin resistance, which is a failed mechanism of these cellular functions to protect themselves from the destructive effects of excess insulin on the cells. In other words, insulin resistance, although a maladaptive response, is a cellular protection mechanism against insulin excess activated primarily by carbohydrate excess. Rather than focus on the para-inflammatory protein in specific, the focus is on the fact that there is an inflammatory process in which cytokines are a major player as they are released from the adipose tissues. What also seems to happen, which may be more of a secondary effect, is the infiltration of the inflamed tissues by immune cells such as neutrophils, eosinophils, and macrophages. This macrophage infiltration of adipose tissue has been described in these para-inflammatory conditions in both mice and humans.[99, 100] This inflammation, from macrophage infiltration of adipose tissue, may have an endpoint of not only increasing insulin resistance but also protecting cells from excess insulin. In any case, we have inflammation (both as a result and a cause of obesity) and as a prime player in diabetes. In the variety of synergies there are also the pathologies of diabetes and inflammation as cross-interacting and associating as a causal factor of obesity.

The bottom line is that there are a variety of inflammatory signals, which disrupt insulin action and result in insulin resistance. For example, the literature finds that insulin uptake in IGF receptors is associated with a receptor tyrosine kinase family, which is connected to a family of insulin receptor substrates (IRS) proteins IRS-126.[101, 102] Insulin initiates this process, creating phosphorylation of IRS proteins, which end up mediating insulin action. This whole metabolic process is beyond the scope of this particular chapter (and even this book), but it gives us a biochemical mechanism for how this is happening. There are other inflammatory kinases, besides IRS-126, which also disrupt insulin signaling.[103, 104] These are just some of the complexities of the system, but one can generally distill the idea that para-inflammation and concomitant insulin resistance is part of the body's effort to reduce the toxic effects of excess nutrition and consequently excessive insulin in response to the excess nutrition.

One other additional mechanism of obesity in its causal relation to diabetes is that obesity causes stress in the endoplasmic reticulum, a system of membranes found in cells—particularly the mitochondria. This stress creates a dysfunctional effect on insulin signaling, leading to insulin resistance. The endoplasmic reticulum is a production site, particularly in mitochondria, for processing proteins and fats and ultimately making new protein. Here additional blood fats are also processed. In the pathology of overnutrition, the endoplasmic reticulum is stressed with too many nutrients. The nutrients need to be processed, stored, and utilized, and so production in the endoplasmic reticulum becomes overworked and sends stress signals, effectively saying, "Hold on! We can't take glucose coming in! You're overloading! So please decrease the power of insulin to bring glucose into this cell (insulin resistance)." In this dynamic the cells become insulin-resistant. The endoplasmic reticulum stress is associated with obesity and is also a signal to trigger para-inflammation and insulin resistance.

The intracellularly occurring endoplasmic reticulum stress observed in obesity and diabetes is a mechanism that gives an additional insight into how overnutritional stress may activate para-inflammation and lead to CDDS and eventually diabetes. This is based on recent research suggesting that endoplasmic reticulum disruption activates the pathways of para-inflammation and consequent insulin resistance and obesity in Type-2 diabetes. There seem to be several minor inflammatory pathways that disrupt insulin function stemming from a stressed endoplasmic reticulum. Without going into elaborate detail, it is possible to postulate that the endoplasmic reticulum might be a location site within the mitochondria that signals metabolic stress from overnutrition and the transformation of that stress into inflammatory signaling. In this context, the endoplasmic reticulum within the mitochondria of the cell might be considered an interface site of integrating between the excess nutrient and general pathogen responses, as it as at this level where there is an interface of glucose-energy metabolism availability, lipids, and pathogen associated components. Recent work suggesting that dietary and genetic obesity are associated with increased endoplasmic reticulum stress in adipose tissue supports this understanding.[105] The bottom line of this discussion is that within cellular systems, at the level of endoplasmic reticulum, when stress increases in the adipose tissues, it may lead to para-inflammatory conditions and to insulin resistance. This is also an additional mechanism for how obesity leads to diabetes by the mechanism of increased insulin resistance.

Within the context of metabolic disease, oxidative stress may also lead to diabetic complications through its pathogenic effect on endothelial membrane function. These interface and support recent evidence that shows oxidative stress and mitochondrial dysfunction have important roles in diabetes.[106, 107] In summary, para-inflammatory mediators, as a response to excess calories from chronic overnutrition (particularly from sugar), can trigger insulin resistance and metabolic dysfunction. This may create a negative synergy, resulting in inflammation and insulin resistance. This process is a probable precursor cocontributing to the development of Type-2 diabetes.

Associated with the general para-inflammation in the tissues (from a variety of endogenous and exogenous reasons, as just explained) are para-inflammation of the arteries and endothelium of the arteries, which many leading cardiologists and holistic physicians now consider the primary causes of cardiovascular disease, rather than cholesterol. Cholesterol is then drawn to these inflamed areas, causing the atherosclerotic plaques, as a secondary phenomenon to the para-inflammation.

In this context, as you will read later in the chapter, this para-inflammation phenomenon gives a possible explanation for why there is no difference in cardiovascular events in people over 50 years of age with cholesterols of 160 to 260[108] or difference in cardiovascular events between those who have a high- or low-fat diet.[109] The exception to this is trans fats, which are pathogenic in every situation, as they specifically cause both a generalized para-inflammatory response as well as a localized para-inflammatory response in the endothelium/intima regions of the arteries. This inflammation and damage of the intima (inner lining of the arteries) draws cholesterol deposits, which creates the plaques. The key to understanding this is that both a low- and a high-cholesterol diet will create the secondary component of the atherosclerotic cardiovascular disease (ASCVD), but the primary cause or variable in ASCVD incidence is the degree of para-inflammation one creates in their life and body. For example, smoking, which inflames the arteries, is associated with increased cardiovascular disease and is a risk factor independent of cholesterol.

This para-inflammation that is part of CDDS, as well as cardiovasospasm from the action of excess insulin and leptin from carbohydrate excess, is primarily responsible for the fact that 75 percent of diabetics die of cardiovascular disease. If we cannot stop this toxic CDDS, the incendiary negative effect on cardiovascular mortality moves relentlessly onward, resulting in a high incidence in cardiovascular disease in diabetes. Unless we decrease or shut off the para-inflammatory process, as well as the carbohydrate surges that express as pathogenic leptin and insulin surges, we will be unable to turn off this toxic metabolic cardiovascular process.

Insulin Metabolism and Insulin Resistance

Having now documented and clarified the significance of para-inflammation and obesity in diabetes, the question arises, "How do we reverse this?" Studies have shown that calorie-restricted diets have been shown to decrease inflammation. Other research has supported this by showing that caloric restriction can decrease inflammation markers such as C-reactive protein.[110, 111] This completely supports my research showing that when one decreases through fasting and through a low-calorie, live-food diet, my 25–45 percent carbohydrate diet (often called "calorie restriction") helps decrease para-inflammation. It is important to again point out that on a live-food diet people naturally eat 40–60 percent less calories without losing nutritional value, as live-food has at least double the bioavailable nutritional density. So in functional caloric restriction with live food, there is no actual functional or experiential restriction, but there is a reduction of active oxygen reactive species, resulting in a decreased oxidized LDL. In other words, calorie restriction (naturally with live-foods) and fasting seem to be very powerful ways to almost immediately decrease inflammation. In my clinical experience, the main lifestyle methods by which to turn off the toxic metabolic genetic and epigenetic inflammatory programs are live foods and fasting. In examining my results, which are more effective compared to any other approaches to ameliorating diabetes, there is a dramatic average 5.3 point drop in C-reactive protein in three weeks, as compared to less than 1 point with other approaches to managing diabetes, even in 22 weeks. In other words, Dr. Cousens's Diabetes Recovery Program—A Holistic Approach has been shown to directly and powerfully decrease the para-inflammatory response initially with green juice fasting and, on a long term basis, with the Phase 1.0 and 1.5

live-food, moderate-low carbohydrate, plant-source-only, organic diet.

Insulin metabolism doesn't only affect many of the body's tissues; in this context, insulin and insulin resistance have significant effects on the global brain glucose metabolism and function, which is mainly in the cerebral cortex, prefrontal cortex, limbic system, and the dentate gyrus part of the hippocampal area in regard to Alzheimer's disease. The data shows that insulin can access the insulin receptors of the brain. Research is also suggesting that in Alzheimer's disease the key brain structures (including the limbic system, hippocampal region, prefrontal cortex, and cortex) begin to suffer from low energy and the consequent degeneration secondary to insulin resistance. As a result, these insulin-resistant brain tissues are unable to get glucose to energize themselves, which contributes to the degeneration of the brain function and thus contributes to Alzheimer's disease. A new approach that seems to ameliorate this is the use of coconut oil, which is directly converted in the liver to ketones. These ketones directly energize the brain tissues and also give energy for brain tissue repair. It is fortunate that brain tissue does not depend solely on glucose for its function but can use ketones, which have been found to supply up to 75–90 percent of the energy necessary for brain function. The use of coconut oil has been shown to dramatically improve Alzheimer's in cases of insulin resistance of the brain is a primary cause.

Insulin has many major effects on our physical functioning, beyond lowering blood sugars. Some additional facts about insulin's metabolic effects demonstrate its significance: When the liver becomes resistant to insulin, T-4 conversion to T-3 is blocked, so that when we decrease insulin resistance with a proper diet, one will naturally have an increase in T-3 function and have better thyroid function. Insulin also controls cholesterol production, as well as estrogen, progesterone, and testosterone levels. Sex hormone binding globulin is also controlled by insulin. When sex hormone binding globulin is high, it creates a higher estrodial to testosterone ratio, because it increases the aromatase, which makes more estrodial. In many cases, as previously discussed, giving testosterone to men with insulin resistance has decreased their insulin resistance. Insulin resistance has also been shown to decrease DHEA and increase osteoporosis. All anabolic hormones are controlled by insulin, which is why insulin resistance is connected to certain specific cancers such as already described as part of the side effects of a higher than 85 FBS and chronic postprandial surges. Insulin resistance also pulls calcium out of the bone, as it attempts to pull sugar from the bones when glucose is unavailable in other tissues. Another reason the high insulin creates osteoporosis is because insulin causes calcium to be excreted in the urine.

Summarily, a key to antiaging and reversing CDDS is decreasing excess insulin secretion, which is primarily caused by a high carbohydrate dietary intake. This helps to decrease insulin resistance because excess insulin creates insulin resistance. Paradoxically, insulin resistance creates a higher insulin secretion, thus increasing the rate of aging, of which prediabetes and diabetes is a symptom.

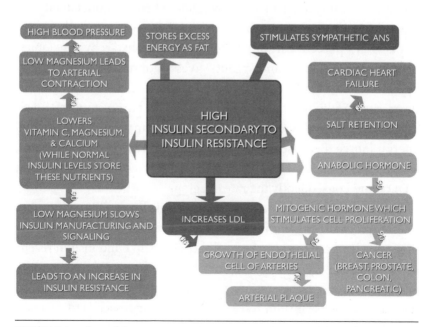

FIGURE 1. Insulin resistance

Fundamental to understanding the ramification of this discussion is that a high-carbohydrate diet creates excess insulin (no matter whether these are simple or complex carbohydrates) and therefore activates CDDS with all its documented pathological degenerative effects. This is explicitly why a 30–50 percent carbohydrate intake is part of an optimal long-term Phase 1.5 dietary strategy to prevent this accelerated aging process. High fructose or galactose also increases insulin levels both indirectly and directly, especially with high-fructose corn syrup. Recently, high-fructose corn syrup has been labeled as a main dietary culprit in activating insulin resistance, and ultimately CDDS, since the 1980s when it was massively introduced into the diet of the general population. The healthiest carbohydrates, as I mentioned previously, are the nonstarchy, fibrous carbohydrates in vegetables, leafy greens, sprouts, and sea vegetables. Insulin resistance, which indirectly raises insulin in the blood as a result, prevents a burning of fats for energy because the role of insulin is to store fat as energy. When I talk about the idea of cutting down on carbohydrates, it helps to understand that, physiologically, there is no absolute essential need for carbohydrates, but a 25–45 percent carbohydrate intake of nonstarchy vegetables, greens, sea vegetables, and sprouts gives an optimal healthy carbohydrate input, therefore minimizing insulin secretion and therefore decreasing insulin resistance. It also helps us shift to an emphasis on fat metabolism instead of carbohydrate metabolism as our fundamental energy source. Because all carbohydrates increase insulin secretion, a high carbohydrate intake essentially accelerates insulin resistance, CDDS, and consequently the rate of aging.

Additional nutrition that best increases insulin sensitivity (reverses insulin resistance) is an intake of high levels of omega-3, because omega-3s increase membrane flexibility and help build insulin receptors and the activity of those receptors. Exercise also builds up receptors and activates them; this is particularly true of resistance training. To decrease or reverse insulin resistance, the best approach is to decrease carbohydrate intake, increase intake of long- and short-chain omega-3 fats, and exercise.

One of two key healthy longevity markers includes an optimal fasting insulin between 4 and 6 but no higher than 10. My clinical experience is that most people who are following my Phase 1.5 diet and are over the age of 50 have fasting insulins between 4 and 6. A good leptin level is normally 2 to 7, and, in women, no higher than 9.5. Other longevity markers are an FBS somewhere between 70 and 85, a normal C-reactive protein, and an A1C of 5.0 or less. In essence, when one looks at the total picture, it appears that insulin resistance is one of the key causes of all chronic aging diseases, metabolic syndrome, and of course CDDS. It is a precursor to many forms of chronic degeneration. A high blood sugar also indirectly decreases immunity. Vitamin C competes with glucose in getting into the cell. When excess sugar goes into system it decreases immune system function because it decreases vitamin C cellular uptake through competitive inhibition. The concentration of vitamin C is 50 times greater inside the cell than outside. When blood sugar goes up to 120, it competes with vitamin C getting into the cell via insulin. Just a little less vitamin C in the cell may decrease the phagocytic index by 75 percent. The phagocytic index is a measure of phagocytic activity. In other words, our phagocyte whole blood cells need vitamin C for optimal function. High insulin is also connected to sodium retention and overstimulation of the sympathetic system and therefore also relates to high insulin as a contributor to high blood pressure.

One little known piece of information is that, contrary to general public understanding, as already hinted at earlier, the incidence of myocardial infarction is approximately 2.5 times greater after a high carbohydrate meal than after a high fat meal. Fat intake does not seem to have any postprandial impact on myocardial infarction.[112] The reason carbohydrates do this (rather than fats) is that carbohydrates stimulate insulin and leptin secretion, which both stimulate the sympathetic system. The sympathetic system stimulation creates arterial spasm, increases clotting, and increases blood pressure. Insulin has also been shown to increase the small pathogenic dense LDLs, which are associated with increased tendency for cardiovascular disease. The body is acting intelligently by becoming insulin resistant because it is protecting itself from the pathogenic qualities of insulin. One other additional fact in understanding the atheroscloteric or atherogenic quality of insulin is that when we're in insulin resistance (which means that there is an increase in the amount of insulin in the blood and the rest of the system), normally healthy macrophage cells become foam cells in arteries and add to creating arterial plaque.

In the complex system of insulin resistance and diabetes, all carbohydrates will stimulate insulin secretion and eventually increase the incidence of insulin resistance and, potentially, further down the line, CDDS. As I share the science on these studies, it becomes more obvious why my emphasis is on a 25–45 percent carbohydrate intake as the best diet for reversing and healing diabetes. The high complex/simple carbohydrate diet, as is currently commonly recommended by the American Diabetes Association (ADA) and most of allopathic medicine, is the most diabetogenic diet, if you understand the scientific information as presented. This helps explain why the ADA, and allopathic medicine in general, believes that diabetes is incurable and irreversible. An old Chinese saying is "When you are going in the wrong direction you will end up in that direction."

Leptin Metabolism and Leptin Resistance

Along with insulin metabolism and insulin resistance, which are the first dysregulation effects, the second aspect of the dynamic duo of hormonal dysregulation in diabetics is a disruption of leptin secretion and leptin signaling. Leptin is a hormone produced by adipose tissue by fat cells (adipocytes). It was discovered in 1985. Its function, when working correctly, is to signal the body to stop storing fat and start burning fat. It also signals us to stop overeating and decreases appetite. It helps us lose our taste for sweets so one does not crave sweets. In this way, it works opposite to insulin. A key cause of insulin resistance and faulty insulin signaling is leptin resistance and faulty leptin signaling. The primary way to decrease insulin resistance and leptin resistance is a moderate-low carbohydrate diet. No allopathically prescribed pharmaceutical drug will do this. There is one African herb that seems to help, however, which I will discuss later. The only diet that is proven to reverse insulin and leptin resistance and dysfunctional signaling is a moderate-low carbohydrate diet.

Leptin is produced in fat cells, and its primary function is regulatory control of the hypothalamus in a way that regulates appetite and body weight. It literally tells your brain when to eat, how much to eat, and (critical to the whole process) when to stop eating. When leptin is secreted in the right levels, it says, "Stop eating, decrease sweet cravings, start burning fat, and get ready to reproduce." Leptin tells your brain what to do with the energy it has. The most important thing in the context of the leptin-insulin dynamic is that leptin plays a key role in the accuracy of insulin signaling and therefore plays a role in the etiology of insulin resistance. Although theoretically one goes into leptin resistance before insulin resistance, my clinical laboratory experience is that in Type-2 diabetics, some are insulin resistant and have normal leptin and vice versa, and some are both insulin and leptin resistant. Interestingly enough, some are neither, as far as can presently be measured in the laboratory. There are some subtleties in the complex dynamics that are not fully enough researched to have a fuller scientific explanation. However, what I have clinically demonstrated is validation of the CDDS theory that a 25–45 percent carbohydrate, plant-source-only, live-food, organic, non-junk-food, non-processed-food, no-white-sugar-or-flour diet will reverse insulin and leptin resistance and will bring the insulin and leptin signaling back into order in a relatively short time. This, of course, is the main point.

The two primary organs in the leptin control complex are the brain and the liver because of their ability to listen to leptin. The ability of the brain and the liver to listen to leptin determines whether one becomes leptin and/or insulin resistant. Simply put, the remedy for insulin and leptin resistance is utilizing a diet that increases the accuracy of insulin and leptin signaling and decreases the overstimulation of insulin and leptin. We should understand the terms *leptin* or *insulin resistance* as indicating disruptions in the flow of signaling and how the signals are listened to. A 25–45 percent carbohydrate diet is a powerful, healthy reorganizing force for the leptin-insulin signaling balance and sensitivity to optimally respond to signals. This is the key to reversing diabetes and part of why Dr. Cousens's Diabetes Recovery Program—A Holistic Approach works. It is the cuisine that will help these things come into proper physiological balance. Leptin resistance causes a variety of problems, and it also acts primarily on the hypothalamic areas in regard to appetite and reproduction and regulation. The condition of leptin resistance desensitizes our taste buds to sugar, and therefore one needs more and more sugar to enjoy a sweet taste. I find that when people move to a Phase 1.0 diet, their taste buds become refined and sensitive to the sweet taste, and people may even find that vegetables and sprouts taste sweet. Most people who are overweight produce too much leptin since it is produced by fat cells, and when there is an excess of leptin, key leptin receptors go into resistance (similar as with insulin). When a person is leptin resistant, similar to insulin resistance, it takes more and more leptin to get the brain to respond and to turn off the appetite drive. Typical symptoms of leptin resistance include one requiring more food to feel satisfied; the brain keeps signaling for more fat to be stored. Normal leptin response is a message to the brain to burn fat and decrease appetite, and it also decreases the desire for sweets. The problem is that the more fat one accumulates through excess insulin, the more leptin one produces. Paradoxically, the more weight one gains, the more leptin one produces in an effort to deal with leptin resistance. When one goes into leptin resistance, it gets a little crazy, as your brain does not know how to tell you to stop eating because of the improperly functioning hypothalamic controls. Carbohydrates trigger a large leptin release at the time of that meal, which also negatively affects the cardiovascular system in the short term and long term. A strong leptin surge has also been found to negatively program the epigenetic program, even as an embryo. Research seems to show that infants who are subjected to embryo starvation associated leptin-surge situations have more leptin imbalance and obesity later on in their lives.[113]

One sign of leptin resistance is the inability to lose weight on a weight-loss diet or rapidly regaining weight after a diet. People who have trouble losing weight on such a diet are most likely already in leptin resistance. Their fat-burning mechanism is not turned on even with a weight-loss, low-calorie diet. This also implies that people who have trouble keeping weight off after dieting may be suffering from leptin resistance. Being always hungry and craving sweets and waking up hungry at night are also signs of leptin resistance. In women, a waist more than 35 inches, and in men, a waist more than 40 inches, suggests insulin and/or leptin resistance. During leptin resistance the body also loses its ability to discriminate when and where to store fat. Much of this fat is stored as subcutaneous fat, causing obesity, especially around the waistline. The stored visceral fat lining the liver also increases insulin resistance. Leptin resistance may also lead to accelerated muscle mass loss, in spite of exercise, because the body burns muscle for glucose and stores fat. Leptin resistance also increases levels of stress hormones and is associated with high triglyceride levels (a factor in cardiac disease) and high blood pressure. High blood pressure is also associated with leptin resistance, as leptin resistance creates an overactive sympathetic system. Leptin resistance, like insulin resistance, can lead to osteoporosis. High levels of leptin will inhibit production of osteoblasts for generating new bone. A high leptin level is also associated with insulin resistance, because insulin resistance blocks vitamin D absorption, creating general acidity, loss of kidney function, and loss of osteoblast function. Leptin resistance is also associated with adrenal stress. High leptin levels are a signal that one has stored enough food. From an evolutionary perspective, the balance of insulin and leptin keeps us in balance with the natural cycles of fast (famine) and feast. When insulin goes down and leptin increases, the leptin signals that one has enough food to biologically reproduce. Leptin, in this context, also affects the biomarkers of the longevity profile.

The heat of the body is a measure of how the body gives energy. Thyroid hormone controls metabolic rate, and leptin controls the thyroid. The lower the body temperature, the longer you live. The heat of the body is a measure of how the body transforms energy. Proper leptin signaling controls the hypothalamus, in terms of overall body functioning, including thyroid function. Beyond regulating the accuracy of insulin signaling and development of insulin resistance, the main role of leptin is its regulating input on the functions of the hypothalamus, including reproduction, thyroid function, adrenal function, and function of the sympathetic nervous system. Excess fat cells and leptin also strongly influence chronic inflammation and are associated with this and all chronic diseases, including diabetes, Alzheimer's, heart disease, and some types of cancer. Normal leptin signaling regulates appetite control centers of the hypothalamus and signals the body to lose its appetite, which is fundamental. One of the things that also happens in leptin resistance is the loss of the ability to know where to store fat. As I pointed out before, one place the fat gets stored is in the abdominal organs and liver, thus further disrupting the liver's ability to listen to insulin signaling. When this happens, the liver cannot listen accurately to insulin, and therefore it cannot turn off the glycogen-to-glucose production metabolism in the liver. It also causes the muscles and bone to make too much glucose from protein, resulting in the breakdown of muscle and bone resulting in weakness and osteoporosis. The body in leptin resistance also gets confused about where to put calcium, so instead of depositing in the bones, calcium ends up going in blood vessels. Unfortunately, the master control center of our sympathetic nervous system in the hypothalamus does not become leptin resistant. Because of this, an elevated leptin, as I previously explained, causes overstimulation of sympathetic nervous system, which leads to diabetes, elevated blood pressure, increased blood coagulation, elevated T-3, heart disease, and para-inflammation.

LEPTIN DYNAMICS

LEPTIN ACTIVATION	LEPTIN RESISTANCE
• REDUCES APPETITE • ACTIVATES FAT BURNING FOR ENERGY • SENSITIZES SWEET TASTE BUDS (LESS DESIRE FOR SWEETS)	• INCREASES APPETITE • STORES MORE FAT TO SUCCESSFULLY REPRODUCE AND LIVE LONG ENOUGH TO DO SO • LOSS OF KNOWLEDGE OF WHERE TO STORE FAT (STORES IN ABDOMEN AND ABDOMINAL ORGANS SUCH AS LIVER, WHICH FURTHER DISRUPTS INSULIN SIGNALING TO THE LIVER)

FIGURE 2. Leptin dynamics

SIGNS OF POSSIBLE LEPTIN RESISTANCE

1. TROUBLE KEEPING WEIGHT OFF AFTER DIETING

2. ALWAYS HUNGRY

3. CRAVING SWEETS: LEPTIN RESISTANCE DESENSITIZES TASTE BUDS TO SUGAR.

4. FAT ACCUMULATION IN THE MIDSECTION WITH A WAIST SIZE GREATER THAN 35 INCHES FOR WOMEN AND 40 INCHES FOR MEN

5. LOSS OF MUSCLE MASS IN SPITE OF EXERCISE

6. FEELING STRESSED OUT

7. HIGH TRIGLYCERIDE LEVELS: ELEVATED TRIGLYCERIDES ARE ALSO ASSOCIATED WITH INSULIN RESISTANCE.

8. OSTEOPOROSIS: HIGH LEPTIN LEVELS INHIBIT PRODUCTION OF OSTEOBLASTS TO MAKE NEW BONE. OSTEOPOROSIS IS ALSO ASSOCIATED WITH ALL INSULIN RESISTANCE, POOR MINERAL ABSORPTION, GENERAL ACIDITY, LACK OF EXERCISE, AND LOSS OF MINERALS THROUGH THE KIDNEYS.

FIGURE 3. Leptin signs

PATHOLOGICAL RESULTS OF LEPTIN RESISTANCE

- DIABETES
- OBESITY
- INCREASED BLOOD PRESSURE
- INCREASED BLOOD COAGULATION
- ELEVATED T-3 LEVELS
- HEART DISEASE
- INCREASED INFLAMMATION
- ACCELERATED AGING

THE SYMPATHETIC CELLS IN THE BRAIN DO NOT BECOME LEPTIN RESISTANT, AND SO ELEVATED LEPTIN CAUSES OVERSTIMULATION OF SYMPATHETIC NERVOUS SYSTEM.

FIGURE 4. Leptin pathology

Normally, leptin is secreted for two reasons: rapidly in response to a high-carbohydrate meal or chronically in response to increased fat stores. In normal, healthy, leptin-sensitive individuals, as previously explained, it reduces hunger and sweet cravings, increases fat burning, and reduces fat storage. In leptin resistance, the leptin signaling messages do not work. However, the sympathetic nervous system is continually aggravated and overstimulated, as it does not go into leptin resistance. As one goes through these intricate mechanisms, the solution to healing diabetes at a hormonal level (however complicated the science) is to simply restore the accuracy of insulin and leptin signaling by eating a 25–45 percent carbohydrate diet. This is why the Dr. Cousens's Diabetes Recovery Program—A Holistic Approach only allows nonstarchy, fibrous carbohydrates from leafy greens, sprouts, vegetables, and sea vegetables.

Although obesity is not the topic of this book, it may help to explain a little bit about obesity and fat intake as part of the general optimal diet discussion. From my perspective, there are two important points to consider. First, people who are obese have usually lost their ability to burn fat because they are often in leptin resistance. As new research is beginning to reveal, a sudden elevated leptin in pregnant women rewires critical areas in the hypothalamus of the fetus and creates dysfunctional patterns, which may lead to obesity later in life.[114] Excess leptin can change our brain structures by changing epigenetic patterns. What researchers are observing is the importance of this epigenetic program shift as a key player in postnatal obesity. When mothers are undernourished, and there is an extra surge of leptin during pregnancy, somehow the newborn fetuses have a higher tendency to later become obese. Researchers seem to have found this pattern also in mice. There is something associated with leptin surges, for the fetus, that affects neural circuitry during development and interferes with leptin signaling to the brain. There has been a causal association that indicates that a leptin surge in the uterus changes the epigenetic pattern in the hypothalamic DNA and that somehow the brain loses its ability to translate leptin signaling, so that it does not know how to handle incoming nutritional energy. Researchers are beginning to understand that the leptin surge in utero is important especially when marked by periods of severe malnutrition. Leptin surges may also affect us as adults. If one eats a meal that gives a postprandial glucose of 140 or above, a leptin surge will occur. This leptin surge lays the foundations epigenetically for chronic degenerative diseases, including diabetes, heart disease, obesity, senility, and accelerated aging.[115] As I have said before, even in this type of situation, a healthy leptin reprogramming is possible through a steady, plant-source-only, 25–45 percent carbohydrate diet. With a proper diet, one can reset leptin hormonal signaling and leptin production back to normal and reverse leptin and ultimately insulin resistance. The bottom line is that a diet high in carbohydrates (simple and complex) may cause surges in leptin. The newer research about surges in leptin after meals for pregnant mothers in a larger context plays an interesting role in what I call the origins of health and disease. Based on my clinical data with 120 people, it appears that the Dr. Cousens's Diabetes Recovery Program—A Holistic Approach has the power to reset a pathogenic epigenetic leptin program back to a healthy one.

Going a little further in depth of the meaning of leptin resistance research has identified a class of proteins that interact with leptin stores, one being associated with C-reactive protein, a high C-reactive protein as a pure marker system of inflammation and a particular cardiac risk. Some research suggests a high C-reactive protein is associated with a 200 percent increased risk of dying within the first 28 days of a heart attack. Other research links elevated C-reactive protein, produced by adipose sites in liver cells, with preobesity and increased plasma leptin, stemming from that obesity.[116, 117] In my study, the C-reactive protein averaged a five-point drop in three weeks, which by any standards is a significant drop. This further supports the healing efficacy of a 25–45 percent moderate-low carbohydrate, live-food diet. This study, other clinical experience, and recent research suggest that a high C-reactive protein counters the balancing effects of healthy leptin. There is an increasing research implication that human C-reactive protein binds to leptin and interferes with leptin signaling.

When I was in Nigeria lecturing on diabetes and setting up a diabetes prevention clinic, I came across an herb called Ugiri (also known as bush mango) and technically known as *Irvingia gabonensis*. It appears to aid in the reversal of leptin resistance. It is the one exception to my statement that there is no medical substance that can reverse leptin resistance, as this herb may just help with this. It was discovered in Cameroon (western Africa) where they discovered a much lower diabetes rate associated with the indigenous people eating large quantities of this herb. Ugiri was discovered by research scientist Julius Oben from Cameroon. It grows throughout western Africa, where I am doing a lot of diabetes prevention education. This herb seems to help people lose weight, and in one study, after 10 weeks consuming the herb, they had a 13 percent decrease in body weight and a total body fat reduction by as much as 18.4 percent. In another study on the herb, markers of inflammation were greatly reduced. There was also a 26 percent reduction in total cholesterol, 27 percent reduction in LDLs, 32 percent reduction in fasting glucose, and a 52 percent decrease in C-reactive protein.[118, 119, 120] This is exciting, and because of my humanitarian antidiabetes work in Ghana and Nigeria,

Cameroon, and Ethiopia, I am encouraging people who live in these regions to start growing these herbs locally for themselves and for export. *Irvingia gabonensis* not only seems to reverse leptin resistance but also positively affects the fat-burning enzyme called glycerol-3-phosphate-dehydrogenase, which is an enzyme needed for the breakdown of body fat. *Irvingia gabonensis* also increases the secretion of the insulin-sensitizing hormone adiponectin, therefore decreasing insulin resistance, and, additionally, inhibiting the digestive enzyme amylase that results in slower carbohydrate assimilation. It is fun to see these herbs in the wild and to know that nature has given us a supportive antidote to leptin resistance as a supplement to the foundational 25–45 percent complex-carbohydrate diet. I conceptualize leptin signaling as a way our fat speaks to our brains to let our brains help our bodies know what energy is available and what to do with it. In that context, we can understand, as I have already explained, how leptin plays a significant role in heart disease, diabetes, heart disease, autoimmune disorders, and rates of aging, as it affects insulin signaling and is associated also with inflammation. While experiencing leptin resistance, one becomes proinflammatory, whereas leptin itself helps mediate the manufacture of other potent inflammatory chemicals that are released from the fat cells.

In summary, leptin regulates our hypothalamic and autonomic nervous system functions, including body temperature, heart rate, hunger, stress, fat-burning, reproduction, fat storage, and osteoblastic activity. There is an interplay here in that extracellular glycosylation is very harmful to the body, and when the body becomes insulin-resistant, cells become protected from intracellular glycosylation but not extracellular glycosylation. As already pointed out, my clinical study of an unrestricted-calorie diet that is 25–45 percent carbohydrate, live, and plant source only has had exceptional results (as compared to the commonly recommended vegan, high-complex carbohydrate, low-fat diet) in reducing high blood sugars and getting people off all medications. This is not to say that any approach that avoids all white sugar, white flour, junk food, GMO foods, and trans fats, as well as all flesh food and animal fat, will not have some positive effects on diabetes. For example,

Dr. Barnard's approach yielded a 46 percent decrease in medication use versus the Dr. Cousens's Diabetes Recovery Program—A Holistic Approach, which had 86.4 percent of all Type-2 diabetics came off all medications and had an overall 70 percent drop in insulin use by the Type-1 diabetics. I would say that in the three-week cycle our results were significantly more effective than the comparative plant-source-only, low-fat, high-complex carbohydrate diets that have been tried and also more effective than the relatively high-animal-protein and low-carbohydrate diets that are available. (At least four such studies have also shown some positive results in reversing diabetes.) In other words, there are many single-focus diets, most of which include no white sugar, white flour, or junk processed foods, which will give some level of efficacy in moderating Type-2 diabetes. The difference in my unmatched, rapid results is the total holistic synergy and overall effectiveness. Even outside of the 21-day program, I have motivated people to follow the Dr. Cousens's Diabetes Recovery Program—A Holistic Approach and got excellent results on a three-month follow-up visit. For example, as I am writing this, I just saw a 69-year-old male outpatient (not in the 21-day program) with Type-2 diabetes, heart disease (with six operations and eight stents), and obesity, whose FBS dropped to normal in three months on the program. His blood pressure and all his abnormal lipid profile also returned to normal in three months. He naturally lost 36 pounds without focusing on weight loss, and he loves the diet and how he feels. My point is that this holistic approach gets great results even outside the 21-day program because it is based on solid integration of scientific and spiritual principles.

A Moderate–Low Carbohydrate Diet: Why FBS of 70–85 Is Important

That leaves some very interesting questions, as generally a high-complex carbohydrate diet is currently recommended for diabetes by the allopathic majority and some of the vegan world as well. When I look at my clients, who started much more out of diabetic control, even with using insulin, and who started the program with much higher FBS compared to those eating the high-complex carbohydrate, low-fat diet, the 25–45 percent carbohydrate approach showed significantly greater drops in overall blood sugars. Why is this important? Why is this the case? What is going on? As I pointed out earlier, the insulin levels, faulty blood sugar regulation, and carbohydrate-driven glucose spikes seem to be correlated with the aging process, and many other chronic degenerative aging symptoms are directly linked to the amount of carbohydrate in the diet. Simple and complex carbohydrates are the most dietarily detrimental in CDDS. Reversing the insulin resistance means creating a fasting insulin in the low, normal range, somewhere between 4 and 6, or at least less than 10. That said, I believe I have found, through my clinical experience, that the most effective way to clinically prevent, reverse, or cure Type-2 diabetes or the variations of prediabetes and glucose dysregulation spikes, and aging in general, is a diet that is high in leafy greens, sprouts, sea vegetables, and low-starch, high-fiber vegetables as the main source of carbohydrates, with no grains or fruits, and a saturated and unsaturated fat intake of approximately 25–45 percent of the diet's calories and a 10–25 percent caloric protein intake. The exact mix depends on the person's constitution. The cuisine's only restrictions are (1) the only source of carbohydrates are leafy greens, sprouts, sea vegetables, and nonstarchy, fibrous vegetables; (2) no animal food of any type; (3) the food is to be whole, fresh, organic, alive, and completely plant source; (4) there is no white flour, white sugar, processed/junk food, or trans-fatty acids. People are asked to stay on this diet for three months after their FBS maintains at less than 100. At that point, they can be graduated to the Phase 1.5 maintenance diet, and they add in some low-glycemic fruits like berries, cherries, lemons, limes, and grapefruit, and also add some grains and beans.

I have presented some of the scientific reasons that theoretically explain these most impressive results. As we go one step deeper than a 25–45 percent carbohydrate diet, when one is fasting and/or on a moderate-low carbohydrate diet and the blood sugar often drops to 85 or less. At this blood sugar level, the body minimizes the secretion of insulin and makes a key shift in its metabolic program to begin to use fat as a source of energy, rather than glucose and fructose as a source of energy. It appears that part of the key metabolic switch is an enzyme called AMPK, which is known as AMP-activated protein kinase. This has a regulating role on the glucose metabolism. It also facilitates the movement of glucose into muscle cells and helps glucose, cholesterol, and triglyceride levels to normalize. This enzyme system gets activated when the amount of energy produced in the cell diminishes, which happens with an FBS less than 85. AMPK works in conjunction with what is known as a fuel-sensing gene SIRT-1, which also is known to also play a role in longevity. The AMPK-SIRT-1 system seems to be activated when people are on a calorie-restricted diet or moderate-low carbohydrate diet, in which their blood sugar goes below 86. This switch to the AMPK-SIRT-1 metabolic pathway also decreases inflammation and improves metabolic function. The AMPK and SIRT-1 causes the fat forming genetic complex, called PPAR-gamma (peroxisome proliferator-activated receptor-gamma), to be blocked. In other words, when the blood sugar goes below 86, AMPK-SIRT-1 is activated and blocks PPAR-gamma, whose job is to store fat. As a result, the system begins to move from a carbohydrate-burning metabolism into fat-burning metabolism for energy. This helps to partially explain why the average weight loss in a short time of 3 weeks on my program is slightly more than 18 pounds versus 12 pounds on Dr. Barnard's high-complex-carbohydrate, vegan, all natural diet over 22 weeks. Additional good news is that fat that may have ended up in the artery plaque is some of the first to be burned as fuel. Based on all research I have reviewed, in addition to my clinical experience, this moderate-low carbohydrate/live-food approach is going to best create a decrease in insulin production and leptin production and therefore is a primary diet for decreasing insulin and leptin resistance and activating the AMPK-SIRT-1 fat-burning pathway. This is one main reason my program is so quickly and effectively able to decrease and heal insulin and leptin resistance, as well as create accelerated weight loss and return the system to normal hormonal signaling. There was a study cited earlier in the book, which showed that people with a fasting insulin of 86 or greater had over 40 percent more heart disease. The findings of this study correlate with the science that shows that if one keeps one's blood glucose 85 and less, one is going to naturally shift to a fat-burning, cardio-protective, and diabetes-protective diet.

So what does a 25–45 percent carbohydrate diet look like? My 120+ clients had no restriction of plant-source fats, nuts, seeds, avocado, coconut oil, and olives, and had an average fat intake of 25–45 percent calories and no restriction on plant protein. Research over the last 70 years does show that humans, with between 20,000 and 30,000 genes and close to 200,000 gene variations, have individual genetic variations as to the right mixture of carbohydrates, protein, and fat needed in our diet for our mitochondrial DNA systems and overall cellular systems to create the optimal biological energy for the system. This is explained in detail in my book *Conscious Eating*.[121]

The Safety of a Mild Ketogenic Diet

Fasting and ketogenic diets, in general, are metabolically similar in that they are usually mildly ketogenic. Ketogenic diets may be mild, moderate, or severe, depending upon the diet. I measured the urine ketones in a group of fasters to examine the actual ketone production on this diet. There were 50 people in the study. They were diabetics and nondiabetics, whom I followed in this informal ketone fasting study.

On a 1-week fast I observed a cycle of urine ketones showing up between 5 and 80 (with some up to 160 and some as low as 0) in mild variation from day 2 to day 8 (after the fast). This was done for the three categories of Type-2 NIDDM diabetics, IDDM diabetics, and nondiabetic people. I observed the effects of a ketogenic diet through fasting ketone production in the urine. I was surprised to note that there did not seem to be any significant difference between the urine ketones of both Type-2 categories of diabetics and also nondiabetic fasters. Neither was greater than an extrapolated urine-to-blood ketone level of less than 2. I want to make a warning that I absolutely do not recommend fasting for Type-1 diabetics. It does not really matter how good one's health is, or the way one's Type-1 diabetes is managed, Type-1 diabetics can slip into diabetic-ketoacidosis in a few hours, even if they have successfully fasted many times before.

As previously noted, diabetics have double the amount of Alzheimer's, which adds a relevance to this ketone discussion. As previously explained, Alzheimer's is associated with insulin resistance in the brain. Diabetics seem to have more insulin resistance in the brain than nondiabetics, and therefore this is part of why there is twice as much Alzheimer's among diabetics. Increased ASCVD in the carotid and cerebral arteries may also play a role, as well as aluminum and mercury, dehydration, B-12 deficiencies, and various causes of brain inflammation. Switching to ketone metabolism is a direct way to antidote this insulin resistance of the brain as one cause of Alzheimer's.

To better understand this discussion, a little information on ketones and ketogenesis would be useful. There are three major ketone bodies—meaning major ketones that are produced in the body. These are acetate (Ac), acetoacetic acid (AcAc), and beta hydroxybutyrate (BHB). BHB appears to be the main ketone involved in brain energy. These three are our normal ketone bodies, which denotes the mix of all three. In our discussion about inflammation and obesity, for a basic background refresher, I also note that there are four primary fuels: (1) glucose and fructose, (2) protein, (3) free fatty acids, and (4) ketones. These four physiological fuels are stored in different ways in the body. This overview will help one understand the discussion. Glucose and fructose are stored in the liver as glycogen and in the adipose tissues (fat) as triglycerides. The second level of fuel storage is glucose as protein. Generally, the body prefers the way it has been trained as a glucose metabolism system versus a lipid metabolism system. The body usually has a one- or two-day reserve of carbohydrate storage. Fasting metabolism, which is actually the switching over to lipid metabolism for energy, begins once one has depleted carbohydrate storage and has moved into more of a lipid metabolism as a way to get energy. In the long run, fat gives twice as much energy per gram and a whole lot more energy storage reserve.

When the body is in this metabolism, where it makes its energy primarily from fats, it is protected against protein being broken down into glucose, which results in muscle wasting (which, to a certain extent, is what happens in uncontrolled diabetes, as well as when one sleeps overnight, even without diabetes). When on a ketogenic diet, which is a fat metabolism diet, the body is trained to burn fat at night for energy rather than to burn muscle protein to get glucose at night. This may be one reason many body builders use a moderate-low carbohydrate diet and why some of us, of age, who use this moderate-low carbohydrate diet do not necessarily suffer from glycopenia (muscle-mass loss)—because one is not losing muscle mass overnight. Switching to lipid metabolism is one of the things that came into public awareness with the East German Olympic athletes in the 1980s, who had better athletic performance because lipid metabolism gives twice as much caloric energy per gram as carbohydrate metabolism and was not catabolic to the muscles. Now, that being said, glucose is preferred in most tissues, if the body is on a high carbohydrate diet. The exception to this is the heart, which uses a mixture of glucose, free fatty acids, and ketones for energy. Although the main source of glucose is dietary intake of simple and complex carbohydrates, one also gets glucose from muscle tissue, and the liver and kidneys, via gluconeogenesis. This is where the term "protein sparing" comes about, because if one has enough carbohydrates there is a "sparing" effect and the body does not breakdown (catabolize) protein in the muscles to make glucose. What most people do not understand is the body can safely use free fatty acids for fuel for many tissues, which include skeletal muscle, the heart, and most of the organs. However, there are certain tissues that cannot use free fatty acids. This includes the brain, red blood cells, renal medulla of kidneys, bone marrow, and type-two muscle fibers. These primarily require glucose or ketones for energy. That brings us to the brain, which is not capable of using free fatty acids but works quite well, contrary to popular belief, on ketones if they are available.

The brain is the most important piece in terms of ketone utilization, especially for the utilization of BHB. As mentioned previously, the brain may derive up to 75–90 percent of its total energy from ketones after it shifts into lipid metabolism. Ketones provide a fuel for the brain whether carbohydrates are available or not. Some research suggests that ketones are the preferred fuel for the brain.[122] The liver does not use ketones for fuel. It relies on free fatty acids. It seems that by the second and third day of a fast that almost all nonprotein fuel comes from free fatty acids and ketones. This only lasts for a few weeks apparently and is followed by a big ketone utilization down-regulation in the brain and body. At this point the tissues move more toward getting the energy from free fatty acids.[123] As I have already explained, the advantage of a ketogenic diet is that there is a metabolic switch to the use of free fatty acids, as well as ketones, for energy, which gives twice as much energy per gram of nutrition, and there is no muscle wasting at night; therefore glycopenia (muscle wasting) with age is minimized.

When one's cell metabolism is dependent on the glucose and fructose, it does not care where it gets the sugar. When one sleeps, the body still requires sugar or glucose to maintain its sugar metabolism addiction while we sleep. When the glycogen in the liver is used up, the cells begin to break down muscle protein into glucose. It even takes glucose from our bones, which is another reason people get osteoporosis, as the body steals sugar from the bone structure. As long as one is in glucose-burning metabolism, the body tells us not to burn fat. The mitochondria will not take from the fat stores, and they focus on sugar for their source of energy. A high complex carbohydrate diet, as I explained before, will both keep us burning sugar and storing fat. The Dr. Cousens's Diabetes Recovery Program—A Holistic Approach helps our body by retraining our brain and our liver to tell our cells to burn fat as the primary fuel. This is best done by eating a diet that creates an FBS of 85 or less. When people switch over to a diet that induces lipid metabolism, they burn fat all the time, even when they are sleeping. Many people may have fat in their arteries, and this ketogenic fat-burning cuisine should help dissolve the fat from the arteries. Although there exists little research on this and its mechanisms, it is highly theoretically suggestible that when one starts burning fat they start cleaning out the arteries.

The picture is a bit complex when one looks at it anthropologically, because there are relatively long-lived indigenous groups eating both high-fat and high-carbohydrate diets, so I have to refine the discussion to the physiology and body types we know in our Western culture today versus indigenous cultures, lifestyles, and their ethno-biological interfaces around the world. When one trains their bodies to become metabolically proficient fat burners, there is a general decrease in muscle wasting throughout the day and night. This may also be why, as a 70-year-old, I do not suffer from glycopenia, as most 70-year-olds do. Just as an experiment, on this diet I have added eight pounds of muscle mass in the past year by increasing exercise simply to make the double point that plant-source-only people do not have to get glycopenia with age. Although this book is not about weight loss or glycopenia, with the moderate-low carb 25–45 percent and 25–45 percent fat dietary approach of the Dr. Cousens's Diabetes Recovery Program—A Holistic Approach, I have had people lose up to 46 pounds in three weeks.

One Inuit Native American shaman from the Bering Strait in Alaska lost 25 pounds in one week and cured his diabetes in two weeks. As pointed out before, the average weight loss in three weeks is slightly more than 18 pounds, but it is not unusual for people to lose 30 to 40 pounds in 21 days with this total holistic approach. In general I do not focus on weight loss, as it is a natural by-product of this healthy holistic cuisine.

The medical use of a moderate-low carbohydrate diet for weight loss goes back at least a few hundred years. In 1825, Brillat-Savarin, author of *The Physiology of Taste*, born in 1775, said, "It can be deduced as an exact consequence that more or less rigid abstinence from everything that is starchy or floury will lead to the lessening of weight." As has been pointed out, obesity and diabetes are connected, so weight loss and avoidance of obesity with a moderate-low carbohydrate diet was actually conventional scientific wisdom up to the 1960s. During the 1960s and 1970s, people went to high-complex carbohydrates in association with antifat diets (a macronutrient shift). This general unfortunate switch can be epidemiologically correlated with the present epidemic of obesity and diabetes. In 1869, to point out the conventional wisdom at that time, British physician Tanner wrote, "Paranatious (starchy) and vegetable foods are fattening and saccharine matters are especially so." In other words, he considered the best diet for weight loss to be a low-carbohydrate diet. Jean Frances Danielle's 1844 writing on obesity or obsessive weight said low-carbohydrate diet was the primary cure for obesity. One of the most famous physicians in Britain, William Harvey, after listening to Claude Bernard (another great physician and researcher) lecture on diabetes in 1856 in Paris, realized to lose weight one had to eliminate starch and sugar. Harvey then successfully treated William Banting. Banting wrote *Letter on Corpulence* in 1864, which became a rather famous book, and instructed people to cut out bread, butter, sugar, milk, and potatoes. One of the great fathers of medicine in North American, Sir William Osler, MD, who wrote *Principles and Practices of Medicine* in 1901, advised obese women to avoid taking too much food and particularly to reduce starches and sugar. Between 1943 and 1952, independent physician researchers from Stanford, Harvard, and Cornell Medical Schools, and Children's Memorial Hospital in Chicago, published separate papers on the power of a low-carbohydrate diet for the treatment of obesity. In other words, the low carbohydrate diet for weight loss is both time tested and medically researched, and it is not a new idea. There are some variations, since people have constitutional variations.

The basic obesity mechanism can be best understood with a simple review of the actions of insulin. Insulin creates the storage of glucose as fat. Insulin is a key regulator of fat metabolism. When there is excess of insulin and sugar in the system, it results in fat storage. It does this by activating LPL (lipoprotein lipase), which sticks out of the cell membrane and pulls fat out of the blood and into the cells. It gives a key in understanding in how men and women distribute fat differently. Areas with more LPL are where people gather more and less fat. The LPL digests the triglycerides into their fatty acid building blocks, which then are absorbed into the cell. Variations of LPL distribution differ in men and women. Men tend to have more LPL in mid-gut area and women have it more below the waist. Insulin is the primary regulator of LPL activity, as it activates the LPL. Insulin also affects HSL (hormone sensitive lipase), which makes our fat cells and us leaner. Insulin suppresses the HSL-complex and activates the LPL-complex. Insulin also signals liver cells not to burn fatty acids but to repackage them as triglycerides and store them again in the fat tissue. It comes down to one main point: anything that's going to increase insulin will increase fat storage, and the main cause for increasing insulin blood levels is carbohydrate consumption. Excess insulin will even make diabetics fatter. I see that all the time when I decrease insulin medication: diabetics go back to a more normal weight. In one study, Type-2 diabetics on intensive insulin therapy gained an average of 8 pounds in less than 1 year, and a third of these people gained more than 20 pounds in 3.5 years.[124]

Another part of this story is that excess dietary carbohydrates usually are converted to fat if they are not used for energy. When one decreases the use of glucose, which is what I describe with the diet of carbohydrate intake less than 100 grams, people often increase the use of fat calories for fuel if they do not want to experience protein excess toxicity. When people move into dietary patterns that support lipid metabolism, they enhance the body's preprogrammed ability to use fatty acids and ketones and decrease body's use of glucose metabolism pathways. One literally must retrain one's body to use the lipid metabolic pathways to optimally make energy that way, which is what I believe the East German Olympians consciously did. Although it happens naturally, when one moves to lipid metabolism, one not only gets twice as much energy per gram but also gets a potentially better fuel source for one's brain and heart from fat metabolism. In the long run, on a 25–45 percent carbohydrate diet diabetes treatment level or a 30–50 percent carbohydrate maintenance diet, one also begins to create the optimal longevity values of blood insulin, leptin, and general energy production.

For a moment let us return to the dangers of insulin excess as part of this comprehensive discussion. When one increases sugar intake, one increases the insulin output to compensate. This insulin increase causes more glucose to be stored as glycogen in liver, muscle, and as triglycerides in fat cells. Insulin also, as I explained earlier, is a fat storage-producing hormone, and it does this by a process of lipogenesis. The free fatty acid release from fat cells is also inhibited by small amounts of insulin. A glucose above 85 will shut off the lipid metabolism energy-producing pathway, and the body switches back over to a glucose energy metabolism. Increasing blood sugar will increase production of insulin. As previously noted, research in 1984 showed that eating a quarter-pound hamburger will raise fasting insulin as much as a quarter pound of white sugar.[125] Looking at the macronutrient mix, neither a high complex carbohydrate nor a high protein diet is the best choice for preventing and healing diabetes. What I have begun to look at, again, depending on one's constitutional type, is a moderate lipid intake of 25–45 percent, which keeps calories from carbohydrates and proteins relatively low to moderate, thus minimizing glucose release from either of these macronutrient groups. Although my personal fat calorie intake is 42 percent, my body mass index is 14, which is low normal for a man. This means that although 42 percent of my calories come from fat, I have a very low fat content in my body, which makes the point that one does not get fat on a 42 percent calorie-from-fat diet. Forty-eight percent of my calories come from carbohydrates as leafy greens, sprouts, nonstarchy and fibrous vegetables, and low-glycemic fruits, and 10 percent of my calories come from plant-source protein. The ratios vary according to one's constitutional type, and some people may need a higher amount of protein and a lower amount of carbohydrates. As a slow-oxidizer/sympathetic type, I do best with a low protein to higher complex carbohydrate ratio. On this relatively low protein diet of about 40–50 grams daily, I did 601 consecutive push-ups at the age of 60.

In other words, my optimal dietary energy production intake according to my mitochondrial DNA requires relatively low protein consumption, and my energy and performance level suggests this works best for, at least, me. On this dietary approach, my FBS is 84–85. Researchers have found exactly this type of result.[126, 127, 128] Research confirms that the body, by regulating its input of carbohydrates, lipids, and proteins, will burn greater amounts of lipids and decrease the amount of glucose burned, which I like to see happen in my dietary approach. This both prevents and treats diabetes, and it also prevents and treats the chronic degenerative diseases associated with aging (essentially all chronic diseases), and it is optimal for longevity. When insulin decreases and fatty acids mobilize, and when the proper leptin signal reaches fat, the stored triglycerides are broken down into glycerol and free fatty acids that travel through the system: that's how we get the free fatty acids that are needed for energy.

To better appreciate the role of a mild ketogenic diet in its role for optimal diabetes prevention and treatment, as well as the optimal longevity diet for our culture, it is useful to understand the difference between starvation, dietary fasting, and diabetic ketoacidosis. The key difference is the amount of ketone concentration in the blood. To have a definition of ketosis, we have to have at least 0.2 ketone bodies per millimol deciliter of blood. After two or three days of fasting on green juices, blood ketone levels in the body rarely go above 0.2–2.0. Postexercise blood ketone may go up to 2. In longer fasting, the blood ketones may go up to 5. With a long-term ketogenic diet, they may go up to 5 to 6. (However, most of my clients and myself on the Phase 1.0 and 1.5 diet rarely get above 0.2–2.0.) For a fast of 3–4 weeks, they may go up to 6 to 7. Those 6–7 values are still ranges of medical safety. Above 7–8 is considered ketoacidosis. Diabetic ketoacidosis starts above 8. In this case, the person would be both acidotic and ketotic. Diabetic ketoacidosis can go up to 35. Minimal ketosis is defined as a ketone concentration above 0.2. Mild ketosis is up to 2, which can happen through exercise. All the Type-2 diabetics and nondiabetics in my 7-day fasting program were between 0.2 and 2.0, which translates to a urine ketone of approximately 15–160. In summary, fasters, Type-2, and Type-1 diabetics on this mild Phase 1.0 ketogenic diet will have normal urine pHs, while having ketones in the urine up to 5–160, which is a safe range, as it is between 0.2 and 2 in the blood. On the Phase 1.5 ketogenic diet, one is closer to 0.2, which is a very mild ketosis.

In my research, I have been using urine ketone levels rather than analyzing the ketones in the blood directly. The conversion rate of ketones into the urine is approximately 10–20 percent of total ketones made in the liver.[129] Interestingly, physiologically, women show higher ketones than men do.[130, 131] In my pilot fasting ketone study, there was a slight trend in that direction. Children also can get higher ketones.[132] The body keeps a normal pH as long as ketone concentration does not exceed 7–10 micromoles. For example, I generally have alkaline urine during fasting even with a urine ketone of 5–15 percent. In diabetics, excretion of ketones is increased, and the ketones create a feedback loop that causes fat cells to slow release of free fatty acids.[133] I hypothesize that Type-1 diabetics do not have strong buffer protection systems, which is what makes them vulnerable to ketoacidosis, usually associated with a blood ketone of less than 8. That is one of the reasons they can so easily go into diabetic ketoacidosis, and why I strongly advise against fasting in the case of Type-1 diabetes. When one looks at fat and ketone use during fasting, the research shows that practically 90 percent of the body's total fuel needs may be met by free fatty acids and ketones.[134] After three weeks of fasting, up to 93 percent of fuel may be from free fatty acids. Interestingly enough, in the first few days of mild ketosis, the brain does not use the ketones for fuel, until it adapts. There are a few tissues in the body that cannot use free fatty acids or ketones. These are leukocytes, bone marrow, and erythrocytes—they still require glucose.

One of the most important components of this discussion is related to both diabetes and Alzheimer's, which is part of where this immediate discussion started. Alzheimer's is the second most feared disease.[135] The incidence of Alzheimer's increases exponentially with age. At the age of 80–85, the prevalence of Alzheimer's rises to 25–30 percent.[136, 137] This discussion of Alzheimer's in relationship to diabetes may give some insight for the general public in terms of Alzheimer's prevention with the use of a 25–45 percent carbohydrate mild ketogenic diet and coconut oil. The brain needs glucose as its fuel, and, in a nonketonic state, the brain uses approximately 100 grams or more of glucose daily.[138, 139]

Research suggests that anything less than 100 grams of carbohydrates daily causes one to enter at least a slight ketosis. The scientific literature also does not suggest that carbohydrates are essential as a source of body energy, and the body can use other sources of fuel (either protein or fatty acid metabolic pathways) to produce the little glucose it needs. That said, I want to be clear that I am not suggesting a no-carbohydrate diet. I am suggesting that people, according to their constitution, need to find the best macronutrient ratio. One needs enough dietary protein (somewhere around 30 to 60 grams daily in a nonpregnant person) and less than 100 grams of carbohydrates to create the mild ketosis, while at the same time eluding a breakdown of muscle for glucose production.

As I have worked on diabetes over the last 40 years, it has become clear to me that a great many people with diabetes develop mental fogginess, lack of clarity, memory loss, and a certain amount of mental confusion. People with diabetes have at least a 65 percent increase in the potential to get Alzheimer's. Decreased brain function is very noticeable in many of my clients, who have these subtle mental signs that I, as a trained psychiatrist, perceive rather acutely. My initial thought was that para-inflammation and atherosclerosis associated with diabetes is affecting and clogging the small arteries of the brain and, therefore, compromising mental functioning, which has to be somewhat the case. But as I researched this further, I began to see a different set of data more primary to that, and these data are suggesting that the brain manufactures its own insulin to convert glucose in the brain blood into energy, and as the whole body begins to become insulin resistant, so does the brain. With time, the brain tissues, particularly noted in the hippocampus, the precortex, the cortex areas, and the limbic system, become more specifically insulin-resistant. That means the brain in these areas is not able to get insulin into the cells in an effective way, and therefore glucose cannot get into those brain areas and brain function is compromised. Without fuel, those brain cells begin to malfunction and ultimately atrophy. This seems to be at least one of several major mechanisms that are associated, from a diabetic perspective, with Alzheimer's. I am not referring to mercury in the brain associated with Alzheimer's; nor am I referring to aluminum in the brain or general brain inflammation such as is secondary to flu vaccinations (all of which contribute), but specifically to diabetes and its effects. In exploring this question, I came across a very interesting article by a case study by Dr. Mary Newport titled, "What If There Were a Cure for Alzheimer's Disease and No One Knew?"[140] This fascinating article opened up my eyes to a very real potential partial solution to this whole story. As her husband's Alzheimer's progressed, she was researching how to help him, and found some commercial pharmaceuticals under exploration. She realized that these were, in essence, ketone bodies or precursors to ketone bodies (also known as midchain fatty acids). She began to experiment with her own husband by giving him coconut oil, which is very high in midchain triglycerides (MCTs). She points out that these MCT oils were handled differently in the body than others. Instead of being stored as fat, research showed they went directly to the liver and were converted into ketone bodies, which could be used as energy. These ketone bodies were available to the brain as energy. At least 75–90 percent of the brain energy can be supplied by ketone bodies. What she reported is that these MCTs caused not only hyperketonemia but a substantial 39 percent increase in cerebral blood flow. She noted that when she administered approximately 4–5 tablespoons a day of coconut oil to her husband, he began to recover a great deal of his mental functioning in the relatively short time of several days. It is an exciting story. The media has suggested that coconut oil is an unhealthy saturated fat. Contrary to this generally accepted myth, in the Philippines, where they consume a great deal of coconut oil, there is the lowest insulin-related cardiovascular disease in the world. Medium-chain triglycerides are also high in human breast milk, which is a 54 percent fat content. This suggests that coconut oil may be rather good for us, provided it is not hydrogenated or heated. Hydrogenated coconut oil is not healthy for anyone. It is a trans fat, which is dangerous. It must be a natural, nonhydrogenated coconut oil, containing no trans fats. This is relevant because some of the early coconut oil was hydrogenated, and people got a wrong impression. It appears hydrogenated trans-fatty acids are a major cause, from a fat point of view, for heart disease, atherosclerosis, and activating diabetes. The world research agrees that trans fats are dangerous to one's cardiovascular and general health. Trans fats are not the same as healthy raw, plant-source, poly-unsaturated, mono-unsaturated, and saturated fats. This is a vital distinction. Some fats are healthy and necessary, but trans fats are pathogenic and unnecessary. They should be avoided 100 percent of the time. The prime ketone for energizing the brain is beta hydroxybutyrate (BHB). It seems to protect and energize the neurons when glucose is unavailable. It is the prime ketone forming from coconut oil being metabolized in the liver.

In conclusion, a major reason for diabetes-associated Alzheimer's (particularly diabetically driven Alzheimer's) is that the brain gets progressively insulin resistant, and as the brain cells cannot get proper glucose fuel, the brain begins to atrophy and lose function particularly in the area of memory loss, speech, movement, and personality. The good news, as pointed out earlier, is that our brains are able to run on ketone energy as well as on glucose energy. A mild ketogenic diet—that is, a 25–45 percent or 30–50 percent carbohydrate (maintenance) diet that includes at least 3–5 tablespoons of coconut oil—produces ketones that specifically energize these atrophied cells and renew brain function. (I suggest 3 tablespoons for prevention and 5, or even 6, tablespoons of coconut oil to increase ketone energy to your brain in presenility, senility, or Alzheimer's.) It restores and renews neuron function even after there has been damage. The mild ketogenic diet also protects against the tendency to develop insulin resistance both in the body and brain in the first place, so it acts on the level of primary prevention as well. There is now a way to actually feed the brain from two angles. One is with glucose, and the other is with ketones. A 25–45 percent or a 30–50 percent carbohydrate diet of less than 100 grams of glucose per day will create a slight to mild ketosis, which will feed and regenerate the brain. The other powerful approach, which creates ketones and solves the insulin resistance of the brain, is to use coconut oil, which converts directly to ketones. When one uses coconut oil, the MCT ketone metabolism almost treats the coconut oil as an energy source, like carbohydrates, in the way it is metabolized in the liver, and like glucose, in the way it is sent out to the rest of the system. It does not cause an insulin spike, because beta hydroxybutyrate does not stimulate insulin. It therefore helps decrease insulin resistance. After as little as 14 days on my program, which is, of course, a fast-track program, I will often see a return of mental clarity, and I will tell people, "Your mind is coming back." It is not something people like to talk about, and it is a little uncomfortable, but people usually say with a smile, "Yes, it's returning." I have seen high-powered businessmen, whose egos were too big to say their minds were going, say, "Yes, it's returning." That is a surprise gift that people get from this program in a relatively short time.

In summary, insulin resistance in the brain is one of the most powerful causes of brain damage and ultimately Alzheimer's. Insulin resistance also creates a significant amount of inflammation, which also prematurely degenerates the brain. The addition of both coconut oil and my mild ketogenic diet helps to minimize, reverse, or prevent this process. A slightly ketogenic diet, in general, will give one the best protection from insulin resistance, diabetes, and Alzheimer's.

Fructose and Diabetes

As part of the overall diabetes discussion, there lurks the misconception that somehow fructose does not contribute to diabetes. This is a major misunderstanding. Fructose is directly associated with diabetes, especially high-fructose corn syrup. When one is cellularly addicted to glucose, sucrose, and/or fructose, they become stuck in sugar metabolism for making energy.

For years, limited and conventional "wisdom" has held that fructose does not affect your blood sugar. This is accurate on a superficial level but unscientific in its assumption that because fructose does not raise blood sugar, it does not affect insulin resistance and cause many metabolic disease problems from the metabolic abnormalities associated with metabolizing an excess amount of fructose. It is therefore falsely deemed a safer sugar than glucose. None of this has been proven to be true. A primary difference is that fructose is metabolized differently than glucose. Fructose is metabolized much more rapidly than any other sugar into fat via the liver. It is also primarily metabolized in the liver. Because of this it has also been associated with a high level of nonalcoholic fatty liver disease (NAFLD) and a rapid accumulation of a particular kind of fat (triglycerides) that is stored in both the liver and general fat tissue. This is related not only to NAFLD but also to heart disease and hypertension. Glucose, when combined with fructose (as in sucrose and high-fructose corn syrup), accelerates fructose absorption. These metabolic differences are further enhanced in light of recent research reported in the March 2011 *Diabetes, Obesity and Metabolism*, which found that cortical areas around hypothalamus in the brain responded differently to fructose than to glucose.[141] They found that in brain scans, glucose raised levels of neuronal activity for 20 minutes, while fructose dropped neuronal activity for about 20 minutes. This is a significant and polar difference; again, making the point that simple sugars are not handled the same. In these two different areas, then, fructose and glucose are handled differently. As one goes a little further with this story, one begins to see some other pieces. The incidence of diabetes increased about 90 percent in the two years, which coincided with the introduction of high-fructose corn syrup into our collective dietary patterns in the 1980s. Another part of the metabolic difference is that fructose is more lipogenic than glucose. High fructose diets have not only been linked to NAFLD, but this rising amount of high-fructose corn syrup use has also been associated with the rising epidemics of obesity, diabetes, and metabolic syndrome.

One of the unique things about fructose metabolism, according to Elizabeth Parks in the *Journal of Nutrition* (2000), is the surprising speed with which humans make fat from fructose.[142] Once the body is trained in the fructose metabolic pathways, it is difficult to turn it off. The body makes a decision when glucose enters the system whether to store it as fat or to burn it. Fructose does not get involved in this decision and bypasses burning, going directly to storage. More and more research is showing that high-fructose corn syrup converts more quickly to triglycerides and adipose tissues than blood glucose. Fructose also interferes with leptin and insulin signaling.[143] That is a problem because insulin and leptin act, as previously discussed, as regulators of food intake. Fructose seems to mix up the signaling, resulting in increased food intake and weight gain. High-fructose corn syrup sweetened foods also contribute to diabetes because they have high levels of complex carbonyls (also high in people with diabetes).[144] Fructose does not contain enzymes, vitamins, or minerals, so it ends up stealing nutrients from the body, particularly magnesium, copper, and chromium.[145] Problematically, fructose has no effect on ghrelin, as compared to glucose, which suppresses ghrelin. Ghrelin is a hormone that signals us to eat. It is called the hunger hormone. Fructose does not turn it off, so it does not suppress the appetite, whereas glucose decreases ghrelin secretion in a feedback loop that decreases appetite. Naturally, if the appetite does not slow down, one will gain weight and become obese. In other words, fructose blocks the leptin message to stop eating and to decrease cravings for sweets. Instead, fructose signals our bodies to keep eating and store fat, which leads to obesity.

Sucrose is 45–50 percent glucose and 50–55 percent fructose. In contrast to this, high-fructose corn syrup can be as high as 80 percent fructose and 20 percent glucose, which is a significant difference. Although they both contain the same calories per gram, there are more differences. Metabolism of excess fructose, which is metabolized differently than glucose, is a general major disaster for human health. High amounts of fructose going to the liver to be metabolized disturbs glucose metabolism in the liver as well as uptake pathways and levels of metabolic pathways that are associated with creating insulin resistance.[146]

Fructose is quite detrimental to us for a number of additional reasons. Taking an overview, the introduction of high-fructose corn syrup in the 1980s has been associated with several major health disasters. In summary, from a holistic perspective beyond diabetes management, excess fructose (over 25 grams daily) and particularly high-fructose corn syrup have been causally associated with increasing rates of high blood pressure, heart disease, diabetes, obesity and insulin resistance metabolic syndrome, gout, kidney stones, NAFLD, brain inflammation, increased cancer, accelerated aging, and increased AGEs. One study in the *British Medical Journal* suggests that sugar, sweetened soft drinks, and fructose were significantly associated with increased risk of gout in men. Fructose encourages, and is connected with, increased kidney stone and, as previously mentioned, a significant increase in cases of NAFLD.[147, 148] Between 1970 and 1990, there was a 1,000 percent increased intake of high-fructose corn syrup in the average American diet, and it comprises 40 percent of the caloric sweeteners added to our foods.[149] Throughout most of human history, as I mentioned before, humans rarely had much fructose in their diets (probably 15 grams daily and it was periodic). It was mostly from fruits and vegetables. Today, there is an estimated 81 grams of fructose daily in the American diet, which is up to five times greater than the amount humans used to have[150] and a serious aberration of fructose intake. Fifteen to 25 grams daily is safe, but people have gone beyond safe limits with 81 grams of fructose daily. As a result of this excess, the body, as I explained earlier, becomes fructose overloaded. The body is not designed to handle three to five times the safe fructose amount. As already pointed out, fructose metabolism is different from glucose in that glucose is a primary source of energy. Glucose goes primarily to ATP production. Excess glucose may go to the liver to be stored in the liver as carbohydrates. By contrast, fructose metabolism takes place primarily in the liver, where it will sludge the metabolic pathways and will increase triglyceride storage in the liver so the overabundance is too much for the liver. It raises triglycerides, activates the atherogenic lipid profile, and therefore increases the cardiovascular pathogenic profile.

Increased dietary fructose, contrary to some earlier teachings, is also associated with insulin resistance and Type-2 diabetes.[151] In 2004, researchers released data correlating refined carbohydrate intake and diabetes. The use of high-fructose corn syrup and other sweeteners was 2,100 percent higher in 1997 than in 1909 and was associated with a higher rate of diabetes. It is thus correlated with the skyrocketing diabetes epidemic.[152] Research was also done to clarify the difference between fructose and glucose in insulin resistance. Controls were compared with high fructose and high glucose diets, and even after one week, those with increased fructose diets significantly increased insulin resistance, as compared to the high glucose group, which had no change.[153] Fructose in excess has also been linked to hypertension,[154] and it does this by inhibiting a key enzyme called *endothelial nitrous oxide synthase*,[155] located in blood vessel walls. In this way, fructose blocks the baso-dilation effect in the arteries.

Contrary to glucose, fructose creates a high concentration of fats and lipoproteins in the body and contributes to unhealthy lipid profiles. One major lipid increase with fructose is the triglycerides.[156] It also converts to activated glycerol 3 phosphate (g-3-p), which is needed to convert free fatty acids into triglycerides. The more g-3-p one has, the more fat one can store. It also increases the activated APOB100, a primary lipoprotein that carries cholesterol to blood vessels and leads to fatty deposits. It decreases the high-density lipoproteins, which help take pathogenic cholesterol away from the vessels and back to the liver.

One of the most serious aspects of fructose excess is NAFLD, which effects up to 30 percent of population; people with NAFLD are found to eat two to three times more fructose. NAFLD is associated with higher rates of cirrhosis and liver cancer. This of course leads to higher death rates from liver disease. A most important aspect of this fructose nightmare is its creation of advanced glycation end products (AGEs), as already stated. Fructose is 10 times more active in creating these AGEs than glucose.[157] Other research shows that cancer cells will use fructose at least 10 times more actively than glucose, which, in itself, is up to 10 to 50 times the normal cell usage for glucose. Data suggests, in general, that long-term fructose consumption increases AGEs and accelerates the aging process.[158]

Should one avoid fructose entirely? No. The body historically is designed to handle 15–25 grams of fructose daily. The question is, what can one do to minimize it since, in the United States, the average intake is 81 grams daily? It is beneficial to minimize sources of dietary fructose, fruit juices, high glycemic fruits, table sugar, and honey; these are your basic and rather simple, straightforward approaches to this. Basically, any packaged product that is not labeled organic will contain high-fructose corn syrup. Additionally, we have a new threat called genetically modified organisms (GMOs). GMO products (which include 86 percent of corn as a source of high-fructose corn syrup) are another very serious concern because they are so hidden in the labeling games. The easy, safe solution is purchase only unpackaged, organic foods. Fifteen to 25 grams of fructose is equivalent to about 2 bananas, 1.5–2 medium-sized papayas, 4 grapefruits, 4 pineapples, 5 kiwis, a few dates, 1 mango, or a half cup of dried figs per day. One of the things to be aware of is that most sweeteners are problematic, including agave, which has often been found to be laced with high-fructose corn syrup. (Some of this was even caught by the FDA.) I recommend avoiding agave, as "organic agave" brands are 59–60 percent fructose, which may be equal to or worse than some high-fructose corn syrup combinations. This is why I recommend avoidance of all fructose products when following a low-carbohydrate diets—not just glucose. I am not recommending substituting fructose for glucose or glucose for fructose. High-fructose corn syrup is an unbound fructose and is therefore more pathogenic than fruit-based fructose, which is bound to other sugars. The strongest and main way to cut down carbohydrates in our intake is simply to cut out all white sugar, all fructose sources (except for 25 grams of fruit), and eat mainly leafy greens, vegetables, nonstarchy, fibrous carbohydrates, sprouts, and sea vegetables. That is the simple way to move away from the dangers of a long-term, high complex carbohydrate diet and high-fructose carbohydrate diet. It is relatively easy to retrain one's body to stop craving sweets. When moving into a Phase 1.0 diet or green juice fasting (no fruit or grains—only nonstarchy vegetables, nuts and seeds, and sea veggies), the body naturally readjusts its programming to a decrease in leptin. Thus we move naturally out of leptin resistance and no longer crave sweets, as we turn off those destructive metabolic pathways. For many, even greens begin to taste sweet, which is nice. When leptin resistance decreases, sweet cravings also decrease immensely. Again, there is no real trick to this other than when one eats less sugar, the body craves less sugar from the epigenetic program down to leptin hormonal programming. The answer on a deeper level is that you have to love yourself enough to want to change your diet.

Holistic Synergy

Now that I have discussed the ideas and concepts involved with a 25–45 percent carbohydrate diet and its importance in reversing Type-2 diabetes, it would not be holistically or scientifically exact or correct to look upon my unusual results in healing diabetes as solely resulting from a 25–45 percent carbohydrate diet. There are other major factors that are part of a holistic synergy associated with the powerful healing results seen in this program. One other major factor is that the cuisine is 100 percent organic, unprocessed, live, and plant source only. The live-food dietary approach creates a natural caloric restriction, which is also a healing force at play here as well. Also white sugar, white flour, all junk processed, and GMO food are 100 percent completely excluded in this diet. Eliminating those substances is extremely powerful for good health in general, as well as diabetes specifically. There is also detox support from pesticides, herbicides, heavy metals, and radiation. I also emphasize adequate sleep, moderate exercise, and emotional and spiritual well-being.

The key part of its antidiabetic effect is the understanding of the healing power of live foods and perhaps, even in a broader way, the importance of the supportive healing power of high-quality, nonprocessed, nonjunk foods. In other words, diet and food understood only as simply carbohydrates, proteins, and fats is a limited perspective; it is important to discuss food in terms of quality. For example, there is a significant difference between cooked trans fat and all natural, plant-based, raw fat (saturated or unsaturated). Not all fats are equal. In the same way, live food has certain qualities that are different from cooked food. As pointed out previously, about 60–70 percent of the vitamins and minerals are destroyed when cooked, up to 95 percent of phytonutrients are destroyed, and about 50 percent of the proteins become coagulated. The simple math is that when one eats live food properly, one literally can consume half the amount of calories because the active quality, nutrient density, and energy of the food are so superior.

The studies on organic foods have shown repeatedly that these foods have significantly more minerals and nutrients than commercial foods (sometimes up to 250 percent more minerals and nutrients). This is compounded by the fact that organic foods are pesticide and herbicide free and that these toxins have been shown to further weaken the body's ability to produce insulin and have been implicated in creating insulin resistance. On a live-food diet, one can take in 50 percent less calories and still get more than adequate nutrition. Earlier I referred to Dr. Spindler's work that showed that by reducing calorie intake by 40 percent, there is a 400 percent increase in antiaging genes function (which is reasonably interpreted as including antiaging, antidiabetic genes). A 400 percent increase in anti-inflammatory genes is essential in our work toward upgrading anti-inflammatory expression and downgrading inflammation, which is a toxic driving force in diabetes and aging. In this context, fasting and a live-food diet is important for turning off the dysfunctional metabolic epigenetic programming and upgrading by 400 percent the antiaging, theoretically antidiabetic, anti-inflammatory, antioxidant, and anticancer genes. Just that fact alone gives a tremendous edge to a properly selected, live-food diet as a healing agent for diabetes. The people in my study had no controls on the volume of food, including fat calories and protein calories taken in, except that, as pointed out previously, carbohydrates were restricted to leafy greens, nonstarchy and fibrous vegetables, sea vegetables, and sprouts. In short, the organic, live-food, plant-source-only diet plays a major healing role because it is a delightful way to get the healing benefits of calorie restriction as well as the healing energy and power of the live-food, plant-source-only diet.

In general, a live food diet is able to deliver the total nutrient density of double the amount of cooked food calories in a delightful, tasty, and enjoyable way. The health, in general, and positive diabetic implications of this is that the properly eaten organic live food diet, as I recommend, creates a genetic upgrade in terms of minimizing diabetic genetic pressure on the system and decreasing inflammation. This is, to some extent, validated by the results of over 120 people in the Dr. Cousens's Diabetes Recovery Program—A Holistic Approach. What I found is that as people observed their FBS, when they ate a lot (especially carbohydrates or protein), or ate too late at night, blood sugars were consistently higher in the morning FBS. The blood sugar, in general, seemed to rise or fall depending on the amount of food (especially carbohydrates and protein) eaten. Part of the training people had throughout the program was not to eat too much after sunset or, in general, to eat less carbohydrates and protein, as both caused the FBS and postprandial blood sugar to increase. In summary, I found that the more calories of carbohydrates and/or protein people ate correlated with increases in blood glucose in the morning. The clear message is "The less you eat, the lower your blood sugar will be." "The less you eat, the better you feel, and the longer you'll live" has been a proven maxim since studies in the 1930s. If properly applied, this plant-source-only, live-food cuisine does not lead to any sort of long-term deficiency or health problems, but actually contributed in my case to an approximately ninefold increase in strength and endurance as well as an increase in flexibility as well as an optimal longevity blood chemistry profile. This fits nicely with Dr. Israel Breckman's research, where he fed mice the same calories, cooked versus raw, and the mice had three times the energy on raw foods.[159] When I wrote *Spiritual Nutrition*, I explained why the live-food diet is superior on many levels. One of the contributing points is increased enzyme assimilation from the live food, as cooking destroys enzymes. Close to 100 percent of diabetics, in general, have about a 50 percent enzyme deficiency. This is why Dr. Cousens's Diabetes Recovery Program—A Holistic Approach adds some important healing components, including natural calorie restriction and the quality and healing power of organic whole, live foods. The increased energy associated with live foods also creates more healing force. That certainly is a component that needs to be factored in to this discussion as to why this diet is so effective. It is not simply a 25–45 percent carbohydrate diet or a plant-source-only diet, but, indeed, an extremely clean, high-quality, organic, healthy, holistic, live-food diet that is low on the food chain with no trans fats, white sugar, white flour, processed or junk food. It is a full holistic synergy.

Comparison of 10 Percent Low Fat with 25–45 Percent Fat

The idea of individualizing your diet also plays an important role in this discussion as well. As already explained, I created a situation where the only sources of carbohydrates, fat, and protein were leafy greens, non-starchy and high-fibrous vegetables, sprouts, sea vegetables, and plant-source fats and protein. It is interesting that with no restrictions on raw plant fat intake, everyone had significant drops in their cholesterol and blood sugar levels. After 21 days on the program, my clients' average triglycerides dropped to 69, which is thought to be cardio-protective, as compared to two publicly well-known 10 percent low-fat studies by Drs. Ornish and Esselstyn. My patients responded well to a 25–45 percent fat diet. Dr. Esselstyn's 11 subjects, who fully participated in his 5-year, all natural, 60-70 percent high complex carbohydrate, 10 percent low-fat diet (with the use of statins), had a high average triglyceride count of 144. Dr. Ornish's 10 percent low-fat, moderately high carbohydrate, moderately low protein (with a touch of low-fat dairy) diet produced an even higher triglyceride average of 232. My clients' average cholesterol was 159 at the end of 3 weeks, and Dr. Esselstyn's approach of 10 percent fat with all his patients being prescribed statins was 137. Dr. Ornish's 10 percent low-fat average cholesterol was 173 (14 points higher than my participants). Contrary to the typical American idea of *bigger is better*, lower levels of cholesterol, particularly below 159, have been found to actually be dangerous to one's nervous system and physical and mental health. I will discuss this in more detail later in this chapter,

TYPE-2 DIABETES

	22 WEEKS ADA	3 WEEKS DR. COUSENS'S PROGRAM	22 WEEKS BARNARD RESEARCH
Fasting Blood Glucose (mg/dl)	Before: 160.4 After: 125.8	Before: 247 After: 86	Before: 163.5 After: 128.0
Total Point Reduction	34.6	161	35.5
Weight Loss (lb)	9.47	18	12.78
Medication Use	26% reduction	97% off ALL medications	46% reduction

DR. COUSENS'S 3-WEEK PROGRAM (TYPE-1 & TYPE-2)

Type-2 Non-IDDM	Type-2 IDDM	Type-1 Diabetics
• 100% off all medication • 61% cure rate	• 86.4% medication reduction • 24% cure rate	• 31.4% off all insulin • Average insulin drop: 67.5% • 21% cure rate

FIGURE 5. Diabetes programs

In this context, it is very important, for the moment, to briefly and dramatically highlight that recent studies including up to 250,000 people have not found any meaningful correlation between a high total cholesterol and heart disease. Contrary to expectations, multiple research studies actually found a higher cholesterol to be correlated to increased longevity and cardio-protection in women. The other side of the discussion, which will be discussed later, is that a cholesterol less than 159 has been found to be detrimental and dangerous, especially to mental, emotional, and physical health. As the literature does not show any meaningful benefits to low cholesterol but does show potential significant pathologies, I feel the risks of a low cholesterol far outweigh the "mythical benefits" of a low cholesterol.

What is interesting in comparing these studies, regardless of whether people were eating 10 percent fat or 25–45 percent fat or low protein or high protein, there was a significant drop in total cholesterol. One problem with the 11-person study done by Dr. Esselstyn is that he also included the allopathic use of statins with every single one of his patients. His study therefore cannot be considered a holistic or natural approach to lowering cholesterol specifically or to a healthy diet in general. Because of this allopathic drug use of statins, Dr. Esselstyn's 10 percent low-fat diet cannot be considered a single cause of his results, but I want to refer to the study anyway because it contains some basics that are true of my and Dr. Ornish's studies that give a key broader insight to the discussion.

The mystery of how all three approaches lowered the cholesterol and triglycerides is a key healing element in my study that is understated but also presents as a healing factor in both Dr. Ornish's and Esselstyn's diets, which is the avoidance of any white sugar; white flour; synthetic, processed, or junk foods; or any trans fats. This is where my diet shares much common healing ground with their approaches. This simple overlap in all three diets may actually be the key, if not even the primary explanation, for why both a 10 percent low-fat and a 25-45 percent fat, raw-food diet would get such similar healthy blood lipid results. My approach gives more importance to the overall healing power of the holistic approach rather than trying to isolate one factor out of the whole picture as the only healing factor. Like Dr. Ornish, I also emphasize the importance of yoga and meditation as a complementary support to the holistic healing process. What is significant in my diet is that no restriction on fats and a 25–45 percent carbohydrate intake gave superior results in triglyceride levels and weight loss and still caused a significant drop to a healthy cholesterol level in normal optimal ranges—neither too high nor, more important, too low.

The Dangers of Statin Drugs

First, a little about why statins, which so many diabetics and "high" cholesterol cardiovascular "risk" people are put on, are unholistic, unnecessary, and potentially dangerous. Obviously, to clarify the dangers of statins, and my objection to using them in 99 out of 100 cases for the use of lowering cholesterol, the reader needs to be informed of the research done on them. They have, however, been shown, likely by their anti-inflammatory effect rather than cholesterol-blocking effect, to decrease the rate of heart attacks to a limited extent, but with a relatively poor risk-to-benefit ratio.

Research scientists reviewed 14 randomized controlled trials funded by the makers of statins (with the exception of one study), which included a total of 34,272 patients between 1994 and 2006. Even with this review of what one would consider a biased study situation, they found that for non-statin users there was a 9 per 1,000 death rate compared to a 8 per 1,000 death rate for statin users. The data suggest that statin use seemed to have prevented 1 death per 1,000 people at a public cost of one million dollars. Earlier studies in regard to statin use show that the life apparently saved from cardiovascular disease, which is 1 per 1,000 people, was nullified by an equivalent number of deaths from statin use for other reasons, such as liver failure, kidney failure, heart failure, suicides, and accidents caused by the statins. In general, collectively speaking, mainstream studies show that 66–75 percent of current statin sales have no useful purpose in terms of public heart health.[160] A conservative conclusion to the statin discussion is that there is no evidence to merit the use of statins preventatively based on simply high cholesterol if there is no accompanying evidence of previous heart attacks or heart disease.[161]

Lifestyle and healthy diet also protect against heart attacks in a much safer and healthier way than statins. The routine use of statins may create several serious and even life-threatening problems. Statins work by blocking HMG-CO-A reductase inhibitors and therefore block the cholesterol producing function of the liver, which unfortunately is also a primary cause of the adverse effects of statins. This liver blockage weakens muscles in general and the heart specifically. Statins also block production of CoQ10, which is needed for optimal heart and muscle strength and function. The Swedish Adverse Drug Reaction Advisory Committee from 1988 to 2010 found the most common negative side effect of statins was statin-induced liver injury, accounting for 57 percent of all statin side effects. The causal link to liver damage is strong.

This included deaths from acute liver failure and jaundice. Given the fact that there is no scientifically established connection between heart disease and diabetes, and that one can reduce cholesterol naturally with an unrestricted fat, unsaturated fat, and 25–45 percent carbohydrate diet, or perhaps simply a diet free of white sugar, white flour, trans fats, pesticides, herbicides, and processed, junk, and GMO foods, it is totally unnecessary to endanger oneself with the risk of statins. The research has shown, in some patients who have recovered from liver damage by stopping statins, that if they started taking them again, similar patterns of liver injury reoccurred. The data from more than two million statin users, ages 30 to 84, in England and Wales, have also identified moderate or increased liver dysfunction as a side effect of statins.

Statins may cause a variety of side effects, including mild to severe memory problems, sleep problems, and mood changes. An ongoing research project at the University of California San Diego called the Statin Effects Study[162] has cited thousands of instances of memory deterioration in patients taking statin drugs. This is a soft suggestion that statins are also associated with brain deterioration. According to the data, impaired memory may be the second most common adverse side effect of statins after muscle aches. Research at Massachusetts General Hospital and Harvard Medical School concluded that people with pre-hemorrhage stroke should not be given statins, as it increased the risk of getting a second one.[163]

In 2007, a meta-analysis of over 41,000 patient records found that people who take statin drugs to lower cholesterol had a higher rate of cancer.[164] There is some indication that statins may also increase the risk of heart failure. This is different than heart attack and atherosclerosis. What I am referring to is that by blocking the CoQ10, there is a decrease in heart muscle strength and energy and, consequently, function and strength, which may lead to heart weakness and failure. One study reported in *Clinical Cardiology* found that heart function was better in the control group, as compared to a statin group.[165] They found statin drug use was associated with "decreased myocardial heart function." Perhaps this supports the wise old advice, "If it's not broken, don't fix it." Loss of CoQ10 also leads to loss of cell energy and increased free radicals, which can further damage mitochondrial DNA.[166] Canada clearly warns about the CoQ10 depletion that could be a result of statin drugs. It is a serious problem, particularly in people who are possibly going into borderline congestive heart failure. Unfortunately, in the United States, there is no FDA warning that CoQ10 depletion will happen after taking statin drugs, and most people are unaware of the problem. Statins may also create dangerously low cholesterol levels, which are those below 159. Symptoms occurring with serum cholesterol levels below 159 include emotional imbalances, including increased depression and suicide, violent behavior, hormonal imbalances, memory loss, stroke, and even Parkinson's disease. It behooves us to keep total cholesterol no lower than 159. In 1990, a meta-analysis of 19 studies showed that men and women with total serum cholesterol levels below 160 exhibited a 10 percent to 20 percent higher mortality rate, compared with those with cholesterol levels between 160 and 199.[167] Statins also increase the incidence of Type-2 diabetes by 9 percent[168] and create a much greater incidence of hyperglycemia, which is associated with a prediabetic state and glycemic postprandial spikes. One particular study reported in *Lancet*, done with a randomized control trial in 1994 ending in 2009, included a total of 91,140 participants taking a statin or placebo and found a 9 percent increase in diabetes. They also found that statin drugs actually increased insulin levels, which of course is not good for health and longevity in general. Increased insulin leads to a cascade of inflammatory cytokines; high cortisol, which leads to increased belly fat; high blood pressure; heart attacks; chronic fatigue; thyroid dysfunction; Parkinson's; Alzheimer's; and cancer. These are serious risks associated with statin use, coupled with insignificant results in terms of cholesterol, since there is no proof of any association between cholesterols of up to 260–270 and increased incidence of heart disease and heart attack.

In 2009, one article showed that statins raised blood sugars in people with or without diabetes.[169] Diabetics do tend to respond differently to foods and drugs (in terms of blood sugar) than nondiabetics. In this study, which involved over 340,000 people, there was a rise in nondiabetic patients' blood glucose of 7 points, but those people who already had diabetes and took statins experienced an average increase of 39.9 in blood glucose points; this fits into the category of the postprandial glycemic spike syndrome.

Statins also decrease vitamin D function because vitamin D production needs cholesterol. We know that sufficient vitamin D also decreases insulin resistance. In fact, a study in *Journal of Clinical Nutrition* found that when we move vitamin D from levels to 25 to 75 micromoles, there is a decrease in insulin resistance up to 60 percent. Vitamin D deficiency is another reason we don't want to have low cholesterol. Statin suppression of CoQ10 also concerns me. It is important nutrient energy for every cell, particularly in the liver. It turns out that CoQ10 is an important antioxidant and helps maintain a normal blood sugar and also protects against the risk of heart failure, high blood pressure, and a weakened heart in general. Hodgson et al. published research in 2002 stating that 200 mg supplemental CoQ10 could decreases your A1C by 0.4 percent.[170] CoQ10 also protects our body from oxidative stress, which contributes to diabetes, metabolic syndrome, and heart attacks. A low CoQ10 is also associated with muscle wasting and is associated with a loss of cell energy and damaged mitochondrial DNA. Muscle wasting and pain is another part of the statin side effect story, which is certain to get worse in people who are older and have a tendency for muscle wasting if they aren't exercising. At this point, there are now more than nine hundred studies proving that statins have adverse effects.

This scientific data directly imply that there is no need to use statins to lower cholesterol. Unfortunately, statins are used routinely on diabetics to protect against high cholesterol, and statins are used by knowledgeable allopathic physicians to decrease inflammation. A live food diet has been shown to have a significant effect in decreasing inflammation, thus abrogating the need to use statins for this purpose.

The Mythological Dangers of
High Cholesterol and High Fat

Clarity is needed on the question of risk/benefit ratio of low cholesterol in general beyond the statin question, as previously discussed,
but especially because 56 percent of Americans have a fear of fat and
cholesterol.[171] On my diet for treatment and prevention of diabetes,
which is plant-based, cholesterol is not a particular concern, as 159
is high enough to be safe. The main reason I am dissecting the "high-
cholesterol danger myth" is that it has resulted in dangerous low-fat
dietary practices. In specific to the Dr. Cousens's Diabetes Recovery
Program—A Holistic Approach and in a larger holistic context, the
increase in healthy fats supports the macronutrient calorie shift away
from carbohydrates. This is additionally important since the research
of the last 30 years shows that a serum cholesterol below 159 is unsafe,
whereas serum cholesterol as high as 260–270 not only is perfectly safe
but actually decreases cardiovascular mortality and increases longevity in women. What exactly is that 56 percent worried about, and are
their worries justified or is it just a fearful, unscientific response to
mythological hype?

As I have made it clear, all forms of carbohydrates in excess, including grains, fruits, and all sugars and sugar substitutes (except stevia and
birch-tree-based xylitol), often result in an increased insulin resistance,
obesity, increased triglycerides and increased levels of pathogenic small
LDL particles. Empowered by the scientifically disproven idea that the
"best way to protect your heart is a low cholesterol diet," we can look
at the whole cholesterol issue from a science-based perspective. Many
people have mistakenly taken the earlier research of the 1950s through
the 1970s to be absolute truth rather than a phase in the research to be
explored in the etiology of heart disease. The high cholesterol–heart
connection is no longer taken as truth in holistic medical circles or
among many progressive allopathic cardiologists and more recently
by the informed public. Serious post-1970s large studies have shown
that the high cholesterol–heart disease correlation is not a valid causal

or even correlative theory. Some of the more recent research that significantly nullifies the earlier speculative research gives us a new perspective of not only why I feel that a 25–45 percent fat diet, depending on constitution, is a safe way of reversing the degenerative process of Type-2 diabetes, but also why I feel (based on my clinical experience and more recent epidemiological scientific studies) that normal cholesterols as well as healthy levels of omega-3s are essential for long-term healthy function. The first thing I would like to point out is that in a 1992 editorial published in the *Archives of Internal Medicine*, Dr. William Pastelli, the former director of the Farmington Heart study, made an amazing statement: "In Farmington, Massachusetts, the more saturated fat one ate, the more cholesterol one ate and calories one ate, the lower the person's serum cholesterol was." It is easier to appreciate Dr. William Pastelli's observation when one understands that the body makes 75 percent of its own cholesterol. The key in helping us understand this process is that the body of research shows that the liver produces three-to-four times more cholesterol than one eats and is always adjusting for the amount of cholesterol taken in orally. A low-cholesterol diet will increase production, and endogenous production decreases with large cholesterol dietary input. There's a homeostasis going on. In addition, when one has a healthy insulin level, one tends to have a healthy cholesterol level because a healthy cholesterol is mediated by a healthy insulin level. This is a remarkable and important statement that is very much validated by the book *The Cholesterol Myths* by Uffe Ravnskov, MD, PhD, which offers many scientific arguments invalidating the idea that saturated-fat and cholesterol intake cause heart disease.[172] His data and the data in general are overwhelming on this point.

The demonization of saturated fat most likely began in 1953 when Dr. Ancel Keys created a mythology in a paper linking saturated fat intake and heart disease mortality. What concerns me is the research, when fully examined, is quite weak. Keys based his theory on a study of six countries in which higher saturated fat was associated with the heart disease theory he was promoting. However, and this is the serious part that I emphatically call *misinformation*, he did not report data from 16 other countries he also studied that did not fit his theory, in which there was no correlation of a high cholesterol intake with heart disease. Combining all data from the 22 countries would have shown that increasing calories from fat actually reduces deaths from coronary heart disease. Many studies have validated this point of the safety of cholesterol since then. It's shocking, but somehow Ancel Keys's misinformation caught on, in spite of the overall poor science.

Now, I believe there is some truth to the fat issue, but it's not about cholesterol, omega-3s, or omega-6s. Looking at recent literature up to 2011, it is about intake of trans fats, which are unquestionably cardio-damaging. Trans fats are found in margarine, vegetable shortening, and hydrogenated vegetable oils, as well as oils that are highly cooked. Trans fats are not the same thing as raw, plant-source-only, unsaturated, or polyunsaturated fats; omega-3s and omega-6s; or saturated fats. Trans fats have definitely been identified as dangerous to health in general for a variety of reasons and should be 100 percent avoided. In contrast to the danger of eating trans fats, the actual data about high and low cholesterol are revealing no danger associated with total cholesterol up to 270. These data, which will be shared, strongly support the currently evolving theory I explained earlier that inflammation, not high cholesterol, is the primary cause of heart disease and cardiac mortality, and it is the amount of cardiovascular inflammation a person has that determines the degree of heart disease and not the level of cholesterol.

Again, to clarify about fats, saturated fats come from animal fats, which are cooked (and not part of the Dr. Cousens's diet) and also from tropical oils, including palm and coconut oils. (Raw palm and coconut oils are not a problem if they are not cooked or hydrogenated.) Polyunsaturated fat from omega-3 and omega-6 sources like nuts and seeds are not a problem. Explicit disease-causing fats are trans fats. Sources of healthy, vegetarian plant-source fats are olives, raw nuts, seeds, almonds, pecans, walnuts, coconut and coconut oil, palm oil, and avocados. Avocados have actually been experimentally shown to be generally healthy, cardio-protective, and to even lower cholesterol in some cases, as previously discussed.[173] I emphasize the importance of eating high omega-3 fat foods, including chia seeds, walnuts, flax seeds, and hemp seeds, because they help shift the ratio between omega-6 to omega-3 toward 2:1 or 1:1, away from the average and pathological ratios of up to 20:1. To minimize the excess of omega-6, I do not recommend high omega-6 fats such as corn, canola, safflower, or sunflower oil, which further imbalance omega-6 to omega-3 ratios and may be associated with increased cardiovascular disease. Raw saturated fats are health promoting and important because they are needed for proper function of cell membranes, especially those of the neuronal cells, heart, bones, liver, immune system, lungs, and hormones, and those that control hunger, calcium balance, and general genetic regulation. I'm not recommending polyunsaturated oils, which are high in omega-6 fats, because they have been associated to a certain extent with accelerated aging.

More than one set of major research has showed that people with high cholesterol developed the same amount of heart disease as people with low cholesterol. One meta-analysis of 21 studies, with a total of 347,747 individuals, showed that people with heart attacks had not eaten any more saturated fat or more polyunsaturated oil than other people.[174] Another fact revealed by several large studies is that women with higher cholesterol live longer and have less cardiac mortality than their lower-blood-cholesterol peers. There are other additional studies that clarify the confusion and myth about the high cholesterol question. For example, there was a study done by Dr. Harlan Krumholz and his coworkers at the Department of Cardiovascular Medicine at Yale on 997 elderly men and women living in the Bronx during a four-year period that showed no difference between lower and higher cholesterol levels in terms of heart disease, except that the women with higher cholesterol lived longer and had less heart disease.[175] Another study reported in *Cholesterol Myths* is that for each 1 percent milligram drop in cholesterol, there is an 11 percent increase in total coronary mortality. The overall results of the studies show that people with blood cholesterols of 160 or less develop just as many cholesterol plaques as those with higher cholesterol—up to at least a total cholesterol of 260.

In all the international studies, out of all the studies, there was only one citing high cholesterol as having a slight association with increased risk of heart disease in men in the United States but no association for men in Canada. Dr. Gilles Dagenais, in Quebec, studying 5,000 men, found the same results as the rest of Canada.[176] Dr. Henry Shanoff at University of Toronto studied 120 men 10 years after they recovered from heart attacks. He found that those with low cholesterol had a second coronary incident just as often as those with high cholesterol.[177] In Russia, low cholesterol is actually associated with increased risk of coronary heart disease. In summary, high cholesterol is said to be possibly slightly pathogenic for American males under 38, but not for Canadians, Stockholmers, Russians, or Maoris at any age. The fact that it is maybe slightly dangerous for men in America (whereas not for men in other nations around the world), or Americans over the age of 38, raises some questions as to the validity of the American study. Once men in the United States are older than 38, a high cholesterol does not seem dangerous. Paradoxically, the American studies suggest it may be questionably marginally pathogenic for healthy men under 38 but not for coronary patients and may even be slightly beneficial for older men. As earlier stated, the protective benefits of a higher cholesterol is clearer for women. In one Norwegian study of 52,087 people between the ages of 20–74, women with cholesterols of 270 or higher had a 28 percent lower mortality rate than women with cholesterols of less than 193.[178] This is a significant finding strongly supporting the cardio-protective and general longevity quality of cholesterol for women.

There is a genetic defect called *familial hypercholesterolemia*. People with this genetic problem do have significantly raised cholesterol, often above 365, and do have a higher risk of heart attack. This genetic subgroup is a genetic exception, and these people may be helped with statins. Including this subgroup in the cholesterol discussion for those without the genetic tendency may have created some distorted data in regard to the cholesterol question. Additional major research contradicting the high-cholesterol danger myth is the Monica Project, monitoring of trends of determinants in trends of cardiovascular disease. This large body of research found that the relationship of blood cholesterol and mortality in coronary disease shows a great variation in coronary mortality in people with the same blood levels of cholesterol.[179] Other contradictions to the myth include the issue of the French Paradox, which basically shows how the French were the most "deviant" to a low-cholesterol diet but still had lower coronary mortality. But it isn't just the French. High-cholesterol intake and lower coronary mortality were observed in Luxembourg and Germany. This supports the point that is critical to the meaning of this discussion: that there are too many paradoxes here. Fundamentally, if a theory is to hold, it can't have exceptions. That is, of course, is what almost all the research is revealing. There are too many discrepancies to give the high-cholesterol/cardio-mortality connection any weight. The key principle is *if a scientific hypothesis is sound, it must agree with all observations.* The formulation of valid, scientific hypotheses should not be like a sports event, where a team with greatest number of points or best public relations wins the game—although the relevant studies showing a disconnect between cholesterol levels and heart morbidity are now in the majority. One observation that doesn't support a hypothesis is enough to disprove it. In this discussion, there are no real exceptions that actually support the "danger" of a high cholesterol–cardiac mortality link.

Another study by Dr. Mama found that Japanese immigrants who became accustomed to the American way of life and gave up their Japanese cultural way of life but preferred lean Japanese food had coronary disease twice as often as those who kept Japanese traditions but preferred high-fat American food.[180] There's a little more to this—I am hinting at stress playing a role, for example. In Wellington, New Zealand, a study of immigrant populations of Tokelau Islands and the Puka-Puka atolls, who had a diet high in coconuts and little chicken in their homelands was also interesting. Coconut is high in saturated fatty acids. It has more saturated than animal fat. When the Tokelau islanders were forced by tornadoes to migrate to New Zealand, their diet changed markedly, and the number of calories from saturated fat was cut in half. Intake of unsaturated fats increased a little bit. What surprisingly happened is the cholesterol levels of the Tokelauans increased by almost 10 percent, even though saturated fat intake was cut in half. It is possible that stress was the main cause for the rise in cholesterol. This data also suggests that, at worst, exogenous cholesterol via the diet has only marginal influence in cholesterol in blood. As previously explained, the body seems to have a cholesterol homeostasis according to our physiological needs. When one eats a large exogenous amount, endogenous production goes down. When one eats a small amount of cholesterol, endogenous production goes up. This may explain that on the Ornish, 10 percent low-fat diet, the cholesterol was 173, whereas on the Dr. Cousens's Diabetes Recovery Diet—A Holistic Approach with 25–45 percent raw fat (with no animal fat but no plant-source-fat restriction), the cholesterol was 159. Cholesterol is internally regulated according to one's needs. Yet one can affect cholesterol to some extent by stress response, and so on. In the three-week, plant-source-only, 100 percent live-food program, there was a 67-point drop in LDLs from 149 to 82, which was a 44 percent decrease and a total cholesterol drop to 159, with no restrictions on fat (except no cooked or animal fat). My theoretical explanation to this is that when people return to a healthy diet including no white sugar; white flour; or junk, processed, and GMO foods, their bodies return to a normal noninflamed physiology and naturally move toward an optimal cholesterol physiology. The main point, however, is that there are many factors affecting cholesterol levels, and although there is a homeostasis corrective factor, diet may have a modest effect on cholesterol.

The safety of a moderate-high fat diet was further confirmed by a study sponsored by The Women's Health Initiative in 1994, wherein they studied 49,000 middle-aged women with 20,000 who were chosen to eat a low-fat diet. After six years, the women who had cut fat consumption and saturated fat by 25 percent did have cholesterols and LDLs somewhat below that of the 29,000 women who did not change their fat consumption, but the change had no effect on the rate of heart disease, stroke, breast cancer, colon cancer, or fat accumulation.[181] It is significant that there was no difference in overall morbidity between the two groups of women. There was no science to support that saturated fats clogged arteries if there was a higher cholesterol in the diet. It is interesting to note that in another women's study, they did find that older women with higher cholesterol lived longer than their lower cholesterol female counterparts.[182] This, of course, supports the efficacy and safety of my dietary system. There have been more than 30 studies, including a total of over 150,000 people, that have shown that people who did not have heart attacks have not necessarily eaten less saturated or unsaturated fats than those who did have heart attacks.[183] Another point to make is that in 1982, the *Wall Street Journal* published the results of a $115 million, decade-long clinical trial conducted by the National Heart, Lung, and Blood Institute to see if less saturated fat intake could cure heart disease. Results in this major study were "not a single heart attack has been prevented."[184]

One of two concluding major points to this cholesterol discussion is the Cochrane Collaboration study, which is known to be free of all corporate pressures and assessed the benefits of eating less fat and less saturated fat in 2001. They reviewed 27 clinical studies back to the 1950s. They concluded, "Despite the efforts and many thousands of people and randomized studies, there is still only limited inconclusive evidence of the effects of modification of a total unsaturated and polyunsaturated diets on cardiac morbidity."[185] This is an important statement for the overall picture that a low-fat diet has not been found to be a significant or even a marginal factor in preventing heart disease.

A final concluding point is a survey of all the literature on this cholesterol topic. In the *Archives of Internal Medicine,* April 13, 2009, a very important study titled "A Systemic Review of the Evidence Supporting the Causal Link Between Dietary Factors and Coronary Heart Disease" was published.[186] It showed several important things. It identified that the most harmful dietary factors usually related to cardiovascular disease included (1) the regular intake of trans-fatty acids and (2) foods that were high glycemic index or high glycemic load. These were the dangerous factors associated with increased heart disease. This systemic review of all the evidence in the literature looked at two kinds of evidence. One is the principle of cohort studies. Cohort studies are epidemiological studies looking at the relationship between specific dietary factors and particular conditions. The second is randomized control, wherein individuals are subject to some kind of dietary change and the result, as compared to individuals who did not make the change. (All the studies I have cited are either one or the other of these two forms.) Looking at the overall picture, they determined that dietary factors created the most heart disease, using a system they called the *Bradford Hill guidelines*, which is a way of measuring causation as opposed to association. The causal levels were highest for diets high in trans-fatty acids and high glycemic diets, which are both cardio-damaging. The diet that was most cardio-protective was a diet high in vegetable consumption and nut consumption. They found that there were no randomized controlled studies that supported the notion that cutting back on saturated fat was good for prevention of heart disease. They also found that there were no cohort studies supporting any link between saturated fat intake and heart disease. Their bottom line conclusion, in looking at all the studies, is that there was no evidence to support the widespread mythical belief that limiting saturated-fat intake is beneficial for heart health.

Researchers also found that an increased consumption of polyunsaturated fats was not associated with relative protection against heart disease. I would like to take this a step further and state that I do not recommend polyunsaturated omega-6 fats, as most of these are damaged trans fats, found in highly processed corn, soy, cakes, biscuits, processed vegetable oils, raisins, package-ready meals, nondairy creamers, soups, salad dressings, fried foods, sauces, and chocolates. Vegetable oils that are not omega-3 vegetable oils were not found to be cardio-protective.

In summary, according to this major 2009 review of the literature, a high carbohydrate and trans-fat intake was found to be bad for heart health, and one need not be afraid of eating the appropriate amount of healthy fat in a diet that feels energetically sustaining.

The overall research is clear that lowering cholesterol does not correlate with a lengthened life or cardio-protection. For women, a low cholesterol actually seems to shorten life-span and increase cardiac mortality rates. A plant-source-only diet yields longevity of 4.42 years longer in women and 7.28 years longer for men, regardless of cholesterol levels.[187]

As I have examined the literature, I feel very confident in prescribing my 25–45 percent carbohydrate diet and 25–45 percent raw fat diet to people because although it lowers cholesterol to normal physiological and healthy levels, it doesn't take it into the danger zone, which is below 159. It also provides the healing, balancing, and building power of long- and short-chain omega-3s for the brain, nervous system, and for healing diabetes. It appears safe in all areas and brings mental and physical good health.

Health Dangers of Low Cholesterol

My biggest concern in this discussion is the significant and pathological dangers with not only statins, as previously explained, but with cholesterol levels under 159. As a psychiatrist, I have been quite aware, for more than 40 years, of the serious mental illness dangers associated with low cholesterol. Recent research has shown that there is a much higher association of depression, suicidability, and anxiety with cholesterols less than 159. Several cohort studies on nondepressed subjects have assessed the relationship between plasma cholesterol and depression. A direct relationship was found between low cholesterol and rates of high depression. It became clear among patients with major depression that there was a strong causative association with low cholesterol. Clinical recovery also was correlated causatively with increases in cholesterol.[188] Several epidemiological studies have shown an increased suicide risks among subjects with lower cholesterol. Although there are a few contradictory studies, the overall relationship has been confirmed by several cohort studies that the same is true with low polyunsaturated acids and low omega-3s and depression. Low polyunsaturated omega-3 fatty acids were associated at different levels with pathology of major depression. The overall hypothesis that emerges in general has to do with maintenance of optimal membrane fluidity and optimal ratios of saturated, mono-saturated, and poly-unsaturated fats in the cell membranes in general and particularly in the neuronal cell membranes. Optimal membrane fat ratios positively affect the quality of neurotransmission and neurotransmitter production. Low cholesterol is also associated with decreased serotonin receptors in the neurons (brain cells).[189] In another study in relationship to cholesterol, called "Low Serum Cholesterol Concentration and Risk of Suicide,"[190] adjusting for age and sex, they found that those with the lowest serum cholesterol concentrations had more than six times the risk of committing suicide. Another study found that if the cholesterol levels were equal to or below the twenty-fifth percentile, the risk of a suicide attempt doubled.[191] Obviously from a holistic and psychiatric perspective, this is highly significant. Researchers found the negative depression effect of low cholesterol persisted for up to five years. In summary, the data indicate that low-serum cholesterol is associated with increased risk of suicide and depression. An article in *Psychology Today* by Emily Deans, MD, on evolutionary psychiatry, links low serum cholesterol to increased suicide, accidents, and violence, as do numerous other papers.[192] It isn't totally proven, but this may be related to the fact that the brain's dry weight is 60 percent fat and cholesterol plays a vital role in neuron signaling and brain structure. One fourth of our cholesterol is found in the nervous system. It makes sense if cholesterol drops too low, our brains and nervous systems can be adversely affected. A low blood cholesterol (less than 159) obviously creates problems from a holistic point of view. One needs cholesterol to make the brain and cell membranes work effectively. To again emphasize the point, neuronal cell membranes, as well as all cell membranes, are constructed from fat, and a proper combination of cholesterol and omega-3 and omega-6 fatty acids is key for optimal cell membrane function. Trans-fatty acids, on the other hand, also significantly disrupt membrane function. Cholesterol depletion is also known to deplete serotonin receptors and reduces serotonin release from the synapse.[193] It is also noteworthy that low serotonin in the spinal fluid is associated with aggression and indeed is also associated with low cholesterol. The cholesterol is needed for formation of synapse to make myelin, which is the insulating cover for nerves and various other signaling processes associated with anxiety and depression. A cholesterol of less than 159 is also associated with an increase of 21 percent premature deliveries, as compared to only 5 percent premature deliveries with a cholesterol of 160 to 261.[194] In general, this is a particularly important consideration for why I recommend a 25–45 percent fat intake for eating plant-source-only, live-food diets, because there's a tendency for lower cholesterol, especially in low-fat, vegan, live-food diets. It is interesting that in both public and private communications, Dr. Neal Barnard has stated that the fat restrictions for his diabetes studies were simply to avoid all animal fats and cooking oils, which is the same protocol as in my study. It is a practical and easy guideline to follow. A higher fat intake, with plenty of coconut oil, is often effective for raising cholesterol; it is an added assurance against the potential of low cholesterol problems or for the treatment of low cholesterol. When people go below 159, the relationship of low cholesterol to mental problems begins to become clearer. As a holistic physician and psychiatrist, I don't want to encourage suicide, depression, aggression, and violence by advising a 10 percent or less low-fat diet.

In summary, on the Dr. Cousens's Diabetes Recovery Program—A Holistic Approach (a 100 percent live-food, plant-source-only unrestricted raw fat diet), one sees significant drops in LDL cholesterol, total cholesterol, and triglycerides to normal healthy levels without going into the low cholesterol danger zone. This low cholesterol concern has been an issue for me since I began to observe many of these mental symptoms in the late 1970s and early 1980s, when I began seeing clients who ate plant-source-only foods with a 10 percent low fat intake. It has been part of my commitment to the plant-source-only world to develop a diet that is generally safe and healthy for everyone.

The Importance of Omega-3s for Health

The same trend is true with the importance of adequate omega-3s versus a low fat and, consequently, low omega-3 diet. General health-protective effects from adequate omega-3s are a reduced risk of death from all causes. In a five-year study, it was discovered that those of an omega-3 index of less than 4 percent aged much faster than those with indexes above 8 percent. The same study also showed that those who had the higher omega-3 levels died at a slower rate or were less likely to die within the study period than the people with low omega-3s. Omega-3 deficiency was considered to maybe be a significant underlying factor of up to 96,000 premature deaths each year, including some of those from coronary heart disease and stroke.[195] Adequate omega-3s decreased risk of premature death by up to 85 percent when at optimal levels.[196]

Adequate omega-3 levels contribute to a healthy brain in a variety of important ways. They are important for maintaining and improving memory, cognition, sleep, neuromuscular control, and slowing the mortality of neurodegenerative diseases. Omega-3s also support new manufacture of acetylcholine, which is an important neurotransmitter needed for memory. They stimulate release of gamma-aminobutyric acid (GABA; which protects against anxiety, depression, pain, and panic attacks). Omega-3s are major components of brain tissue. They also help with brain and eye development in babies. An adequate long-chain omega-3 supply helps prevent and treat postpartum depression.[197] These are essential for prevention and treatment of all depression, including bipolar disorder. Recent studies investigating the epidemic of military suicides in Iraq and Afghanistan found that those who committed suicide had the lowest omega-3 levels in the military population. In specific, low DHA was associated with a 60 percent increase in suicide, making a clear point that adequate brain DHA is necessary for healthy brain and mental health function.[198] Adequate omega-3s improve mood regulation and ameliorate and treat impulsivity, hostility, and aggression.[199] They improve dysfunction of monoaminergic systems including 5-hydroxytryptamine and serotonin.[200] They help prevent cortisol, epinephrine, and norepinephrine elevations in biological and emotional stress. They reduce the risk of Parkinson's disease and help proper nerve signaling.[201] Lower omega-3 fatty acids contribute to many disease dysfunctions including increased heart disease,[202] liver-[203] and kidney-function instability,[204] and general mental disturbances,[205] specifically ones that result in suicide.[206] The proinflammatory cytokines associated with increased omega-6s also disturb neurotransmission.

It becomes obvious that another danger of the 10 percent low-fat diet is that it's highly probable to create omega-3 deficiency syndromes, which I will now briefly review. For heart health, omega-3s are antiarrhythmic and help counteract or prevent cardiac arrhythmia.[207] Adequate omega-3s are antiatherosclerotic in that they prevent fatty deposits and fibrosis of the inner layer of the arteries from forming.[208] Adequate omega-3s lower triglyceride concentrations.[209] They improve endothelial function.[210] They are a major factor in promoting the growth of new blood vessels.[211] They tend to prevent thrombosis (a blood clot within a blood vessel),[212] and they decrease cardiovascular risk factors. People with atrial fibrillation with high omega-3 levels have 85 percent lower risk of dying from all causes.[213] Adequate omega-3 lowers blood pressure.[214]

Omega-3s also have some anticancer benefits: They protect skin cells from cancer-causing effects of the sun and help decrease prostate cancer risks. In premenopausal women, a high omega-3 to omega-6 ratio resulted in a decreased rate of breast cancer by 50 percent. Omega-3s constitute 50 percent of our cell membranes and give our cells optimal stiffness, flexibility, integrity, and function. They improve liver health and protect the liver from toxins. Long-chain omega-3s, EPA, and DHA are independent nutrients for preventing and treating nonalcoholic fatty liver disease (NAFLD). Men with the greatest EPA and DHA consumption had a 52–56 percent reduction in NAFLD.[215] They help build a strong immune system. They contribute to healthy lungs and also have an anti-inflammatory in counteracting inflammation (heat, pain, swelling, etc.). They protect organs and tissues from inflammation in general. They are associated with protection against kidney damage in adults. (People with the highest amount of omega-3s had a 31 percent less chronic kidney disease.)[216]

From an Ayurvedic perspective, deficient omega-3s, as well as inadequate cholesterol, create an imbalanced "vata" mental state with poorer cognition, memory, and functioning. This results in lower life-force, lower vitality, and generally a lower reserve of vital life-force and sexual energy. Along with this there may be depression, violence, anxiety, and even suicide. The Ayurvedic term for this is vital reserve is *ojas*, which means deep primordial vigor and reserve. Low *ojas* results in a generally weakened physical, emotional, mental, and spiritual condition. In this larger context, the overall effect of a low-fat diet has serious, global, negative ramifications for quality of life. To balance the vata Ayurvedic dosha, and specifically for calming a vata dosha imbalance (which, in essence, is the clinical description I have given of an omega-3, long- and short-chain deficiency, as well as a cholesterol deficiency), I highly recommend adequate raw plant-source-only fat consumption in one's diet to prevent Ayurvedically described "vata" physical and mental imbalances.

In summary, low-cholesterol and low-omega-3s have been shown through overwhelming scientific evidence to be a danger to the general health and longevity of the individual. The "extremely low cholesterol is good for your heart" and extreme low-fat mythology campaign is based on bad science and fear, which has, by 2011, been disproved. Saturated fat and omega-3 intake from plant-based fat is actually cardio-protective, brain- and mental-health protective, general-health protective, and life-force protective. This higher fat intake creates a macronutrient balance with the 25–45 percent carbohydrate direction, with its higher vegetable and nut and seed fat. A higher fat diet allows the potential for a lower protein in the diet, which is important when one understands about the glycemic impact of excess protein intake. Research more strongly suggests that high insulin is more linked to cardiovascular disease than the "cholesterol link." There is a distinction between association and causal effect. *Causal* means a direct link and thus a stronger effect. There's a causal link between high insulin and high leptin and heart disease and diabetes. There is neither an association nor a causal relationship between cholesterol and heart disease. The key to cardiovascular disease and diabetes is an imbalanced, dysfunctional insulin and leptin signaling secondary to excess carbohydrates, which of course is perhaps the key to all chronic diseases but particularly coronary disease.

Dr. Cousens's Diabetes Recovery Diet—A Holistic Approach diet is not just for diabetes but optimal for overall well-being. What I am describing for diabetics is a lifelong enhancement diet for optimal health and longevity in general. That is also a distinction that I make when people focus too much on a detox diet. People who stay on a detox diet too long may become metabolically imbalanced if they don't transition to a healthy holistic diet. That's why part of my progressive protocol is that once former diabetics are at least three-months reestablished in a relatively normal physiology, which is a blood sugar under 100 (though an FBS of 70–85 is optimal) and A1C blood tests of 5.7 or less, then they can move to the Phase 1.5 diet that I outline in detail in my book *Rainbow Green Live-Food Cuisine*. The Phase 1.5 diet includes the use of cherries, berries, low-glycemic fruits, and moderate use of cooked grains and beans. It is a slight move from 25–45 percent carbohydrates to 30–50 percent, allowing for 20 percent high-quality cooked food if one so desires.

The Protein-Glucose Relationship

To further clarify the protein-glucose relationship and importance of a low-to-moderate protein intake is a study I previously referred that found that a quarter pound of hamburger raises your fasting insulin as much as a quarter pound of white sugar. The two main sources of glucose production in the body are from simple and complex carbohydrates and protein. Protein is needed in various amounts, depending on one's constitutional type, for maintenance and repair of tissues, but excess protein may convert to glucose and raises the blood sugar. In my research, I was able to show clients that, after taking a high protein meal, which I ask people to do, there is a significant increase in blood sugar. My approach not only decreases the amount of sugar in the system but also guides one to decrease protein to the point that one still gets maintenance repair and reproduction energies, as well as strength, vitality, and general health, but not any more than required (which would create more glucose in the system). This is a very important statement because generally speaking even with people eating high amounts of meat, with age, they tend to get a slight and progressive muscle mass wasting with age, which is called glycopenia. This does not need to happen if you're getting adequate protein and exercising. With this approach, I do build muscle mass and do not suffer from glycopenia, which, up until recently, was thought to happen to everyone with age, regardless of eating habits (meat eater or plant source only). These are some considerations for the perennial question: How do you know that you're getting enough protein? If hair, skin, nails, tissues, and, in general, muscle mass, and vitality are not compromised, you are getting enough protein. These are general clinical considerations. I have found clients in their 60s, whom I follow very closely, also have the same sort of very positive anabolic vitality and increased flexibility results on this holistic, plant-source-only diet and lifestyle. The Dr. Cousens's Diabetes Recovery Program—A Holistic Approach reflects a larger holistic view of diabetes and the treatment of it and has been highly successful for all levels of general physical, emotional, mental, and spiritual healing.

The Dr. Cousens's Diabetes Recovery Program—A Holistic Approach diet in Phase 1.0 is a plant-source-only, live-food cuisine of no grains, fruits, white sugar, white flour, or fructose in the diet, with unrestricted consumption of nuts, seeds, avocados, and other fatty plant-source foods and moderate amounts of high-quality omega-3 fats and saturated fats. Although the results on this diet are unusually successful and rapid, that doesn't mean that there aren't studies available where people were able to significantly modify, or even in some cases, reverse their diabetes over a period of time on basically low-carbohydrate diets alone, even if they were eating flesh foods. There are even studies (such as Dr. Barnard's) that show that diabetes can be at least modified, but not necessarily reversed, on a high-complex carbohydrate diet, but the results are not comparable to the consistency, rapidity, and efficiency on a constant large scale with my synergistic approach. Those are some of the thoughts in this larger discussion that I choose to include, which is why this particular diet appears to be so successful.[217, 218] The key common denominator of these moderate-low-carbohydrate or high-carbohydrate diets, and low- or high-fat diets, is that almost all these approaches share a commonality of no white sugar, white flour, junk food, GMOs, irradiated foods, processed foods, or trans fats. This seems to be a baseline for even marginal success in healing CDDS.

Meat Consumption Increases Diabetes

Research also shows that adding smoked and processed meats into the diet increases the risk of diabetes by at least 30 percent.[219] Perhaps the best assessment of diabetes and meat intake correlation was a meta-analysis of 12 studies published in *Diabetologia* in 2009. Previous studies have associated diabetes with processed meat,[220, 221, 222, 223, 224, 225, 226] red meat,[227, 228] and total meat.[229, 230] In these 12 cohort studies, 6 were from the United States, 3 were from Europe, 2 were from Asia, and 1 was from Australia, giving their assessment an international perspective. The total number of people involved in the 12 studies was more than 1,259,000 people. Their overall assessment was that a Type-2 diabetes risk for vegetarians was 35–50 percent lower than for omnivores. This meta-analysis clearly established that high intakes of red meat and processed meat are risk factors for type 2 diabetes. I believe that the plant-source-only component plays an additional special survival role because the regular meat, fish, chicken, and dairy available, consumed by the majority of the public, is very high in pesticides, herbicides, heavy metals, hormones, and radiation. Some research suggests that pesticides and radiation are concentrated up to 30 times more in flesh foods, and therefore it is important to eat lower on the food chain.

Benefits of Live Foods

The general healing and rejuvenative effects of a 100 percent live-food diet is another key diabetes healing factor in the Dr. Cousens's Diabetes Recovery Program—A Holistic Approach. In general, on a live-food, plant-source-only diet, people's sense of well-being greatly improves, which is already well described in the results of one of my master students' thesis, where 525 people who'd been on at least 80 percent live foods for at least two years had significant improvements.[231]

Her study found that overeating was decreased by five times. Eighty-two percent of people moved closer to their optimal weight. Quality of sleep increased 19 percent for participants since transitioning to live foods. Blood pressure normalized, cholesterol levels normalized, and postmeal symptoms including indigestion, bloating, fatigue, and weakness diminished. Bowel functions improved. Participants experiencing two or more bowel movements per day increased from 25 percent to 78 percent. Laxative use dropped from 36 percent to 2 percent. The immune system improved, with a 93.4 percent decrease in reports of getting sick easily. Seventy-three percent reported improvement in flexibility. Fifty-eight percent reported improvement in muscular strength. Participants experienced threefold improvement in overall energy levels. Arthritis and joint problems showed an 88 percent improvement. Exercise became more regular (67 percent exercised 3–6 times a week versus 46 percent before live foods). Teeth conditions improved, and "good or excellent" teeth and gum evaluations rose from 51 percent to 68 percent. Addictions diminished, with 62 percent of those who were suffering from food addiction feeling addiction free after switching to live foods.

There was a general decrease in medication use after two years on 80 percent live foods: Antacids use dropped from 20.3 percent to 1.3 percent. Antibiotics use dropped from 31.6 percent to 0.6 percent. Antidepressants use dropped from 15.1 percent to 6.9 percent. Antifungal use decreased 16-fold from 9.6 percent to 0.6 percent. Aspirin/ibuprofen use dropped 7-fold from 34.9 percent to 5 percent. Recreational drug use dropped approximately 2-fold from 20.9 percent to 11.3 percent.

Tylenol/acetaminophen use decreased greater than 4-fold: 18.7 percent to 3.8 percent. Thyroid medication use was an exception, with an increase from 8.5 percent to 14.5 percent. Reports of no chronic illness increased by 68 percent, including reports of reductions of the following chronic conditions: Chronic fatigue dropped from 16 percent to 3.6 percent. Candida dropped 4-fold from 21 percent to 5 percent. Depression dropped from 27 percent to 7 percent (a 400 percent decrease). Anxiety dropped from 22 percent to 2.6 percent (an approximate 900 percent decrease).

Experiences of a weak immune system went from 17 percent to 0.2 percent. Hypoglycemia symptoms decreased greater than 5-fold from 15 percent to 2.6 percent. Fibromyalgia decreased 3.5-fold from 5.6 percent to 1.5 percent. Osteoarthritis decreased approximately 4.8 percent to 2.8 percent. Cancer decreased from 2.7 percent to 0.4 percent. Other benefits include normalization of sex drive, a reduction of stress levels from 56 percent down to 20 percent, and improved menstrual cycles from 27 percent of women to 53 percent of women reporting comfortable cycles after 2 years on live foods.

There was significant improvement in mental well-being with 68 percent reporting intellectual development of "quite a bit" or "tremendously." Eighty-one percent felt more emotionally balanced in general. Approximately 87 percent reported improved mental/emotional/spiritual well-being, including increases in general sense of well-being from 36 percent to 91 percent. Enthusiasm and optimism more than doubled from 43 percent to 91 percent. Patience/tolerance increased from 29 percent to 84 percent. A feeling of self-sufficiency increased from 54 percent to 88 percent, and openness to change/flexibility increased from 53 percent to 89 percent. Memory/focus/clarity improved from 36 percent to 82 percent. Creativity expanded from 48 percent to 82 percent. The ability to multitask increased from 53 percent to 82 percent.

Relationships dynamic improved from 37 percent to 80 percent. Occupational satisfaction increased from 34 percent to 71 percent. Faith/hope increased from 47 percent to 85 percent. Passion (for anything) increased from 53 percent to 88 percent. Intuition increased from 52 percent to 91 percent. Compassion and love increased from 55 percent to 90 percent. Social comfort increased from 36 percent to 77 percent. Comfort being alone increased from 61 percent to 89 percent. Depth of meditation increased from 28 percent to 68 percent (3 times increase). Spiritual desire and interest increased from 50 percent to 85 percent. Quietness of mind tripled from 25 percent to 74 percent. Non-causal contentment increased from 30 percent to 80 percent. Noncausal peace increased from 32 percent to 80 percent. Noncausal joy more than doubled from 31 percent to 79 percent. Ecstatic bliss increased from 32 percent to 51 percent. Based on these results, it was concluded that people who have been on raw foods for two years or more experienced significant improvements emotionally, mentally, and spiritually.

There is an interesting, yet relatively unknown, aspect of the health quality of live food. Research published at Mount Sinai Hospital in New York City found high levels of advanced glycation end products (AGEs) where glucose was unnaturally combined with protein and/or lipids to form dysfunctional accelerated aging glucose-protein (or glycolipids) compounds in the body. These toxic components were high in infants. They discovered these glycation end products were high in both maternal breast milk and baby formulas. (Note that conventional baby formula is a highly cooked food.) They raised the risk that the tendency toward diabetes could be affected if people were exposed. The first studies were published in *Diabetes Care* in December 2010 and shows that AGEs can be elevated even at birth. These AGEs are inflammatory and are associated with increased insulin resistance and can be passed on from the mother.[232] In a study of 60 infants exploring passive transfer of AGEs from mother to the baby through the blood, they found that AGEs in the pregnant mother apparently had transferred to the babies, and their level of concentration in their infant blood was as high as their adult mother's. They also found that when babies switched from breast milk to commercial formula, their AGEs doubled in baby's blood to levels similar to diabetics. These children also had elevated insulin levels. Their finding was that formulas that were processed under high heat had at least a hundred times more AGEs than breast milk. These formulas are therefore more toxic to the baby.

There is a second piece of research published in 2011 in *Diabetes Care*, showing that people who cut down on foods that were high in AGEs (which come from the way the cooked foods are prepared) had a correlative decrease in insulin resistance.[233] They discovered that AGEs were found to be high in grilled, fried, and baked foods. In essence, all foods that were processed were higher in AGEs. They found there was an improvement in the insulin level and general health of the patients when foods with less AGEs were consumed. The study included 36 people, 18 overweight people, and 18 healthy adults. They were assigned according to a standard diet, with the same calories, and a diet of AGE-restricted intake. These studies give another reason why live food is important, because the results showed that subjects with diabetes assigned to the AGE-restricted diet group had a 35 percent decrease in blood insulin levels, which was significantly better than when they were on their previous non-AGE-restricted diet. They also found there was decreased inflammation and improved immune systems. This is the first clinical study to show in humans that AGEs promote insulin resistance and possibly diabetes. And, more important, it showed for the first time that restricting the amount of AGEs, which we minimize by eating live, uncooked foods, may restore the body's immune system and decrease insulin resistance. In summary, when you cook food, you increase AGE production in the food, which stimulates insulin resistance and aging.

There is really no question that a live-food, plant-source-only diet with all high-quality, organic nutrients, increased life-force, and energy can improve people's health, vitality, and healing force in general and also works specifically for diabetes. So in my opinion, the live food, for all those reasons, plays an important part in the healing process.

Individualizing the Diet

The next consideration in this "Why does the Dr. Cousens's diet work so quickly and powerfully?" discussion is the science of individualizing your diet. Although it is clear that the baseline constant in the

Dr. Cousens's diet is organic, live-food, plant-source-only food, there are variables in all the balance of the macronutrients that need fine tuning for maximal effect: (1) 25–45 percent carbohydrates, with no white sugar, white flour, junk food, processed food, or trans fats; (2) 25–45 percent fat; and (3) 10–25 percent protein. The variable is the percentage of fat, carbohydrate, or how much protein was in the diet, within these general ranges. Finding the right mix of these variables optimizes the vital life and healing force of the overall diet.

Why Does Dr. Cousens's Diabetes Recovery Program—A Holistic Approach Work for Type-1 Diabetics?

Type-1 diabetes, which is considered an autoimmune disease, that for diagnosis generally requires a positive beta cell antibody test and a fasting insulin of less than 2, is not the focus of this book. However, I had some surprising and seemingly unbelievably positive results with Type-1 diabetics. It is almost unbelievable to me that about 21 percent of these people have completely reversed their Type-1 diabetes in three weeks, and a total of 31.8 percent were off all insulin after three weeks. As equally important as that, the average Type-1 diabetic that comes into the program and is still on some insulin by the end of the 21 days, decreases their insulin need by approximately 70 percent. This is of course completely contrary to what is taught in any medical school in the world and completely unexpected from my point of view. However, just because I didn't expect it doesn't mean it's not true. The question is, how do we explain those results? In *Diabetologia* in 2005, research showed that insulin secretion is detectable in some Type-1 diabetics with long-standing diabetes.[234] The authors also suggested there is a small population of surviving beta cells or a continuing regeneration of beta cells. Now that alone tells me something, because I believe that my diet at least reduces the need for insulin and therefore if one is producing some insulin, even if it is less than 2 units, there still may be enough insulin if the insulin need is low enough on the 25–45 percent moderate-low carbohydrate, anti-inflammatory, live-food, organic diet. Some postmortem research has shown that when 42 Type-1 diabetics and 14 nondiabetics were compared, 88 percent of people with Type-1 diabetes still had functioning beta cells, even postmortem.[235] It appeared that the number of beta cells remaining was unrelated to the duration of the Type-1 diabetes disease, which, in the range of this research, was between 4 and 67 years. They also found that beta cell apoptosis (meaning death of beta cells) was twice as high in people with Type-1 diabetes. And they also saw that there was a marked increase in periductal fibrosis, which implies chronic inflammation over many years and also implies that ducts, which carry insulin from beta cells to the blood stream, had become fibrotic and insulin could not get through.

That leads me to several possibilities to discuss. But there's one more point, which was revealed in *Diabetologia*: one research paper showed direct evidence that beta cell regeneration through the mechanism of beta cell replication was found in 89-year-old Type-1 diabetic in which there was a hundredfold increase in beta cell production.[236] This study documents that beta cell regeneration by actual beta cells themselves replicating in the diabetics is a possibility and also does not exclude the option that there are other sources of beta cell production such as neogenesis. The overall suggestion, however, is that the beta cell formation in humans is probably by beta cell replication. This is very important and provides an additional explanation why I may be seeing these provocative and intriguing results of the healing of Type-1 diabetics. I also want to point out that what I'm theorizing as an explanation for these positive results was hypothesized by Warren and Root in *American Journal of Pathology* in 1925 in regard to Type-1 diabetics.[237] What they suggested, from a theoretical position, and what I am again suggesting from a clinical experience, are some possible reasons for why complete reversal can happen in Type-1 diabetics.

My theory is that since Type-1 is an inflammatory, autoimmune disease, by decreasing the amount of inflammation and the amount of autoimmune reactivity in the system, which is what my approach appears to do, I have created an upgraded condition in which more beta cells would survive and produce insulin. Second, if I were able to stimulate beta cell production, which is possible with herbs and possibly with live foods, then I am able to increase insulin production. The third consideration is that by decreasing the need for insulin in the system with a 25–45 percent carbohydrate, anti-inflammatory diet, such as a live-food, 25-45 percent fat, calorie restricted diet, the need for insulin significantly decreases, and the little that is produced by the Type-1 beta cells may be sufficient to produce normal FBS values. My program also adds a fourth healing factor to mine and Warren and Root's hypothesis, which is the use of very high potency proteolytic enzymes. These have been noted to actually help Type-1 diabetics because they help dissolve the peri-ductal fibrosis, which consequently increases the availability of the little insulin there is in the system to reach the blood. These high-intensity enzymes seem to reverse scarring and inflammation in IDDM Type-2 as well.

In summary of the theoretical understanding based on the clinical results of the efficiency of this program for Type-1 diabetics, I propose several synergistic explanations for the unusual results in the healing and amelioration of Type-1 diabetes: (1) decreased auto-immune inflammation, because the live-food, plant-source-only diet is anti-inflammatory and specifically reduces C-reactive protein, which is a marker of inflammation; (2) a 25–45 percent carbohydrate diet that decreases insulin needs and therefore (if one is producing even a little insulin, as suggested in the research) supports the possibility that 88 percent may be producing enough insulin to come off their insulin medication and have a normal FBS and minimal spikes; (3) as all these small factors converge, some beta cell production in some Type-1 diabetics, enhanced by the overall healthy diet of live, plant-source-only food, aided with the use of specific herbs, which increase the production of beta cells; and (4) the use of high-intensity proteolytic enzymes, which dissolve the peri-ductal fibrosis and decrease the destructive anti-inflammatory process that destroys beta cells. Presently, I am not able to tell in advance who is going to respond with a total healing (as some with the highest beta cell antibodies have healed), and so I make it clear to all patients on this approach that it is highly likely they will need less insulin and by itself that is important because insulin is an aging hormone and is directly associated with a variety of problems, including metabolic syndrome, cancer, heart disease, and obesity. By decreasing that, even if Type-1 is not healed, I have a potential way to expand the long-term healthy prognosis for Type-1 diabetics. Some of the Type-1 diabetics who are off all insulin, but with an FBS greater than 100, often slowly decrease their FBS to under 100 over the next year.

In summary, this chapter has attempted to explain the theoretical reasons behind the extraordinary clinical results in reversing and healing Type-2 IDDM and NIDDM in three weeks and the exciting results with ameliorating Type-1 diabetes and even having some return to a non-insulin-dependent, normal physiology. Practitioners have been using live foods to heal Type-2 diabetes since the 1920s, as mentioned previously. In 1925, Warren and Root hypothesized that Type-1 diabetes could also be healed via live foods. This suggests that my success with Type-1 and Type-2 diabetes may not be anything new.

The Healing Synergy in Summary

In summary, a review of the results for reversing diabetes in 120 clients is that in NIDDM Type-2 diabetics, there's a 61 percent cure rate in three weeks, which means 100 percent of people were off all medication and 61 percent had a blood sugar less than 100. For IDDM Type-2s, 86 percent were off all medication and 24 percent were off all diabetic medications and had a blood sugar of less than 100 in three weeks. In total, 97 percent of all Type-2s were off all diabetic medication in three weeks. Twenty-one percent of IDDM Type-1 diabetics and 31.4 percent of NIDDM Type-1 diabetics were medication free in three weeks. Sixty-nine percent of NIDDM Type-1 diabetics were able to reduce their medication intake by an average of 70 percent. After the three-week cycle, the percentages of those cured increased for all types of diabetic conditions, the longer patients stayed on the diet. As I've attempted to explain, there is a multifaceted, holistic synergy of reasons for these extraordinary results in the 120 people. This basic healing synergy (in order of probable importance) is as follow:

1. The avoidance of all carbohydrates except leafy greens, non-starchy and fibrous vegetables, sprouts, and sea vegetables in the diet. This included the avoidance of all grains, all sorts of sugars, white sugar, white flour, sweets, and sweeteners (except for stevia and birch-tree, natural xylitol). This is a 25–45 percent carbohydrate, slightly ketogenic diet. This moderate-low carbohydrate diet either significantly decreased and/or seemed to heal both insulin resistance and leptin resistance, which are the two driving hormonal imbalances in diabetes, and also helped to ameliorate or heal the metabolic syndrome of prediabetic state.

2. The power of a 100 percent live-food, plant-source-only, organic diet in the healing of diabetes

3. An anti-inflammatory live-food diet in decreasing the metabolic para-inflammatory condition. The use of live food decreased the para-inflammation by as much as fivefold in three to four weeks. The use of Culture of Life Intenzyme, which is a high-potency proteolytic enzyme to decrease inflammation, peri-ductal scaring, and beta cell scaring and destruction, also aided in healing.

4. Significant weight loss, on the 25–45 percent carbohydrate diet, of an average of slightly more than 18 pounds in 21 days, with some losing up to 25 pounds in 1 week and 46 pounds in 3 weeks. In *JAMA* (2007),[238] Stanford research produced the A–Z weight-loss diet. They showed that a high-fat, moderate-low-carbohydrate diet was superior to the Dean Ornish low-fat diet. These Stanford researchers made a very interesting statement: "Many concerns have been expressed that low-carbohydrate weight loss diet, high in total saturated fats, will adversely affect blood levels and cardiovascular risk. These concerns have not been

unsubstantiated in previous weight loss studies." This is exactly what I found in my study with 120 people. In fact, as I point out in my study, I saw a 24 percent drop in total cholesterol and also a drop in LDLs by 44 percent. This *JAMA* 2007 research makes me feel very comfortable that the diet that I'm suggesting to reverse and/or cure Type-2 diabetes also raises HDLs, lowers triglycerides, lowers LDLs, improves circulation, and helps the LDLs in Type-1 diabetes become larger and more fluffy, therefore actually lowering the risk of heart attack and decreasing the risk of developing metabolic syndrome, which is prediabetic syndrome.

5. A plant-source-only diet, as described in Genesis 1:29, itself had an important effect, as highlighted by the 12-study meta-analysis of 1,259,000 people that showed a 35–50 percent smaller risk for vegetarians versus omnivores for developing diabetics.

6. The use of all organic food, which minimizes negative effects of pesticides and herbicides, radiation, and heavy metals on insulin resistance and pancreas function

7. Moderate exercise

8. In a sense, it's a sleeper! People need to get adequate sleep. People who had nights without enough sleep, or minimal sleep, had blood sugars go up, even in one night. There's correlation between lack of sleep and increased FBS. I noticed it in myself as well. My FBS is usually in the low 80s and increased after several nights of limited hours sleeping by as much as 10 points.

9. The healing effects of meditation

10. Individualizing the diet type and phase type for optimal healing effects and long-term 90-percent compliance. In Phase 1.0, I recommend using approximately 25–45 percent calories from fat, approximately 25–45 percent from carbohydrates, and 10–25 percent protein in a live-food, plant-source-only diet (dependent upon individual constitution)

for three months of confirmed healing. I then recommend Phase 1.5, an 80–100 percent live-food, plant-source-only maintenance diet with 30–50 percent carbohydrates, including some grains, beans, and low-glycemic fruit but no junk or processed foods, white flour, white sugar, or trans fats.

11. The overall holistic effect of a 25–45-percent fat-intake diet, including a drop in total cholesterol to a safe, cardio-protective, mentally protective level of 159, and a cardio-protective triglyceride count of 82. The use of all raw fats except for trans fats creates an excellent macronutrient balance for minimizing carbohydrate intake and finding the best protein intake for repairing and rebuilding the tissues and enzyme replacement. The global long-term risks associated with a low-fat diet far outweigh any theorized and unsubstantiated scientifically potential benefits of a low-fat diet.

12. Loving yourself enough to want to heal yourself and the use of a psycho-spiritual approach to activate this

As I look at the overall clinical picture in the last 120 patients, my final thoughts are that the Dr. Cousens's Diabetes Recovery Program—A Holistic Approach has become a way of life in which people feel healthier and happier on every level of their lives. The Dr. Cousens Diabetes Recovery Program—A Holistic Approach gives the most efficacious results ever recorded in the literature at this time. It is my intention in future research to apply this program to at least two hundred Type-2 diabetics while using much more rigorous monitoring in a full scientific research paradigm. After this, I am considering doing a study with Type-1 diabetics.

The data collected from 120 participants (in this second edition) are certainly more significant than the data collected from 11 participants (in the first edition). I feel that there is enough data and that the issue is important enough, given the pandemic nature of diabetes, to release my results at this time. I do so with an awareness that more research is needed to validate this theory and the results.

The big question is the human question: Can people sustain themselves in the Culture of Life with a high degree of success? With highly motivated people there is a high success rate, but as this is applied to a pandemic level in many cultures and economic realities, I am looking very closely at support programs that will be desirable and thus successful for all circumstances. This will require a lot of creativity to apply this logical, common-sense breakthrough to national cultures worldwide, as I am now doing in Ghana, Nigeria, Ethiopia, Cameroon, New Guinea, Peru, Argentina, and Mexico; with migrant farm workers in the United States; with some Native Americans; and also in Israel. It is one thing to develop a successful health program in a volunteer clinical setting like the Tree of Life Rejuvenation Center U.S. but something else to create a program that is feasible for all on a national basis.

The Culture of Death and corresponding diet causes diabetes and leads people to a place where they feel at a point of no return once CDDS manifests as Type-2 diabetes and the negative epigenetic and genetic programs have been activated. The sensible and important awareness is that there is always the potential of a return. Paracelsus said, "No physician can ever say that any disease is incurable. To say so blasphemes God, blasphemes Nature, and depreciates the great architect of Creation. The disease does not exist, regardless of how terrible it may be, for which God has not provided the corresponding cure."

In this context, the current so-called normal standard American diet is immoderate and detrimental, as it directly contributes to the manifestation of diabetes. Previous "moderate" diets have been shown to ameliorate and control diabetes to a limited degree. The dramatic changes that result from my program do not come as the results of practicing the conventional moderation approach of the Culture of Death, which in essence is a way of making denial seem reasonable in this case. To make this kind of significant change requires a lifestyle and diet that is dramatically and excitingly different, resulting in powerful results in a short period of time. This requires leading a life of love, purpose, meaning, and self-value, and choosing a diet and lifestyle that reflect these values. This is the diet and lifestyle being taught in my program.

The essential question that is asked of participants is, Do you love yourself enough to want to heal; and potentially add 10 to 19 healthy years to your life? The results revealed in this book, for those who have answered this question in the affirmative, show that the conventional paradigm for diabetes—as labeled by the ADA and most medical schools as incurable—is a self-defeating myth. In all fairness, the conventional paradigm also teaches that proper diet and exercise help slow the progression of this "incurable" disease, but those adhering to the conventional paradigm do not offer the proper diet and intensity to do the job. I have activated a new paradigm that previous research has pointed toward by taking the next logical step, going deeper into the underlying causes by seeing diabetes as a symptom of the Culture of Death. In this book I have validated that there is an option if one is ready to take it.

By the Culture of Death, I am talking about a culture founded on predatory competition in which people are economic commodities. The focus is on wealth for the few versus health for the many. It is a culture of separateness, domination, and resulting exploitation. In this culture, people have lost their soul connection and life purpose. This is connected to the approximate 80 percent obesity rate in diabetics, for as previously stated, there is never enough food for a hungry soul. The Culture of Death spawns a food environment characterized by the heavy marketing of excitotoxin-rich processed junk foods that are high in white sugar, white flour with alloxan, and refined carbohydrates, and the heavy use of cooked animal fats and hydrogenated trans fats, agrochemical-laden foods, radiation, and heavy-metal toxicity. These characteristics combine to result in a negative synergy that has precipitated Type-2 diabetes at pandemic levels, compared with its relative rarity before 1940. This is not an accident—the Culture of Death diet is an active and thoughtless Crime Against Wisdom.

The Culture of Life manifests as cooperation, health, harmony, and compassion, combined with production of healthy, natural, organic foods that preserve soil and minimize the pollution of both people and planet. The Culture of Life helps us reconnect to our heart and soul in a way that brings the presence of light, love, and the divine back into the core of our human experience. Instead of a "moderate" diet, the Culture of Life cuisine is a common-sense diet of low-glycemic, moderate-low high-quality carbohydrate, low-insulin-index foods that are organic, high in minerals, hydrating, and live, with no animal, hydrogenated, or trans fats, 25–45 percent high EFA plant-based fats, high fiber, 10–25 percent plant-source protein, and thoughtful food intake.

The healing of diabetes at the pandemic level requires the healing of the ecology of the planet and the consciousness of the people. To heal oneself requires the ability to love oneself enough to have the intention to reconnect with the Culture of Life, which is our birthright. In that way, one performs an act of love for oneself as an individual person and as part of the living planet. This results in the healing of the planet and all species. The healing of diabetes in this context is an act of love, compassion, and consciousness.

How to Self-Screen for Possible CDDS, Prediabetes, or Diabetes*

Fasting Blood Sugar (FBS)

- One needs a glycometer to do this. They are about the same quality, although prices vary.
- To find your FBS, test your blood with a glycometer when you wake up in the morning before you have eaten anything. This is called FBS. It must be taken before eating or drinking.
- If your FBS is above 85, it is best to be on a Phase 1.0 diet until it has dropped to 85 or below. If the FBS is 86 to 99, you have entered the first phase of CDDS. At this stage, it is a preventative health and warning diagnosis. It is, however, a strong suggestion to go to a Phase 1.0 diet and maybe just green juice for dinner.

*All definitive diagnoses should be made by your personal physician.

- If FBS is 100 to 125, it suggests that you are prediabetic, like a third of all Americans.
- If your FBS is 126 and above two days in a row, it suggests that you may be diabetic.
- No definitive diabetes diagnosis should be made without a full diabetes work-up by your personal physician. If you get an A1C test, from my higher standard perspective, 5.0 or less is optimal, 5.3 is good, and above 5.7 is considered diabetes. Others suggest that the diabetes diagnostic cut off point should be 6.0.

Test Blood Sugar (BS) One and Two Hours after Meals

- A second part of CDDS evaluation is your postprandial spike, which is your blood sugar value one hour after finishing your meal.
- If your blood sugar is above 125 or 40 points higher than your before meal blood sugar, it indicates that you need to go back to the Phase 1.0 diet until the blood sugar level is less than 125 or less than 40 above your premeal blood sugar.
- If your blood sugar is greater than 140 one hour after eating, it is a probable sign that you are a prediabetic and need to go on a Phase 1.0 diet. You should have a diabetes work-up by your physician, including at least a five-hour glucose-tolerance test and an A1C test.
- If your blood sugar is above 180, you are most likely a diabetic and should immediately arrange with your personal physician for a more complete diabetic work-up and begin a Phase 1.0 diet. The Phase 1.0 recipes listed in Chapter 7 will serve you well.

Daily Chart

(One Meal Example)		Mon	Tues	Wed	Thurs	Fri	Sat	Sun
		MEAL 1	MFBS (Morning Fasting Blood Sugar)			85	B or C – A = S (Spike value)	
			A (Blood Sugar BEFORE Meal)				100	
			B (Blood Sugar 1 hr AFTER Meal)			125	(125 - 100 =) 20	
			C (Blood Sugar 2 hrs AFTER Meal)			130	(130 - 100 =) 30	

MFBS		S		S	S	S	S	S	S
MEAL 1	A								
	B								
	C								
MEAL 2	A								
	B								
	C								
MEAL 3	A								
	B								
	C								
MEAL 4	A								
	B								
	C								

MFBS – Morning Fasting Blood Sugar
BS – Blood Sugar
A – BS **BEFORE** Meal
B – BS **1 hr AFTER** Meal
C – BS **2 hrs AFTER** Meal
B or C – A = **S (SPIKE)**
(Spike value should not be higher than 40)

FIGURE 6. Daily chart

Notes

1. Piccardo, C, Cai, W, Chen, X, Zhu, L, Striker, G E, Vlassara, H, and Uribarri, J. "Maternally transmitted and food-derived glycotoxins." *Diabetes Care*, doi:10.2337/dc10-1058.

2. Centers for Disease Control and Prevention. "Number of Americans with diabetes rises to nearly 26 million." http://www.cdc.gov/media/releases/2011/p0126_diabetes.html.

3. Batty, G D, Kivimaki, M, Smith, G D, Marmot, M G, and Shipley, M J. "Post-challenge blood glucose concentration and stroke mortality rates in non-diabetic men in London: 38-year follow up of the original Whitehall prospective cohort study." *Diabetologia*, July 2008, 51: 1123–26.

4. Pan, W H, Cedres, L B, Liu, K, et al. "Relationships of clinical diabetes

and symptomatic hyperglycaemia to risk of coronary heart disease mortality in men and women." *Am J Epidemiol*, March 1986, 123(3): 504–16.

5. Coutinho, M, Gerstein, H, Poque, J, Wang, Y, and Yusuf, S. "The relationship between glucose and incident cardiovascular events: A metaregression analysis of published data from 20 studies of 95, 783 individuals followed for 12.4 years." *Diabetes Care*, February 1999, 22(2): 233–40.

6. Wilson, P W F, Cupples, L A, and Kannel, W B. "Is hyperglycaemia associated with cardiovascular disease? The Framingham Study." *Am Heart J*, February 1991, 121(2, part 1): 586–90.

7. De Vegt, F, Dekker, J M, Ruhe, H G, et al. "Hyperglycaemia is associated with all-cause and cardiovascular mortality in the Hoorn population: The Hoorn study." *Diabetologia*, August 1999, 42(8): 926–31.

8. DECODE Study Group 200, the European Diabetes Epidemiology Group. "Glucose tolerance and cardiovascular mortality: Comparison of the fasting and the 2-hour diagnostic criteria." *Arch Intern Med*, February 12, 2001, 161(3): 397–404.

9. Saydah, S H, Miret, M, Sung, J, Varas, C, Gause, D, and Brancati, F L. "Post-challenge hyperglycemia and mortality in a national sample of U.S. adults." *Diabetes Care*, August 2001, 24(8): 1397–402.

10. Held, C, Gerstein, H C, Zhao, F, et al. "Fasting plasma glucose is an independent predictor of hospitalization for congestive heart failure in high-risk patients." *American Heart Association 2006 Scientific Sessions*, November 13, 2006, abstract 2562.

11. Lin, H J, Lee, B C, Ho, Y L, et al. "Postprandial glucose improves the risk prediction of cardiovascular death beyond the metabolic syndrome in the nondiabetic population." *Diabetes Care*, September 2009, 32(9): 1721–26.

12. Cukierman-Yaffe, T, Gerstein, H C, and Williamson, J D. "Relationship between baseline glycemic control and cognitive function in individuals with Type-2 diabetes and other cardiovascular risk factors: The action to control cardiovascular risk in diabetes-memory in diabetes (ACCORD-MIND) trial." *Diabetes Care*, March 2009, 32(2): 221–26.

13. Cheng, Y J, Gregg, E W, and Geiss, L S. "Association of A1C and fasting plasma glucose levels with diabetic retinopathy prevalence in the U.S. population: Implications for diabetes diagnostic thresholds." *Diabetes Care*, November 2009, 32(11): 2027–32.

14. Sumner, C J, Sheth, S, Griffin, J W, Cornblath, D R, and Polydefkis, M. "The spectrum of neuropathy in diabetes and impaired glucose tolerance." *Neurology*, January 14, 2003, 60(1): 108–11.

15. Gastaldelli, A, Ferrannini, E, Miyazaki, Y, Matsuda, M, and De Fronzo, R A. "Beta-cell dysfunction and glucose intolerance: Results from the San Antonio metabolism (SAM) study." *Diabetologia*, January 2004, 47(1): 31–39.

16. Polhill, T S, Saad, S, Poronnik, S, Fulcher, G R, and Pollock, C R. "Short-term peaks in glucose promote renal fibrogenesis independently of total glucose exposure." *Am J Physiol Renal Physiol*, August 2004, 287(2): F268–73.

17. Bash, L D, Selvin, E, Steffes, M, Coresh, J, and Astor, B C. "Poor glycemic control in diabetes and the risk of incident kidney disease even in the absence of albuminuria and retinopathy: Atherosclerosis risk in communities (ARIC) study." *Arch Intern Med*, December 8, 2008, 168(22): 2440–47.

18. Hemminki, K, Li, X, Sundquist, J, and Sundquist, K. "Risk of cancer following hospitalization for Type-2 diabetes." *Oncologist*, May 17, 2010, 15: 548–55.

19. Aleksandrova, K, Boeing, H, Jenab, M, et al. "Metabolic syndrome and risks of colon and rectal cancer: The European Prospective Investigation into Cancer and Nutrition Study." *Cancer Prev Res (Phila)*, June 22, 2011.

20. Czyzyk, A, and Szczepanik, Z. "Diabetes mellitus and cancer." *Eur J Intern Med*, October 2000, 11(5): 245–52.

21. Vigneri, P, Frasca, F, Sciacca, L, Pandini, G, and Vigneri, R. "Diabetes and cancer." *Endocr Relat Cancer*, December 2009, 16(4): 1103–23.

22. Cust, A E, Kaaks, R, Friedenreich, C, Bonnet, F, et al. "Metabolic syndrome, plasma lipid, lipoprotein and glucose levels, and endometrial cancer risk in the European Prospective Investigation into Cancer and Nutrition EPIC." *Endocr Relat Cancer*. September 2007, 14(3): 755–67.

23. Rosato, V, Tavani, A, Bosetti, C, et al. "Metabolic syndrome and pancreatic cancer risk: A case-control study in Italy and metaanalysis." *Metabolism*, May 5, 2011.

24. Stocks, T, Lukanova, A, Bjorge, T, et al. "Metabolic factors and the risk of colorectal cancer in 580, 000 men and women in the metabolic syndrome and cancer project (Me-Can): Metabolic Syndrome Cancer Project (Me-Can) Group." *Cancer*, December 17, 2010.

25. Kato, M, Noda, M, Suga, H, Matsumoto, M, and Kanazawa, Y. "Fasting plasma glucose and incidence of diabetes—for the threshold for impaired fasting glucose: Results from the population-based Omiya MA cohort study." *J Atheroscler Thromb*, 2009, 16(6): 857–61.

26. El-Osta, A, Brasacchio, D, Yao, D, Pocai, A, Jones, P L, Roeder, R G, Cooper, M E, and Brownlee, M. "Transient high glucose causes

persistent epigenetic changes and altered gene expression during sub-sequent normoglycemia." *J Exp Med*, September 29, 2008, 205(10): 2409–17.

27. Ibid.

28. Ibid.

29. Ibid.

30. Ibid.

31. Bland, J S. *Genetic Nutritioneering*. New York, NY: McGraw-Hill, 1999.

32. El-Osta, Brasacchio, Yao, et al. "Transient high glucose causes persistent epigenetic changes."

33. Li, Q, Chen, A H, Song, X D, et al. "Analysis of glucose levels and the risk for coronary heart disease in elderly patients in Guangzhou Haizhu district." *Nan Fang Yi Ke Da Xue Xue Bao*, June 2010, 30(6): 1275–79.

34. Matthews, C E, Sui, X, LaMonte, M J, Adams, S A, Heebert, J R, and Blair, S N. "Metabolic syndrome and risk of death from cancers of the digestive system." *Metabolism*, August 2010, 59(8): 1231–39.

35. Gerstein, H C, Pais, P, Pogue, J, and Yusuf, S. "Relationship of glucose and insulin levels to the risk of myocardial infarction: A case-control study." *J Am Coll Cardiol*, March 1999, 33(3): 612–19.

36. Sumner, Sheth, Griffin, et al. "The spectrum of neuropathy in diabetes."

37. Bjornholt, J V, Erikssen, G, Aaser, E, et al. "Fasting blood glucose: An underestimated risk factor for cardiovascular death. Results from a 22-year follow-up of healthy nondiabetic men." *Diabetes Care*, January 1999, 22(1): 45–49.

38. Zeymer, U. "Cardiovascular benefits of acarbose in impaired glucose tolerance and Type-2 diabetes." *Int J Cardiol*, February 8, 2006, 107(1): 11–20.

39. Ibid.

40. Minatoguchi, S, Zhang, Z, Bao, N, et al. "Acarbose reduces myocardial infarct size by preventing postprandial hyperglycemia and hydroxyl radical production and opening mitochondrial KATP channels in rab-bits." *J Cardiovasc Pharmacol*, July 2009, 54(1): 25–30.

41. Frantz, S, Calvillo, L, Tillmanns, J, et al. "Repetitive postprandial hyper-glycemia increases cardiac ischemia/reperfusion injury: Prevention by the alpha-glucosidase inhibitor acarbose." *FASEB J*, April 2005, 19(6): 591–93.

42. Donahue, R P, Abbott, R D, Reed, D M, et al. "Postchallenge glucose concentration and coronary heart disease in men of Japanese ancestry.

Honolulu Heart Program." *Diabetes*, June 1987, 36(6): 689–92.

43. Fuller, J H, Shipley, M J, Rose, G, et al. "Coronary-heart-disease risk and impaired glucose tolerance. The Whitehall Study." *Lancet*, June 28, 1980, 1(8183): 1373–76.

44. Jackson, C A, Yudkin, J S, and Forrest R D. "A comparison of the relationships of the glucose tolerance test and the glycated haemoglobin assay with diabetic vascular disease in the community. The Islington Diabetes Survey." *Diabetes Res Clin Pract*, August 1992, 17(2): 111–23.

45. Singleton, J R, Smith, A G, and Bromberg, M B. "Increased prevalence of impaired glucose tolerance in patients with painful sensory neuropathy." *Diabetes Care*, August 2001, 24(8): 1448–53.

46. Sumner, Sheth, Griffin, et al. "The spectrum of neuropathy in diabetes."

47. Singleton, Smith, and Bromberg. "Increased prevalence of impaired glucose tolerance."

48. Tavee, J, and Zhou, L. "Small fiber neuropathy: A burning problem." *Cleve Clin J Med*, May 2009, 76(5): 297–305.

49. Beckley, E T. "ADA scientific session: Retinopathy found in pre-diabetes." *DOC News*, August 2005, 2(8): 1–10.

50. Stattin, P, Bjor, O, Ferrari, P, et al. "Prospective study of hyperglycemia and cancer risk." *Diabetes Care*, March 2007, 30(3): 561–67.

51. Gleason, C E, Gonzalez, M, Harmon, J S, and Robertson, R P. "Determinants of glucose toxicity and its reversibility in pancreatic islet Beta-cell line, HIT-T15." *Am J Physiol Endocrinol Metab*, 2000, 279: E997–E1002.

52. Yokoi, T, Fukuo, K, Yasuda, O, et al. "Apoptosis signal-regulating kinase 1 mediate cellular senescence induced by high glucose in endothelial cells." *Diabetes*, June 2006, 55(6): 1660–65.

53. Kato, Noda, Suga, et al. "Fasting plasma glucose and incidence of diabetes."

54. Yamagata, H, Kiyohara, Y, Nakamura, S, et al. "Impact of fasting plasma glucose levels on gastric cancer incidence in a general Japanese population: The Hisayama study." *Diabetes Care*, April 2005, 28(4): 789–94.

55. Gerstein, Pais, Pogue, et al. "Relationship of glucose and insulin levels to the risk of myocardial infarction."

56. Pereg, D, Elis, A, Neuman, Y, Mosseri, M, Lishner, M, and Hermoni, D. "Cardiovascular risk in patients with fasting blood glucose levels within normal range." *Am J Cardiol*, December 1, 2010, 106(11): 1602–5.

57. Gastaldelli, Ferrannini, Miyazaki, et al. "Beta-cell dysfunction and glucose intolerance."

58. Ibid.

59. Butler, A E, Janson, J, Bonner-Weir, S, et al. "Beta-cell deficit and increased beta-cell apoptosis in humans with Type-2 diabetes." *Diabetes*, January 2003, 52(1): 102–10.

60. Pehuet-Figoni, M, Ballot, E, Bach, J F, and Chatenoud, L. "Aberrant function and long-term survival of mouse beta cells exposed in vitro to high glucose concentrations." *Cell Transplant.* September–October 1994, 3(5): 445–51.

61. Zhou, Y P, Marlen, K, Palma, J F, et al. "Overexpression of repressive camp response element modulators in high glucose and fatty acid-treated rat islets. A common mechanism for glucose toxicity and lipo-toxicity?" *J Biol Chem*, December 19, 2003, 278(51): 51316–23.

62. Ceriello, A, Falleti, E, Bortolotti, N, et al. "Increased circulating intercel-lular adhesion molecule-1 levels in Type-2 diabetic patients: The pos-sible role of metabolic control and oxidative stress." *Metabolism*, April 1996, 45(4): 498–501.

63. Folli, F, Corradi, D, Fanti, P, et al. "The role of oxidative stress in the pathogenesis of Type-2 diabetes mellitus micro- and macrovascular complications: Avenues for a mechanistic-based therapeutic approach." *Curr Diabetes Rev*, August 15, 2011.

64. Bucala, R, Cerami, A, and Vlassara, H. "Advanced glycosylation end products in diabetic complications. Biochemical basis and prospects for therapeutic intervention." *Diabetes Rev.* 1995, 3: 258–68.

65. Barlovic, D P, Soro-Paavonen, A, and Jandeleit-Dahm, K A. "RAGE biology, atherosclerosis and diabetes." *Clin Sci (Lond)*, July 2011, 121(2): 43–55.

66. Miura, K, Kitahara, Y, and Yamagishi, S. "Combination therapy with nateglinide and vilda gliptin improves posterprandial metabolic derangements in Zucker fatty rats." *Horm Metab Res*, September 2010, 42(10): 731–45.

67. Monnier, L, and Colette, C. "Glycemic variability: Should we and can we prevent it?" *Diabetes Care*, February 2008, 31(suppl. 2): S150–S154.

68. Monnier, L, Colette, C, and Owens, D R. "Glycemic variability: The third component of the dysglycemia in diabetes. Is it important? How to measure it." *J Diabetes Sci Technol*, November 2008, 2(6): 1094–1100.

69. Pan, Cedres, Liu, et al. "Relationships of clinical diabetes and symptom-atic hyperglycaemia."

70. Wilson, Cupples, and Kannel. "Is hyperglycaemia associated with car-diovascular disease?"

71. De Vegt, Dekker, Ruhe, et al. "Hyperglycaemia is associated with all-cause and cardiovascular mortality."

72. Saydah, Miret, Sung, et al. "Post-challenge hyperglycemia and morality."

73. Coutinho, Gerstein, Poque, et al. "The relationship between glucose and incident cardiovascular event."

74. Donahue, Abbott, Reed, et al. "Postchallenge glucose concentration."

75. Batty, Kivimaki, Smith, et al. "Post-challenge blood glucose concentration."

76. Hemminki, Li, Sundquist, et al. "Risk of cancer following hospitalization Type-2."

77. Cust, Kaaks, Friedenreich, et al. "Metabolic syndrome, plasma lipid, lipoprotein and glucose levels."

78. Rosato, Tavani, Bosetti, et al. "Metabolic syndrome and pancreatic cancer risk."

79. Shoen, R E, Tangen, C M, Kuller, L H, et al. "Increased blood glucose and insulin, body size, and incident colorectal cancer." *J Natl Cancer Inst*, July 7, 1999, 91(13): 1147–54.

80. Aleksandrova, Boeing, Jenab, et al. "Metabolic syndrome and risks of colon and rectal cancer."

81. Healy, L, Howard, J, Ryan, A, et al. "Metabolic syndrome and leptin are associated with adverse pathological features in male colorectal cancer patients." *Colorectal Dis*, January 20, 2011.

82. Tali Cukierman-Yaffe, T, Gerstein, H C, and Williamson, J D. "Relationship between baseline glycemic control and cognitive function in individuals with Type-2 diabetes and other cardiovascular risk factors: The action to control cardiovascular risk in diabetes-memory in diabetes (ACCORD-MIND) trial." *Diabetes Care*, February 2009, 32(2): 221–26.

83. Sonnen, J A, Larson, E B, and Brickell, K. "Different patterns of cerebral injury in dementia with or without diabetes." *Arch Neurol*, March 2009, 66(3): 315–22.

84. Polhill, Saad, Poronnik, et al. "Short-term peaks in glucose."

85. Sumner, Sheth, Griffin, et al. "The spectrum of neuropathy in diabetes."

86. Hoffman-Snyder, C, Smith, B E, Ross, M A, Hernandez, J, and Bosch, E P. "Value of the oral glucose tolerance test in the evaluation of chronic idiopathic axonal polyneuropathy." *Arch Neurol*, August 2006, 63(8): 1075–79.

87. Medzhitov, R. "Origin and physiological roles of inflammation." *Nature*, July 24, 2008, 454: 428–35, doi:10.1038/nature07201.

88. Ibid.

89. Hotamisligil, G. "Inflammation and metabolic disorders." *Nature,* December 2006, 444, 14, doi:10.1038/nature05485.

90. Lamon, B, and Hajjar, D. "Inflammation at the molecular interface of atherogenesis: An anthropological journey." *American Journal of Pathology,* 2008, 173: 1253–64, doi:10.2353/ajpath.2008.080442.

91. Sorensen, L B, Raben, A, Stender, S, and Astrup, A. "Effect of sucrose on inflammatory markers in overweight humans." *American Journal of Clinical Nutrition,* August 2005, 82(2): 421–27.

92. Lopez-Garcia, E, Schulze, M B, Meigs, J B, Manson, J E, Rifai, N, Stampfer, M J, Willett, W C, and Hu, F B. "Consumption of trans fatty acids is related to plasma biomarkers of inflammation and endothelial dysfunction." *The American Society for Nutritional Sciences J Nutr,* March 2005, 135: 562–66.

93. International Diabetes Federation. "Presidential address ahead of *New Diabetes Atlas, 5th ed.*" Presented at European Association for the Study of Diabetes (EASD) 47th Annual Meeting, September 13, 2011 (Lisbon, Portugal).

94. Hotamisligil, G S. "Inflammation and metabolic disorders." *Nature,* December 2006, 444, 14, doi:10.1038/nature05485.

95. Wellen, K E, and Hotamisligil, G S. "Inflammation, stress, and diabetes." *J Clin Invest,* 2005, 115: 1111–19.

96. Cummings, D E, and Schwartz, M W. "Genetics and pathophysiology of human obesity." *Annu. Rev. Med,* 2003, 54: 453–71.

97. Miller, C, et al. "Tumor necrosis factor-alpha levels in adipose tissue of lean and obese cats." *J Nutr,* 1998, 128(suppl. 12): 2751S–2752S.

98. Xu, H, et al. "Chronic inflammation in fat plays a crucial role in the development of obesity-related insulin resistance." *J Clin. Invest,* 2003, 112: 1821–30, doi:10.1172/JCI200319451.

99. Weisberg, S P, et al. "Obesity is associated with macrophage accumulation in adipose tissue." *J Clin Invest,* 2003, 112: 1796–808.

100. Xu, H, et al. "Chronic inflammation in fat plays a crucial role."

101. Taniguchi, C M, Emanuelli, B, and Kahn, C R. "Critical nodes in signaling pathways: Insights into insulin action." *Nature Rev Mol Cell Biol,* 2006, 7: 85–96.

102. White, M F. "IRS proteins and the common path to diabetes." *Am J Physiol Endocrinol Metab,* 2002, 283, E413–E422.

103. Beutler, B. "Innate immunity: An overview." *Mol Immunol,* 2004, 40: 845–59.

104. Tuncman, G, et al. "Functional in vivo interactions between JNK1 and JNK2 isoforms in obesity and insulin resistance." *Proc Natl Acad Sci USA*, 2006, 103: 10741–46.

105. Ozcan, U, et al. "Endoplasmic reticulum stress links obesity, insulin action, and Type-2 diabetes." *Science*, 2004, 306: 457–61.

106. Lin, Y, et al. "The hyperglycemia-induced inflammatory response in adipocytes: The role of reactive oxygen species." *J Biol Chem*, 2005, 280: 4617–26.

107. Houstis, N, Rosen, E D, and Lander, E S. "Reactive oxygen species have a causal role in multiple forms of insulin resistance." *Nature*, 2006, 440: 944–48.

108. Anderson, K M, Castelli, W P, and Levy, D. "Cholesterol and mortality. 30 years of follow-up from the Framingham Study." *Journal of the American Medical Association*, 1987, 257: 2176–80.

109. Kannel, W B, and Gordon, T. "The Framingham diet study: Diet and the regulation of serum cholesterol." In *Nutrition Research Reviews*, 1994, 7: 43–65, doi:10.1079/NRR19940006.

110. Choi, Y S, Goto, S, Ikeda, I, and Sugano, M. "Age-related changes in lipid metabolism in rats: The consequence of moderate food restriction." *Biochim Biophys Acta*, 1988, 963: 237–42.

111. Holloszy, J O, and Fontana, L. "Caloric restriction in humans." *Exp Gerontol*, 2007, 42: 709–12.

112. Jakobsen, M U, Dethlefsen, C, Joensen, A M, Stegger, J, Tjonneland, A, Schmidt, E B, and Overvad, K. "Intake of carbohydrates compared with intake of saturated fatty acids and risk of myocardial infarction: Importance of glycemic index." *Am J Clin Nutr* 2012, 91: 1764–68.

113. McMillen, I C, Adam, C L, and Mühlhäusler, B S. "Early origins of obesity: Programming the appetite regulatory system." *The Journal of Physiology*, May 2005, 565(1): 9–17.

114. Ibid.

115. El-Osta, B, et al. "Transient high glucose causes persistent epigenetic changes." *JEM* 205(10), doi:10.1084/jem.20081188.

116. Chen, K, Li, F, Li, J, et al. "Induction of leptin resistance through direct interaction of C-reactive protein with leptin." *Nat Med*, Apr 2006, 12(4): 425–32.

117. Kuch, B, et al. "Differential impact of admission C-reactive protein levels on 28-day mortality risk in patients with ST-elevation myocardial infarction (from the Monitoring Trends and Determinants on Cardiovascular Diseases [MONICA]/Cooperative Health Research

in the Region of Augsburg [KORA] Augsburg Myocardial Infarction Registry)." *Am J Cardiol*, November 1, 2008, 102(9): 1125–30.

118. Oben, J E, Ngondi, J L, Momo, C N, Agbor, G A, and Sobgui, C S. "The use of a Cissus quadrangularis/Irvingia gabonensis combination in the management of weight loss: A double-blind placebo-controlled study." *Lipids Health Dis*, 2008, 712.

119. Ngondi, J L, Oben, J E, and Minka, S R. "The effect of Irvingia gabonensis seeds on body weight and blood lipids of obese subjects in Cameroon." *Lipids Health Dis*, May 25, 2005, 412.

120. Ngondi, J L, Matsinkou, R, and Oben, J E. "The use of Irvingia gabonensis extract (IGOB131) in the management of metabolic syndrome in Cameroon." 2008. Submitted for publication.

121. Cousens, G. *Conscious Eating*. Berkeley, CA: North Atlantic Books, 2000, p. 43.

122. Robinson A M, and Williamson, D H. "Physiological roles of ketone bodies as substrates and signals in mammalian tissues." *Physiol Rev* (1980) 60: 143–87.

123. Ibid.

124. Action to Control Cardiovascular Risk in Diabetes Study Group. "Effects of intensive glucose lowering in Type-2 diabetes." *New England Journal of Medicine*, June 12, 2008, 358 (24): 2545–59.

125. Nuttall, F Q, Mooradian, A D, Gannon, M C, Billington, C, and Krezowski, P. "Effect of protein ingestion on the glucose and insulin response to a standardized oral glucose load." *Diabetes Care*, September/October 1984, 7(5): 465–70, doi:10.2337/diacare.7.5.465.

126. Fery, F, et al. "Hormonal and metabolic changes induced by an isocaloric isoprotienic ketogenic diet in healthy subjects." *Diabetes Metab*, 1982, 8: 299–305.

127. Phinney, S D, et al. "The human metabolic response to chronic ketosis without caloric restriction: Physical and biochemical adaptations." *Metabolism*, 1983, 32: 757–68.

128. Swendseid. M E, et al. "Plasma amino acid levels in subjects fed isonitrogenous diets containing different proportions of fat and carbohydrate." *Am J Clin Nutr*, 1967, 20: 52–55.

129. Mitchell, G A, et al. "Medical aspects of ketone body metabolism." *Clinical and Investigative Medicine*, 1995, 18: 193–216.

130. Merimee, T J, et al. "Sex variations in free fatty acids and ketones during fasting: Evidence for a role of glucagon." *J Clin Endocrin Metab*, 1978, 46: 414–19.

131. Merimee, T J, and Fineberg, S E. "Homeostasis during fasting II:

Hormone substrate differences between men and women." *J Clin Endocrin Metab*, 1973, 37: 698–702.

132. Haymond, M W, et al. "Effects of ketosis on glucose flux in children and adults." *Am J Physiol*, 1983, 245: E373–E378.

133. Porte, D, and Sherwin, R, eds. *Ellenberg and Rifkin's Diabetes Mellitus: Theory and Practice*. 5th ed. New York: Appleton and Lange, 1997.

134. Elia, M, et al. "Ketone body metabolism in lean male adults during short-term starvation, with particular reference to forearm muscle metabolism." *Clinical Science*, 1990, 78: 579–84.

135. Laino, C. "Alzheimer's feared, misconceptions common." Accessed August 1, 2011. http://www.webmd.com/alzheimers/news/20110720 /alzheimers-feared-misconceptions-common.

136. Ott, A, Breteler, M M, van Harskamp, F, et al. "Prevalence of Alzheimers disease and vascular dementia: Association with education. The Rotterdam study." *BMJ*, April 15, 1995, 310(6985): 970–73.

137. Hebert, L E, Scherr, P A, Bienias, J L, Bennett, D A, and Evans, D A. "Alzheimer disease in the U.S. population: Prevalence estimates using the 2000 census." *Arch Neurol*, August 2003, 60(8): 1119–22.

138. Cahill, G. "Starvation in man." *N Engl J Med*, 1970, 282: 668–75.

139. Felig, P, et al. "Blood glucose and gluconeogenesis in fasting man." *Arch Intern Med*, 1960, 123: 293–98.

140. Newport, M. "What if there was a cure for Alzheimer's disease and no one knew?" A case study by Dr. Mary Newport, July 22, 2008. http:// www.coconutketones.com/whatifcure.pdf.

141. Purnell, J Q, Klopfenstein, B A, Stevens, A A, Havel, P J, Adams, S H, Dunn, T N, Krisky, C, and Rooney, W D. "Brain functional magnetic resonance imaging response to glucose and fructose infusions in humans." *Diabetes, Obesity and Metabolism*, March 2011, 13(3): 229–34, doi:10.1111/j.1463-1326.2010.01340.x.

142. Parks, E J, and Hellerstein, M K. "Carbohydrate-induced hypertriacl-glycerolemia: Historical perspective and review of biological mechanisms." *Amer J Clin Nutr*, 2000, 71.

143. Basciano, H, Federico, L, and Adeli, K. "Fructose, insulin resistance, and metabolic dyslipidemia." *Nutr Metab (Lond)*, February 21, 2005, 2(1): 5.

144. American Chemical Society. "Soda warning? High-fructose corn syrup linked to diabetes, new study suggests." *ScienceDaily*, August 23, 2007, http://www.sciencedaily.com/releases/2007/08/070823094819.htm.

145. American Society of Nephrology. "High fructose intake from added

sugars: An independent association with hypertension." *ScienceDaily*, October 29, 2009, http://www.sciencedaily.com /releases/2009/10/091029211521.htm.

146. Basciano, Federico, and Adeli. "Fructose, insulin resistance, and metabolic dyslipidemia."

147. Ouyang, X, Cirillo, P, Sautin, Y, et al. "Fructose consumption as a risk factor for non-alcoholic fatty liver disease." *J Hepatol*, June 2008, 48(6): 993–99.

148. Thuy, S, Ladurner, R, Volynets, V, et al. "Nonalcoholic fatty liver disease in humans is associated with increased plasma endotoxin and plasminogen activator inhibitor 1 concentrations and with fructose intake." *J Nutr*, August 2008, 138(8): 1452–55.

149. Bray, G A, Nielsen, S J, and Popkin, B M. "Consumption of high-fructose corn syrup in beverages may play a role in the epidemic of obesity." *Am J Clin Nutr*, April 2004, 79(4): 537–43.

150. Gaby, A R. "Adverse effects of dietary fructose." *Altern Med Rev*, December 2005, 10(4): 294–306.

151. Basciano, Federico, and Adeli. "Fructose, insulin resistance, and metabolic dyslipidemia."

152. Gross, L S, Li, L, Ford, E S, and Liu S. "Increased consumption of refined carbohydrates and the epidemic of Type-2 diabetes in the United States: An ecologic assessment." *Am J Clin Nutr*, May 2004, 79(5): 774–79.

153. Beck-Nielsen, H, Pedersen, O, and Lindskov, H O. "Impaired cellular insulin binding and insulin sensitivity induced by high-fructose feeding in normal subjects." *Am J Clin Nutr*, February 1980, 33(2): 273–78.

154. Hsieh, P S, Tai, Y H, Loh, C H, Shih, K C, Cheng, W T, and Chu, C H. "Functional interaction of AT1 and AT2 receptors in fructose-induced insulin resistance and hypertension in rats." *Metabolism*, February 2005, 54(2): 157–64.

155. Avramoglu, R K, Qiu, W, and Adeli, K. "Mechanisms of metabolic dyslipidemia in insulin resistant states: Deregulation of hepatic and intestinal lipoprotein secretion." *Front Biosci*, January 1, 2003, 8: D464–d476.

156. Elliott, S S, Keim, N L, Stern, J S, Teff, K, and Havel, P J. "Fructose, weight gain, and the insulin resistance syndrome." *Am J Clin Nutr*, November 2002, 76(5): 911–22.

157. McPherson, J D, Shilton, B H, and Walton, D J. "Role of fructose in glycation and cross-linking of proteins." *Biochemistry*, March 22, 1988, 27(6): 1901–7.

158. Dunn, W, Xu, R, Wingard, D L, et al. "Suspected nonalcoholic fatty liver

disease and mortality risk in a population-based cohort study." *Am J Gastroenterol*, August 5, 2008.

159. Cousens, G. *Rainbow Green Live-Food Cuisine*. Berkeley, CA: North Atlantic Books, 2003, p. 117.

160. Taylor, F, Ward, K, Moore, T H M, Burke, M, Davey Smith, G, Casas, J-P, and Ebrahim, S. "Statins for the primary prevention of cardiovascular disease." *Cochrane Database of Systematic Reviews* 2011, 1, art. no.: CD004816, doi:10.1002/14651858.CD004816.pub4.

161. Ibid.

162. University of California San Diego. "Statin effects study." http://www.statineffects.com/info.

163. Westover, M B, Bianchi, M T, Eckman, M H, and Greenberg, S M. "Statin use following intracerebral hemorrhage—A decision analysis." *Arch Neurol*, 2011, 68(5): 573–79, doi:10.1001/archneurol.2010.356.

164. Alsheikh-Ali, A A, Maddukuri, P R, Han, H, et al. "Effect of the magnitude of lipid lowering on risk of elevated liver enzymes, rhabdomyolysis, and cancer." *Journal of the American College of Cardiology* 2007, 50: 409–18.

165. Rubinstein, J, Aloka, F, and Abela, G S. "Statin therapy decreases myocardial function as evaluated via strain imaging." *Clin Cardiol*, December 2009, 32(12): 684–89.

166. Hippisley-Cox, J, and Coupland, C. "Unintended effects of statins in men and women in England and Wales: Population based cohort study using the Q Research database." *BMJ*, May 20, 2010, 340: C2197, doi:10.1136/bmj.c2197.

167. Meilahn, E. "Low serum cholesterol hazardous to health?" *Circulation*. 1995, 92: 2365–66, doi:10.1161/01.CIR.92.9.2365.

168. Byrne, C D, and Wild, S H. "Increased risk of glucose intolerance and type 2 diabetes with statins." *BMJ*, August 8, 2011, 343: D5004. Medline 21824907.

169. Sukhija, R, Prayaga, S, Marashdeh, M, Bursac, Z, Kakar, P, Bansal, D, Sachdeva, R, Kesan, S, and Mehta, J. "Effect of statins on fasting plasma glucose in diabetic and nondiabetic patients." *Journal of Investigative Medicine*, March 2009, 57(3): 495–99, doi:10.231/JIM.0b013e318197ec8b.

170. Hodgson, J M, et al. "Coenzyme Q10 improves blood pressure and glycaemic control: A controlled trial in subjects with type 2 diabetes." *Eur J Clin Nutr*, 2002, 56: 1137–42.

171. Ravnskov, U. *The Cholesterol Myths: Exposing the Fallacy That*

Cholesterol and Saturated Fat Cause Heart Disease. Washington, DC: NewTrends Publishing, 2002.

172. Ibid.

173. Bazzano, L A, He, J, Odgen, L G, et al. "Dietary intake of folate and risk of stroke in U.S. men and women: NHANES I Epidemiologic Follow-up Study." *Stroke*, May 2002, 33(5): 1183–89.

174. Siri-Tarino, P W, Sun, Q, Hu, F B, and Krauss, R M. "Meta-analysis of prospective cohort studies evaluating the association of saturated fat with cardiovascular disease." *Am J Clin Nutr*, January 2010, ajcn.27725.

175. Krumholz, H M, et al. "Lack of association between cholesterol and coronary heart disease mortality and morbidity and all-cause mortality in person older than 70 years." *Journal of the American Medical Association*, 1994, 272: 1335–40.

176. Dagenais, G R et al. "Total and coronary heart disease mortality in relation to major risk factors: Quebec cardiovascular study." *Canadian Journal of Cardiology*, 1990, 6: 59–65.

177. Shanoff, H M, Little J A, Csima A. "Studies of male survivors of myocardial infarction: XII. Relation of serum lipids and lipoproteins to survival over a 10-year period." *Canadian Medical Association Journal*, 1970, 103: 927–931.

178. Jostein Holmen, Kristian Midthjell, Øystein Krüger, Arnulf Langhammer, Turid Lingaas Holmen, Grete H. Bratberg, Lars Vatten, and Per G. Lund-Larsen. "The Nord-Trøndelag Health Study 1995–97 (HUNT 2): Objectives, contents, methods and participation." *Norsk Epidemiologi* 2003, 13 (1): 19–32.

179. Evans, A, Tolonen, H, Hense, H-W, Ferrario, M, Sans, S, Kuulasmaa, K, for the WHO MONICA Project. "Trends in coronary risk factors in the WHO MONICA Project." *International Journal of Epidemiology*, 2001, 30: S35–S40.

180. Marmot, M G, Syme S L. "Acculturation and coronary heart disease in Japanese-Americans." *American Journal of Epidemiology*, 1976, 104: 225–247.

181. Howard B, Manson J, Stefanick M, et al. "Low-fat dietary pattern and weight change over 7 years: the Women's Health Initiative Dietary Modification Trial." *JAMA*, 2006, 295: 39–49.

182. Petursson, H, Sigurdsson, J A, Bengtsson, C, Nilsen, T I, and Getz, L. "Is the use of cholesterol in mortality risk algorithms in clinical guidelines valid? Ten years prospective data from the Norwegian HUNT 2 study." *J Eval Clin Pract*, September 25, 2011, doi:10.1111/j.1365-2753.2011.01767.x.

183. Ravnskov, U. *The Cholesterol Myths.*

184. Bishop J R. "Heart Attacks: A Test Collapses." *Wall Street Journal,* October 6, 1982.

185. Hooper, L, Summerbell, C D, Thompson, R, Sills, D, Roberts, F G, Moore, H, and Smith, G. "Reduced or modified dietary fat for preventing cardiovascular disease." *The Cochrane Collaboration,* July 6, 2011, doi:10.1002/14651858.CD002137.pub2.

186. Andrew Mente, PhD; Lawrence de Koning, MSc; Harry S. Shannon, PhD; Sonia S. Anand, MD, PhD. "A Systematic Review of the Evidence Supporting a Causal Link Between Dietary Factors and Coronary Heart Disease." *Arch Intern Med.,* 2009, 169(7): 659_669. doi: 10.1001/archinternmed.2009.38.

187. Fraser, G E, and Shavlik, D J. "Ten years of life: Is it a matter of choice?" *Arch Intern Med,* July 9, 2001, 161(13): 1645–52.

188. Colin A, Reggers J, Castronovo V, and Ansseau, M. "Encephale." *Lipids, depression and suicide.* January–February 2003, 29(1): 49–58.

189. Ruljančić, N, Malić, A, and Mihanović, M. "Serum cholesterol concentration in psychiatric patients." *Biochemia Medica* 2007, 17(2): 197–202.

190. Ellison, L F, and Morrison, H I. "Low serum cholesterol concentration and risk of suicide." *Epidemiology,* March 2001, 12(2): 168–72.

191. Golier, J A, Marzuk, P M, Leon, A C, Weiner, C, and Tardiff, K. "Low serum cholesterol level and attempted suicide." *Am J Psychiatry,* March 1995, 152(3): 419–23.

192. Deans, E. "Low cholesterol and suicide: Your brain needs cholesterol—don't go too low." *Evolutionary Psychiatry,* March 21, 2011. http://www.psychologytoday.com/blog/evolutionary-psychiatry/201103/low-cholesterol-and-suicide.

193. Shrivastava, S, Pucadyil, T J, Paila, Y D, Ganguly, S, and Chattopadhyay, A. "Chronic cholesterol depletion using statin impairs the function and dynamics of human serotonin receptors." *Biochemistry,* 2010, 49(26): 5426–35.

194. Mario Merialdi, MD, and Jeffrey C. Murray, MD. "The Changing Face of Preterm Labor." *Pediatrics,* October 1, 2007.

195. Starling, S. "Omega-3 deficiency causes 96, 000 U.S. deaths per year, say researchers." *NutraIngredients,* June 26, 2009.

196. Macchia, A, Monte, S, Pellegrini, F, et al. "Omega-3 fatty acid supplementation reduces one-year risk of atrial fibrillation in patients hospitalized with myocardial infarction." *Eur J Clin Pharmacol,* June 2008, 64(6): 627–34.

197. Golding, J, Steer, C, Emmett, P, et al. "High levels of depressive symptoms in pregnancy with low omega-3 fatty acid intake from fish." *Epidemiology*, July 2009, 20(4): 598–603.

198. Lewis, M D, Hibbeln, J R, Johnson, J E, Lin, Y H, Hyun, D Y, and Loewke, J D. "Suicide deaths of active-duty U.S. military and omega-3 fatty-acid status: A case-control comparison." *J Clin Psychiatry* 2011, 72(12): 1585–90.

199. Garland, M R, and Hallahan, B. "Essential fatty acids and their role in conditions characterized by impulsivity." *Int Rev Psychiatry*, April 2006, 18(2): 99–105.

200. Ibid.

201. Bousquet, M, Saint-Pierre, M, Julien, C, Salem, N, Cicchetti, F, and Calon, F. "Beneficial effects of dietary omega-3 polyunsaturated fatty acid on toxin-induced neuronal degeneration in an animal model of Parkinson's disease." *The FASEB Journal*, 2007, 22 (4): 1213–25.

202. Pottala, J V, Garg, S, Cohen, B E, Whooley, M A, and Harris, W S. "Blood eicosapentaenoic and docosahexaenoic acids predict all-cause mortality in patients with stable coronary heart disease: The Heart and Soul Study." *Circ Cardiovasc Qual Outcomes*, July 2010, 3(4): 406–12.

203. Masterton, G S, Plevris, J N, and Hayes, P C. "Review article: Omega-3 fatty acids—a promising novel therapy for non-alcoholic fatty liver disease." *Aliment Pharmacol Ther*, April 2010, 31(7): 679–92.

204. Gopinath, B, Harris, D C, Flood, V M, Burlutsky, G, and Mitchell, P. "Consumption of long-chain n-3 PUFA, alpha-linolenic acid and fish is associated with the prevalence of chronic kidney disease." *Br J Nutr*, May 2011, 105(9): 1361–68.

205. McNamara, R K, Jandacek, R, Rider, T, et al. "Deficits in docosahexaenoic acid and associated elevations in the metabolism of arachidonic acid and saturated fatty acids in the postmortem orbitofrontal cortex of patients with bipolar disorder." *Psychiatry Res*. Sep 30, 2008, 160(3): 285–99.

206. Sublette, M E, Hibbeln, J R, Galfalvy, H, et al. "Omega-3 polyunsaturated essential fatty acid status as a predictor of future suicide risk." *Am J Psychiatry*. 2006, 163(6): 1100–1102.

207. De Caterina, R, Madonna, R, Zucchi, R, and La Rovere, M T "Antiarrhythmic effects of omega-3 fatty acids: From epidemiology to bedside." *American Heart Journal*, 146(3): 420–30.

208. Din, J N, Newby, D E, and Flapan, A D. "Fish oil and heart disease." *British Medical Journal*, January 3, 2004, 328: 30–35.

209. Kabir, M, Skurnik, G, Naour, N, et al. "Treatment for 2 mo with n 3 polyunsaturated fatty acids reduces adiposity and some atherogenic factors but does not improve insulin sensitivity in women with Type-2 diabetes: A randomized controlled study." *Am J Clin Nutr*, December 2007, 86(6): 1670–79.

210. Chin, J P, and Dart, A M. "How do fish oils affect vascular function?" *Clin Exp Pharmacol Physiol*, 1995, 22: 71–81.

211. Sapieha, P, Stahl, A, Chen, J, Seaward, M R, Willett, K L, Krah, N M, Dennison, R J, Connor, K M, Aderman, C M, Liclican, E, Carughi, A, Perelman, D, Kanaoka, Y, SanGiovanni, J P, Gronert, K, and Smith, L E H. "5-lipoxygenase metabolite 4-HDHA is a mediator of the antiangiogenic effect of –3 polyunsaturated fatty acids." *Science Translational Medicine*, 2011, 3(69): 69ra12, doi:10.1126/scitranslmed.3001571.

212. Mori, T A, Beilin, L J, Burke, V, et al. "Interactions between dietary fat, fish, and fish oils and their effects on platelet function in men at risk of cardiovascular disease." *Arterioscler Thromb Vasc Biol*, 1997, 17: 279–86.

213. Macchia, A, Monte, S, Pellegrini, F, et al. "Omega-3 fatty acid supplementation."

214. Gleijnse, J M, Giltay, E J, Grobbee, D E, Donders, A R, and Kok, F J. "Blood pressure response to fish oil supplementation: Metaregression analysis of randomized trials." *J Hypertens*, August 2002, 20(8): 1493–99.

215. Oya, J, Nakagami, T, Sasaki, S, et al. "Intake of n-3 polyunsaturated fatty acids and non-alcoholic fatty liver disease: A cross-sectional study in Japanese men and women." *Dur J Clin Nutr*, October 2010, 64(10): 1179–85.

216. Gopinath, Harris, Flood, et al. "Consumption of long-chain n-3 PUFA, alpha-linolenic acid and fish."

217. Mercola, J. *Take Control of Your Health: Your Proven Guide to Peak Wellness and Ideal Weight.* Hoffman Estates, IL: Mercola.com, 2007.

218. Rosedale, R. *The Rosedale Diet.* New York, NY: William Morrow, 2004.

219. Aune, D, Ursin, G, and Veierod, M B. "Meat consumption and the risk of Type-2 diabetes: A systematic review and meta-analysis of cohort studies." *Diabetologia*, 2009, 52: 2277–87, doi 10.1007 /s00125-009-1481-x.

220. Fung, T T, Schulze, M, Manson, J E, Willett, W C, and Hu, F B. "Dietary patterns, meat intake, and the risk of Type-2 diabetes in women." *Arch Intern Med*, 2004, 164: 2235–40.

221. Schulze, M B, Manson, J E, Willett, W C, and Hu, F B. "Processed meat

intake and incidence of Type-2 diabetes in younger and middle-aged women." *Diabetologia*, 2003, 46: 1465–73.

222. Song, Y, Manson, J E, Buring, J E, and Liu, S. "A prospective study of red meat consumption and Type-2 diabetes in middle-aged and elderly women: The women's health study." *Diabetes Care*, 2004, 27: 2108–15.

223. van Dam, R M, Willett, W C, Rimm, E B, Stampfer, M J, and Hu, F B. "Dietary fat and meat intake in relation to risk of Type-2 diabetes in men." *Diabetes Care*, 2002, 25: 417–24.

224. Villegas, R, Shu, X O, Gao, Y T, et al. "The association of meat intake and the risk of Type-2 diabetes may be modified by body weight." *Int J Med Sci*, 2006, 3: 152–59.

225. Simmons, R K, Harding, A H, Wareham, N J, and Griffin, S J. "Do simple questions about diet and physical activity help to identify those at risk of Type-2 diabetes?" *Diabet Med*, 2007, 24: 830–35.

226. Vang, A, Singh, P N, Lee, J W, Haddad, E H, and Brinegar, C H. "Meats, processed meats, obesity, weight gain and occurrence of diabetes among adults: Findings from adventist health studies." *Ann Nutr Metab*, 2008, 52: 96–104.

227. Lee, D H, Folsom, A R, and Jacobs, D R. "Dietary iron intake and Type-2 diabetes incidence in postmenopausal women: The Iowa Women's Health Study." *Diabetologia*, 2004, 47: 185–94.

228. Schulze, M B, Hoffmann, D, Boeing, H, et al. "An accurate risk score based on anthropometric, dietary, and lifestyle factors to predict the development of Type-2 diabetes," *Diabetes Care*, 2007, 30: 510–15.

229. Hirayama, T. *Life-Style and Mortality: A Large-Scale Census-Based Cohort Study in Japan.* Basel, Switzerland: Karger, 1990.

230. Montonen, J, Jarvinen, R, Heliovaara, M, Reunanen, A, Aromaa, A, and Knekt, P. "Food consumption and the incidence of type II diabetes mellitus." *Eur J Clin Nutr*, 2005, 59: 441–48.

231. Lenka, J Z. "Living examples survey: An investigation of people who have eaten a raw foods diet for over two years." Master of arts in live food nutrition thesis, Dr. Cousens' Culture of Life Institute, February 2006.

232. Mericq, V, Piccardo, C, Cai, W, Chen, X, Zhu, L, Striker, G E, Vlassara, H, and Uribarri, J. "Maternally transmitted and food-derived glycotoxins: A factor preconditioning the young to diabetes?" *Diabetes Care*, October 2010, 33(10): 2232–37.

233. Uribarri, J, Cai, W, Ramdas, M, Goodman, S, Pyzik, R, Chen, X, Zhu, L, Striker, G E, and Vlassara, H. "Restriction of advanced glycation

end products improves insulin resistance in human Type-2 diabetes: Potential role of AGER1 and SIRT1." *Diabetes Care*, 2011, 34(7): 1610, doi:10.2337/dc11-0091.

234. Meier, J J, Bhushan, A, Butler, A E, Rizza, R A, and Butler, P C. "Sustained beta cell apoptosis in patients with long-standing Type-1 diabetes: Indirect evidence for islet regeneration?" *Diabetologia*, 48(11): 2221–28, doi:10.1007/s00125-005-1949-2.

235. Ibid.

236. Bonner-Weir, S, Li, W-C, Ouziel-Yahalom, L, Guo, L, Weir, G C, and Sharma, A. "Cell growth and regeneration: Replication is only part of the story." *Diabetes*, October 2010, 59.

237. Warren, S, and Root, H F. "The pathology of diabetes, with special reference to pancreatic regeneration." *The American Journal of Pathology*, 1925, 1(4): 415–30.

238. Gardner, C D, Kiazand, A, Alhassan, S, Kim, S, Stafford, R S, Balise, R R, Kraemer, H C, and King, A C. "Comparison of the Atkins, Zone, Ornish, and LEARN diets for change in weight and related risk factors among overweight premenopausal women: The A to Z Weight Loss Study: A Randomized Trial." *JAMA*, 2007, 297(9): 969–77, doi:10.1001/jama.297.9.969.

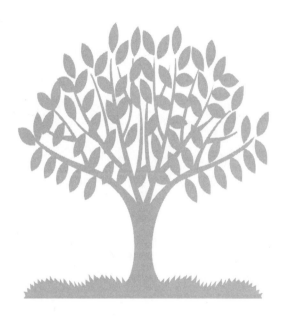

CHAPTER 6

Happy Continuation:
Living in the Culture of Life

Loving yourself enough to continually heal yourself into your highest octave of holistic health is the life- and spirit-affirming way of the Culture of Life. Breaking the four-minute mile of diabetes by reversing diabetes completely will require continued positive healing action at home after the Dr. Cousens's Diabetes Recovery Program—A Holistic Approach. This is what everyone with or without diabetes benefits from to maintain optimal health on every level. By the time your blood sugar has reached nondiabetic levels, your cholesterol, triglycerides, and C-reactive protein levels most likely will have normalized. Your weight, depending on where you started, may not yet be optimal. Returning home, you will be taking with you the gift of fearlessness and an enthusiastic and deep knowing that you have the ability to succeed in the next and perhaps most crucial step in this healing process of becoming a healthy human being—stabilizing in the antidiabetogenic, pro-Culture of Life diet and lifestyle. You recognize that life does not have to be lived in a diabetogenic wasteland, that complications can be reversed, and that you can achieve a level of health that is well beyond what you have been experiencing for yourself.

For all of us, as we move into a healthy physiology, this positive state has an ascending effect on the higher levels of our being, right up through our mind, emotions, and spirit. Healing from years of diabetes and complications means that something that has taken up such a large space in our lives is now gone. As your own life potential opens up, others will begin to see you as the vibrant example of humanity you have become. Any attachment one had to diabetes, and the diet and lifestyle of the Culture of Death that created it, is in the process of dissolution and transformation.

After the 21-day program, living in a protected environment in the shade of the Tree of Life, you return home to familiar surroundings, and the next phase of your sustained healing begins. What you are about to learn is how to live in the Culture of Life in your old world. An immediate challenge is how to establish a physiology (cellular memory) that does not continue to ask for the familiar yet diabetogenic foods of the old culture that helped create the chronic diabetes degenerative syndrome (CDDS) and ultimately full-blown diabetes. One will begin to learn how to respond to the compliments, questions, skepticism, and enthusiasm of friends and coworkers. It is good to allow time for the mind to adapt to your new healthy diet of plant-source, nutrient-dense foods. You will naturally become more conscious of how living in the Culture of Life illuminates every aspect of your new life.

Sustainable Diet, or a Fad?

> All of this is much easier to implement than it seems. The biggest hurdle is not the physiological but psychological aspects. As Walter Bagehot once remarked, "The pain of a new idea is one of the greatest pains in human nature. . . . Your favorite notions may be wrong, your firmest beliefs ill founded." And your favorite foods may be the root cause of your greatest pains! It's a fact of life that people find it easier to believe a lie they've heard a thousand times than a fact they've never heard before.
>
> Daniel P. Reid, *The Tao of Sex, Health, and Longevity*

The Dr. Cousens's organic, 80–100 percent raw, plant-source-only, holistic lifestyle has been our cultural Biblical foundation for approximately 5,700 years and is clearly stated in Genesis 1:29 and Deuteronomy 7:15. The history of eating a diet of plant foods, abstaining from meat eating, fasting and drinking plant juices, and using herbs to heal goes back possibly further than recorded history itself. Hippocrates, the father of medicine (460–357 BC) said, "He who does not know food, how can he understand the diseases of man?" *The Ethics of Diet* by Howard Williams outlines an entire recorded history of abstaining from flesh eating and returning to a natural diet, citing more than 50 major Western thinkers such as Hesiod (eighth century BC), Pythagoras (570–470 BC), Plato, Ovid, Seneca, Plutarch, Thomas More, Voltaire, Rousseau, Leonardo da Vinci, Schopenhauer, Dr. Albert Schweitzer, and Albert Einstein. A plant-source-only diet is advocated by most every major world religious tradition, as illustrated in *Food for the Gods* by Rynn Berry. This reality is also concisely stated in the chapter "Vegetarianism in the World's Religions" in my book *Conscious Eating* and also in *Spiritual Nutrition*, two books containing arguably the best scientifically documented case for a lifelong plant-source-only diet of live foods. The reader has seen evidence that a processed diet, high in white sugar and flour, is a diabetogenic diet. The Culture of Death way of eating and living creates far more suffering and sickness worldwide than just diabetes. It also bears repeating that the Dr. Cousens's antidiabetogenic cuisine, adopted globally as our true potential, would make enough food available for all the people of the world to be fed at least seven times over at current agricultural production levels. Again, this is no fad; it is rooted deeply in our cultural, spiritual, and genetic heritage and is truly a diet and lifestyle that significantly meet the needs of our times, individually and collectively.

With approximately one out of two or three children born today in the United States projected to develop Type-2 diabetes and the spiraling worldwide pandemic threatening the economies of nations, it is important to have simple and serious solutions that are not simply palliative but do the job effectively. As has been made abundantly clear, the Culture of Death diet and lifestyle are the underlying causes of Type-2 diabetes, which comprises 95 percent of all diabetes. I offer a wise, historically valid, simple, and practical cuisine and lifestyle solution to this nightmare of the CDDS and full diabetes pandemic. It might appear an extreme antidote, but in reality, the conditions that have created diabetes are themselves ridiculously extreme. At the turn of the 1900s, people ate about 15 pounds of sugar per year; now we eat up to 150 pounds per year. It is so extreme that eating just 15 pounds per year, which is relatively normal, may itself seem radical. It is important to see clearly through the conventional denial thinking with such ineffective approaches as "moderation"—a term itself that gives an illusion of wisdom—in your decision to reverse diabetes. Consumption of 150 pounds of sugar per year (approximately 52 teaspoons per day) is an active Crime Against Wisdom.

Moderation Kills!

> If your friend had been a smoker all of his or her life and looked to you for advice, would you tell them to cut down to only two cigarettes a day, or would you tell them to quit smoking all together? It's in this way that I'm telling you that moderation, even with the best intentions, sometimes makes it more difficult to succeed.
>
> **T. Colin Campbell,** *The China Study*

> Moderation? It's mediocrity, fear, and confusion in disguise. It's the devil's reasonable deception. It's the wobbling compromise that makes no one happy. Moderation is for the bland, the apologetic, for the fence sitters of the world afraid to take a stand to live or die. Moderation is lukewarm tea, the devil's own brew!
>
> **Dan Millman,** *The Way of the Peaceful Warrior*

CDDS and diabetes are benign diseases and are therefore reversible, via a Culture of Life cuisine and lifestyle. For many who are new to eating plant-source foods, this diet can seem unusual until one adjusts to it. As one moves toward an organic, live-food diet, one also moves from low-nutrient to high-nutrient-dense foods; from the suffering of disease symptoms to their dissolution; from dead food to vibrant, living food; from maximum to minimum health care costs; from below-average to above-average life-span; from millions dying of starvation to almost none; from a translative diet of eating for comfort alone to a transformative diet of eating as a means and support for personal growth and spiritual evolution. Research and cultural data worldwide show that moving to a plant-source diet means the enhanced prevention and eventual elimination of obesity, heart disease, diabetes, arthritis, hypertension, depression, and constipation, to name a few. It is a shift from an egocentric way of eating for oneself to a world-centric way of being as an act of love for all plants, animals, and people, as well as oneself.

When it comes to prevention of disease, and particularly reversal of diabetes, the conventional understanding of moderation, with its attractive appearance of intelligent balance, is anything but prudence and wisdom. A strong intention and determination to completely reverse the diabetic physiology and lifestyle back to a nondiabetic and healthy one is a key component.

Once you recognize that Type-2 diabetes, properly addressed, can be a benign disease and that CDDS and even full-blown diabetes, with all its complications, need not exist and can be reversed, a sense of determination will permeate your being, driving you toward a realization of a healthy physiology and lifestyle that is beyond what you may have ever imagined. This journey is an inner revolution toward loving yourself enough to heal yourself. You may pass through three typical internal realizations and useful affirmations as you make this life-saving transition:

1. I am not eating my standard, comfort-zone diet anymore, but I am not deprived.
2. I feel good, have more energy, and my fasting blood sugar (FBS) is normal. I now eat at least 80 percent live, organic, moderate-low carbohydrate, plant-source-only cuisine and live a holistic lifestyle and love the transition.
3. I eat and live this wonderful way and enjoy the pleasure of being healthy and free from diabetes and enjoy an abundance of health and spiritual well-being.

At first, you may perceive the changes in your life as deprivation, because the Culture of Death diabetogenic foods and lifestyle choices available are ubiquitous. The Culture of Death version of modern living will be a constant reminder to you that you have left the conventional paradigm of the Culture of Death. Your friends and family may also be an outward sign that you are in another mode of existence, and either applaud you, counsel you, or be skeptical and defensively in denial. The Roman stoic Lucius Seneca wrote in his essay, "On the Happy Life," "For it is dangerous to attach oneself to the crowd in front, and so long as each one of us is more willing to trust another than to judge for himself, we never show any judgment in the matter of living, but always a blind trust, and a mistake that has been passed on from hand to hand finally involves us and works our destruction. It is the example of other people that is our undoing; let us merely separate ourselves from the crowd, and we shall be made whole."

Seneca was describing the importance of recognizing the power of the shadow of the Culture of Death, how one may become entrapped in it and how to disentangle from it. One's healthy and happy life depends on understanding this. With success, you naturally will be able to inspire others to also succeed in their healing. Although some friends may become distant, many new friends will come who see your growing light and want to be around it.

Living in the Culture of Life requires a revolution involving an internal and external geographical reorientation. We have existed in a poor food environment for so many years and our choices in it have been making us sick and squandering our potential. This book is a doorway, not only to heal diabetes, but also to reclaim excellent health for oneself, regardless of the environment, the actions of others, or one's past history.

Externally, it includes looking at shifting away from conventional restaurants and out of the center aisles of the grocery store with its processed, adulterated foods and into the farmer's markets, the co-ops, and the produce section of the grocery store. As pointed out in Chapter 2, buying cheap, calorie-rich, nutrient-poor processed foods in the center aisles of the grocery store seems associated with the diabetogenic process. As you recall, Drewnowski found that a dollar could buy 1,200 calories of cookies or potato chips but only 250 calories of carrots; that his dollar bought 875 calories of soda but only 170 calories of orange juice.[1] According to the USDA Economic Research Service, between 1982 and 1997, the cost increases for these (diabetogenic) foods were as follows: dairy products, 47 percent; fats and oils, 47 percent; meat, poultry, and fish, 49 percent; and sugar and sweets, 52 percent. The cost increase for your Culture of Life healthy, antidiabetogenic foods went up a staggering 93 percent, making eating a healthy diet the most costly thing at the register—but not in terms of your health, which is the main point. This economic reality of high-priced fresh foods is going to encourage you to frequent farmer's markets, co-ops, and locally grown food suppliers, where the costs are much lower for higher-quality foods because the prices are not controlled by agribusiness, which tends to organize the commercial price structures to favor Culture of Death high-calorie, diabetogenic junk foods.

Buying local food straight from the farmer puts you in closer touch with the origin of the food, cuts a significant portion of the time and money spent transporting and "selling" the food, saves you money, and places more dollars in the pocket of those who produce your food. Eating in the Culture of Life is about more than feeling good because of the food itself, but involves the impact of your dietary choices on supporting the economic, agricultural, ecological, political, social, cultural, and spiritual realities of your community, your nation, and even the world.

This external shift creates a change internally, as we are reorienting ourselves to who we really are, away from what we have been told we are. The following quotes come from an agenda of economics, not conscious health concerns. Junk food, empty calories, low nutrient density, high-sugar content, and low-fiber foods can never be considered healthy by the wildest stretch of the imagination. It is time we stop listening to the economic propaganda of the Culture of Death that leads the American Diabetes Association (ADA) and conventional medicine to incorrectly label diabetes as incurable:

> It is the position of the American Dietetic Association that all foods can fit into a healthful eating style.
>
> **ADA position statement**

All foods and beverages can fit into a healthy diet.
National Soft Drink Association

Policies that declare foods "good" or "bad" are counterproductive.
Grocery Manufacturers of America[2]

Despite the myths we have been told and sold, we are not by genetic constitution Mars-Bar eaters, Super-Big-Gulp drinkers, or Big-Mac snackers, nor do we suffer from a deficiency of these junk foods. None of us is suffering from a deficiency of Red Dye #40, Blue Lake #5, disodium inosinate, MSG, aspartame, or any of the other excitotoxins that have been deliberately placed in our foods to seduce and addict us for profit. For millions of years we have been physiologically, biochemically, and genetically designed to eat a diet of organic living plant foods. The overwhelming medical, sociological, and historical data corroborate this. Food is a fundamental way that we interface with our home, the living planet, with our cultural ancestry (which existed with rare mention of diabetes), and is a most important and subtle way we acknowledge an association or dissociation with who we truly are.

Living in the Culture of Life is an invitation to go on a journey to find ourselves and our God-given right to vibrant, durable health. Committing to a plant-source-only diet because we are determined to remove the causes of diabetes and ill health is an act of love and consciousness. In this liberating and transformative process, we naturally move beyond the false identity that has been given us by advertising, including the so-called health education we have received in our schools that has been primarily financed by the dairy and meat industries so we will buy their products. Please know that this "education" we take as the truth is directly contrary to our 3.2 million years of history of the human diet (until 10,000 years ago), the message of the Bible in Genesis 1:29, and teachings through the ages. All these and many modern sources that are not motivated by profit say the same thing: a plant-source-only diet is the healthiest and most natural diet for human beings. A plant-source diet helps us reconnect with our fundamental nature and helps heal the ecology of the planet, because it does not create a hoarding of resources, and it frees up the resources to feed everyone on the planet seven times over. In order to do this, we need the means, motivation, and support necessary to reclaim our most basic right of health and well-being.

Part of the Diabetes Recovery Program Includes Green Juice Fasting

Five effects of green juice fasting are: cleansing, rebuilding, rehydrating, alkalizing, and resetting and reestablishing your holy rhythm (including the genetic and epigenetic programs) by reconnecting to your soul and its purpose.

Two of the Seven Stages of Disease associated with CDDS and diabetes are toxemia and inflammation. Green juice fasting helps reverse the toxemia (including sugar toxicity) and inflammation. It can also help reverse hypoglycemia. It most rapidly upgrades the toxic epigenetic program.

Cleanse

Cleansing is associated with weight reduction, but toxicity exists on many physical levels as well as emotional, mental, and spiritual levels. There is heavy-metal toxicity; uneliminated waste matter in our blood, lymph, cells, intestinal tract, and colon; toxic buildup in our organs, such as arterial plaque in our heart, calcifications in our kidneys, and stones in our liver and gallbladder; and many of us have edema, or excess water weight from the body trying to hold toxins in solution to protect the tissues. While this is not explicitly a weight loss program, juice fasting will accelerate your coming back in a natural way to a normal weight and eliminate one of the major cofactors in diabetes, obesity.

Supporting the organs of elimination is a key part of the detoxification process. There is waste matter coming forth from all over the body, and fasting shows them the exit door in a timely manner. Otherwise one eventually gets a buildup of toxins leading to cleansing reactions and healing crises, which appear as headaches, muscle or joint pain, skin eruptions, emotional imbalance, fever, and so on. Support of the organs of elimination (lymph, blood, skin, liver, kidney, tongue, lungs, and bowel) is part of the green juice fasting protocol and helps to move toxins out quickly while minimizing or avoiding any healing crises.

Colon hygiene (either through enemas or colonics) is essential for fasting. Most of the toxins you release are going to come through your bowel. I recommend doing an enema or colonic each day of fasting. Enema kits are available at most drug stores; I suggest you purchase one that is multiuse, not the single-use variety that does not hold enough liquid, is inefficient, and wasteful in its throw-away design. Colonics may be of benefit as well, as a colonic employs a deeper cleansing action with more water. Please consult your health professional about the appropriateness of this excellent method for moving out old matter, particularly if you are overweight and have been constipated for many years. Generally I do not recommend colonics regularly outside of fasting, as they weaken the downward eliminative energy.

Skin brushing is also an effective method of cleansing. The skin is one of the five main elimination channels of the body, throwing off up to one pound of toxic material each day in the form of perspiration and dead skin. The skin has been called the third kidney because of its ability to rid the body of toxic waste material. Skin brushing moves lymphatic fluid under the skin. This involves using a natural-bristle brush with a long handle. The whole body (except the face) should be brushed in a circular motion toward the heart before your morning shower. It takes two to three minutes to do this. At first, you will see something powdery coming off your skin as you brush. According to Dr. Bernard Jensen, "these are crystals of uric acid and other dried waste products that came out with the perspiration." Jensen continues:

> Always brush the skin when it is dry, and never expose the brush to
> water. Although the bristles may seem a bit stiff at first, this is because
> the brush is new and your skin is not yet used to the brushing. If you
> find the brush is too stiff, you may, just once, hold the bristles in hot

water for no longer than one minute and no deeper than one-half inch. This will soften the bristles a little. However, it will not be long before you desire a stiffer brush! Your skin will love you for brushing it regularly, and you will love the way your skin feels and looks, too.[3]

The brushing motion is circular and from the feet and hands toward the heart. The skin needs to be brushed with enough pressure to create a comfortable pink color to the skin.

A hot/cool treatment is also highly effective. This is easy and goes back for thousands of years. If you have ever been to a Japanese spa or to a sauna, you will experience the use of hot and cold to invigorate and help the body to cleanse. What you are achieving with the transition from hot to cold is a movement of lymphatic fluid and blood to the surface of the skin with heat, then toward the center of the body with cold, back again to the surface with heat, and so on. A way to do this at home is in the shower. Stand in the hot water for five to eight minutes until you are nice and warm and have rinsed off. Then begin to crank the water back toward cool for about one minute, then to hot for one minute, and so forth, three to seven times, ending on cool water. This will invigorate you first thing in the morning and do wonders for helping the lymphatic fluid in your body to move, thus improving the elimination of old wastes from your system.

Detox supplements include zeolite, or natural cellular defense (discussed in Chapter 4), for the removal of heavy metals and environmental toxins, Tachyon Fasting Elixir, for a liver-gallbladder and kidney cleanse and reenergizing, and Rad Neutral for our excessive radiation exposure, post-Fukushima.

Lastly, exercising is a very important part of the cleansing process. The benefits of moderate exercise for diabetics are well known. During your green juice fast, I suggest a light yoga routine. This means simple stretches just to loosen up and move your body. Then add walking longer distances: up to 30 minutes each day. When the body is in a state of cleansing, it is best to conserve most of your energy to build the vital force in order to stimulate cellular detox, but moderate exercise that moves the lymph and blood and leaves the body stimulated but not exhausted is excellent. Don't overtax your body with activity.

Rebuild

Our body replaces its tissues and cells every one to seven years. This wide range of time depends on physiology and varies with the sources we read.

Muscles get replaced every 6 months to 3 years. The pancreas replaces every 5 to 12 months. The liver replaces every 3 months. Our bones replace every 8 months to 4 years. Red blood cells replace every 90 to 120 days. The intestinal lining replaces every 5 to 30 days. One has the opportunity to completely rebuild the physical structure to its highest genetic potential. A healthy body helps support your optimal emotional balance, highest intelligence, and increased spiritual awareness. I recommend 7–10 days of green juice fasting at least two times yearly to detox and cleanse from the great increase in environmental toxin exposure we face today.

Rehydrate

The human adult body is approximately two-thirds water and 50–70 percent of our body weight. In utero, the fetus body is 90 percent water and an infant's body is 75–80 percent water. If we don't hydrate appropriately, our water content may drop as low as 50 percent with age. Water is one of the main components of other body tissues and cells: fat is 20 percent water, blood is 80 percent water, bone is 25 percent, kidneys are 80 percent, the liver is 70 percent, muscles are 75 percent, the skin is 70 percent, and the brain is 85 percent. Unfortunately, many people are dehydrated. This is very important when you realize that 85 percent of the brain is water, and when the brain starts to dehydrate, the neurons dehydrate and shrink. This is potentially a significant contributor to senility.

Water acts as a universal solvent and antioxidant, and that is partly how it produces life on the planet. Water's ability to act as a solvent is what makes nutrition work for all living substances. Plants absorb nutrients when they are watered, just like water dissolves nutrients so they can enter our bloodstream. This is basic information, but it becomes clearer, as research has shown, that water acts as a medium that transfers and relays the tiny frequencies of information of DNA from one cell to another. If our water is polluted, meaning that what is entering our body is polluted with a set of negative frequencies such as in pesticides and herbicides, the water can't effectively relay accurate intracellular and extracellular information. If I am consuming water that is contaminated, it not only brings in poisons but it blocks adequate frequency information extracellularly and intracellularly to and from the DNA.

Water, acting as the solvent, has an electrical and mineral content that helps to regulate all the functions in the body. This is disrupted by dehydration and toxic wastes, which block the information transfer. This disturbance causes a distinct loss of electrical flow and breakdown of the cellular reactions. Dehydration also creates a buildup of extracellular acidity and toxemia, which greatly impairs the electrical energy differentiation between the cells. Because of this, it disorders the intra- and extracellular gradient. Toxemia and extracellular acidity leads to oxygen starvation, damages the DNA, and accelerates aging. It increases free-radical damage and the extracellular acidity blocks the flow of hydrogen into the cells.

It is important to understand what we call the symptoms of dehydration. One is dyspepsia, or stomach pain. This results because the cells in the lining of the stomach need to be hydrated and flushed between meals to get rid of acids and to develop a certain level of alkalinity. When we are dehydrated, or we don't drink before meals, we actually cause a thinning of the stomach cell membrane buffer zone, and it does not adequately protect our stomachs from the acidity that is naturally secreted. Another symptom of dehydration is rheumatoid pain, or arthritic pain, which has to do with any sort of joint pain because the joints are lubricated by water. The water creates a small film of water that helps lubricate the interface of the joint. With dehydration, this lubricating film of water evaporates and the joints rub right on each other. Back pain, particularly lower back pain, and sciatica are often the result of the intervertebral discs becoming dehydrated. These discs normally create a space cushion between the vertebrae by virtue of how much water they can hold. When the discs are dehydrated, 75 percent of the upper body weight that they cushion against begins to bear down on the intervertebral spaces and put pressure on the intervertebral nerves. This often causes muscle spasms. Usually a few days after we rehydrate, the pressure on the nerves begins to alleviate. Relief from sciatic pain, in fact, may happen within an hour of rehydrating. Heart pain, or angina, is another symptom. When the body is dehydrated, the blood flow to the heart is reduced. Headaches, from toxic buildup and contracted blood vessels, are another symptom, along with dry tongue and constipation. One of the main causes of death in airplanes is dehydration, which may cause clots in the legs, which then can migrate to the lungs as pulmonary embolisms.

It is estimated by some scientific sources that 75 percent of Americans are chronically dehydrated. In 37 percent of Americans, the thirst mechanism is so weak from the dehydration that it is mistaken for hunger. One of the best ways to lose weight is to drink water when you are hungry. One glass of water at bedtime can shut down midnight hunger pangs for close to 100 percent of dieters. This both treats the dehydration and helps to alleviate the cause of excess appetite, or mistaking the thirst mechanism for hunger. The disruption of the metabolic system in the body is so significant when we become dehydrated that even with mild dehydration, the metabolism will slow down as much as 3 percent. Dehydration is probably the number one trigger of fatigue in the daytime. A 2 percent drop in body water can so significantly dehydrate the neurons and the passage of neurotransmitters in brain function that we can become fuzzy headed, develop short-term memory difficulties, have trouble with basic math, and lose focus on the computer screen. This is with only a 2 percent drop. A glass of water can significantly reverse some of the process of dehydration. A study at the University of Washington showed that drinking five glasses of water a day decreases the risk of colon cancer by 35 percent, the risk of breast cancer by 79 percent, and the risk of bladder cancer by 50 percent. This is a significant statement about the importance of water. Dehydration is something that is more likely to happen with age if we are not paying attention, so one of the main important antiaging treatments is drinking adequate water. A good sign of adequate hydration is urinating every one to two hours during the day.

Alkalize

This is a central healing principle. Acidity, as in diabetes, brings illness, and alkalinity brings health. We are constantly generating acidic waste products of metabolism that must be neutralized or excreted in some way if life is to be possible. Humans, therefore, need a constant supply of alkaline food to neutralize this ongoing acid generation. Our very life and health depend on the body's physiological power to maintain the stability of blood pH at approximately 7.46, which is also optimal for mental wellness, through a process called homeostasis. At this slightly alkaline pH, the chemical processes of the body function most efficiently and all waste products are more easily eliminated.

The normal pH for all the tissues and fluids in the body, except the stomach, is alkaline. For example, the digestive secretions from the liver and liver bile range between 7.1 and 8.5. Bile from the gall-bladder ranges from 5.0 to 7.7. If any of these pH systems are not at the optimal pH range, the digestive and metabolic enzymes in those areas and organs will function suboptimally and we will suffer from decreased health. With the exception of the blood, all these systems have a wide range of pH, in part so they can shift pH to maintain a balance of the blood pH. In my 40 years of experience, the healthiest blood pH is between the narrow range of 7.42 and 7.50. It is in this range that the cells operate most efficiently, especially for the brain cells. Being too alkaline can throw off body and brain function as much as being too acidic can. I focus on acidity because most people are too acidic in their blood, but we need to be mindful of both directions. The optimal urine pH for the first urine of the morning (which is the most accurate) is 6.4 to 7.2. However, if too much acidic food is eaten and the body, blood, and urine become acidic instead of alkaline, then the spleen, liver, heart, and kidneys, which are the blood-purifying organs, become overworked and ultimately weakened and susceptible to disease. Then the waste poisons can no longer be properly eliminated and instead collect in the joints, causing arthritis and/or gout. Or they seek elimination through the skin, causing eczema, acne, sores, and boils. The condition of acidity thus may be a contributing factor to many different syndromes, including piles, cancer, kidney and liver trouble, gallstones and gall bladder infections, impotency, high blood pressure and heart disease, strokes, asthma, and allergies. If the morning urine is consistently above 7.2, it is suggestive that the blood is too alkaline. Typical symptoms of excess alkalinity are muscle spasms, cramps, hyperreactivity, spaciness, a sense of ungroundedness, and mental imbalance.

The Culture of Death diet and lifestyle are themselves acid forming—they rob the body of alkalinizing foods and their minerals. The biggest offenders are white sugar, white flour, all processed and junk foods, animal foods, soft drinks, alcohol, medical drugs, and stress. To remedy the inability of the body to maintain proper acid-alkaline balance, and thus support the resolution of many diseases, it is important to increase in the diet the amount of plant-source foods that provide alkaline minerals such as organic sodium, magnesium, calcium, and potassium.

Reestablishing One's Holy Rhythm

The first four effects of the juice fast naturally lead us to reestablish our holy rhythm and life purpose. As we fast and purify, the aggravating toxicities of the body and mind subside. When the mind is quiet, we begin to transcend the mind and naturally reconnect to our life purpose.

Juice Recipes

I suggest drinking low-glycemic, Phase 1.0 juices made fresh at home with either a press-style juicer (such as a Green Star) or even a high-speed blender (Vitamix) and a cloth filter. The juice can also be separated from the pulp by straining with a fine mesh bag and contain the following elements:

- Base—celery, cucumber
- Leafy greens—spinach, parsley, kale, collards, Swiss chard, bok choy, watercress, beet green, cabbage, herbs (use sparingly, to avoid bitterness), dandelion, grasses, all other leafy greens
- Other vegetables—tomato, bell pepper (red, yellow, orange), nopal cactus, string beans, burdock root, Jerusalem artichoke, radish, any green sprouts
- Sweetener—stevia and xylitol (the only safe sweeteners for diabetics)
- Condiments—lemon and lime juice, cayenne powder, ginger root juice, juiced garlic, Transformational Salts, Himalayan salt, turmeric (powder or juice)

Role Models Thriving on a Plant-Source-Only, Live-Food Diet

You may have never encountered live-food, plant-source-only nutrition before. Many nutrition and diet books are written by people who aren't exactly the picture of health, and this could be an indication of the authenticity of their approach. I have eaten a near 100 percent plant-source-only diet of live, organic foods for more than 30 years and enjoy vibrant health, flexibility, strength, and energy.

It is important that you seek out people who are doing well living in the Culture of Life, and you will find the names of such people in the acknowledgments at the beginning of this book. My graduate masters students from our Vegan Live Food Spiritual Nutrition Mastery Program are able to provide excellent support for anyone who would like extra support. (Go to DrCousens.com for a list of these in your area or country.)

In addition, seek out raw-food potlucks in your area, and go online using the resources suggested throughout this book. At this very moment, you are drawing into your life the best things possible. You are a vortex of positive energy, and you have the opportunity to begin anew, becoming more than you ever thought possible. Become the continuation of those who are living the lifestyle that is achieving what you want so much to have as your daily life reality. The community of people living in the Culture of Life are some of the most vibrant, alive, and loving people on the planet.

Further Support

The Dr. Cousens's Diabetes Recovery Program—A Holistic Approach is a one-year program that often becomes a way of life with a minimum of a 21-day on-site experience. It includes medical personnel check-ins one to two times monthly, via phone or email, according to need, and a 30-minute teleconference check-in with Dr. Cousens each month. See DrCousens.com for a list of such groups globally. This support is not just nutrition focused but addresses in a practical way one's emotional and spiritual life as well.

I like to measure the HgbA1c levels of participants three months into the program and every three months thereafter. My program activates the antidiabetogenic genes and brings most people to a normal FBS in close to 21 days: greater than 61 percent of Type-2 non-insulin-dependent diabetes mellitus (NIDDM) participants, 24 percent for Type-2 insulin-dependent diabetes mellitus (IDDM) participants, and 21 percent of Type-1 diabetic participants, with 31 percent off insulin. The real task is how to stabilize participants in this new diet and lifestyle. For on-site intellectual, emotional, and spiritual support and growth, at the Tree of Life we offer several valuable retreat programs in addition to the 21-day program; these are arranged to support people's needs.

The crucial reason for a one-year follow-up is that breaking free from the Culture of Death is difficult without support. We live in a society that surrounds us by the shadow of the Culture of Death. My 40 years of clinical experience has shown that it may take people one to two years to transition emotionally, psychologically, and physiologically to stabilize into the Culture of Life. My experience is that this most likely cannot be accomplished in one day. On a more humorous side, Neal Barnard, MD, relates in *Breaking the Food Seduction* that an April 2000 survey of 1,244 adults showed that when offered $1,000 to stop eating meat for a week, 25 percent of those asked would not "swap meat for cash." It was interesting that people from Hispanic and Asian backgrounds were more willing to accept this hypothetical offer (probably because fruits and vegetables are more a part of their indigenous diet), with less than 10 percent turning it down, but Caucasians and African Americans turned down the $1,000 approximately 25 percent of the time.

What is the issue here? Why does meat seem so addictive? Because indeed it is.

Meat, as we pointed out earlier, has a high insulin index. A quarter pound of meat creates the same insulin response in the body as a quarter pound of sugar. Meat appears to be involved in the release of dopamine, which is the pleasure-stimulating neurotransmitter that is also activated by the opiates, nicotine, cocaine, alcohol, amphetamines, and dairy. (As pointed out earlier, dairy has a particular casomorphin that is one-tenth the strength of pure morphine.) When researchers from Edinburgh, Scotland, blocked meat's opiate effect, it cut the appetite for ham by 10 percent, salami by 25 percent, and tuna by a whopping 50 percent.

As previously, mentioned, not only do humans become addicted to animal products, but sheep, which are herbivores, and parrots, which are frugivores, can also become habituated to a diet of flesh. During their long sea voyages, the Nordics discovered that when the lambs on board the ships were induced to eat meat and fish, they became habituated to it. Upon arriving on land the lambs no longer desired their natural diet of grass. Horses are often fed fish and can be habituated to enjoy it, even though this is an unnatural food for them. Frugivorous parrots can be taught to eat and relish animal foods, as well. In other words, these animals that were on a natural live-plant-only diet became physiologically addicted to a diet of flesh foods.

As pointed out in *Breaking the Food Seduction*, sugar, as well as chocolate, releases natural opiates in the brain. In this case endorphins are released, which are relatives of opiates in their chemical structure. These endorphins activate the dopamine neurotransmitter system, which activates the pleasure centers of the brain. The opiate effect of sugar, according to the general research, may be triggered even by the mere taste of sugar, before the meat-dopamine response occurs. Carbohydrate-rich foods boost another neurotransmitter, serotonin, which helps with elevating mood, relaxation, and sleep.

Wheat, and particularly the gluten part of the wheat, is metabolized into at least 11 different opiates. It is for these reasons that this year of support to break our addiction to the Culture of Death lifestyle and its food is so crucial.

Zero Point Process Intensive

As an internationally recognized spiritual teacher, psychiatrist, and family therapist who developed and teaches the Zero Point Process Intensive, I have this to say about it:

Zero Point assists clients in learning how to clear emotional and mental blocks, psychosomatic problems, food addictions, and other addictions. It helps us to love ourselves enough and overcome the subtle resistance to healing from diabetes. We are empowered with the ability to dissolve codependent and unhealthy relationship patterns and ultimately align with our sacred design, so to become the full authentic living truth of we are. The Zero Point Process Intensive opens the door to clarity and freedom from the mind's preoccupation with its own addictive psycho-emotional patterns. Zero Point helps participants awaken from the dream state that one is separate from One. It helps one to understand that the personality is a case of mistaken identity and to be able to open to all life. Although it is not taught as a spiritual path, it is a powerful spiritual process that supports the spiritual process of all paths and religious traditions.

The fundamental understanding that we gain in Zero Point is that the personality is a case of mistaken identity. To be free, we must transcend our personal, cultural, archetypical, and even our spiritual identities. We are not our thoughts, minds, or bodies. This awareness gives one the option to choose a completely new orientation in life, resulting in the freedom to move into our expression of the Culture of Life. The process allows us to enter in the dual/nondual synchronicity in which we have our personalities and archetypes without being them.

Once one understands that one's thoughts have no power over us, one is free to dissolve them as needed. In this way, one becomes fearless in addressing their emotional blocks and issues. By dissolving what one is not, we come to the indescribable awareness of whom one is. This internal change in one's cosmic world perspective opens the way to enter into the flow of a God-centered life if one so chooses. Life's struggles then cease to have any impact. One is free to follow the flow of one's destiny in a way that manifests our sacred design, our true expression in the world, including being diabetes free. Zero point opens the option for us to discover and choose to be present as our authentic self.

Being present gives us the freedom not to be captured by the mind and its preoccupation with itself, the past, present, or future, or its relationship with the world. We are awakened from the entrapment of our stories and our pain.

With these tools, one is now empowered to embrace their destiny and their lives without fear, hesitation, or resistance. Freed from the slavery of the mind, one can live their life in celebration, subtle noncausal joy, inner contentment, and the bliss of freedom. This holistic transformation on every level is a supportive cornerstone for helping one heal from diabetes and all the negative projections that are often associated with a diabetes prognosis.

Conscious Eating Training

The foundation of the Conscious Eating Training at the Tree of Life Rejuvenation Center U.S. is to create food for the support of consciousness awakening. Conscious Eating begins with conscious food preparation. Studies have shown that our intentions influence the smallest particles of creation. In living food, water crystalline structures take on the energy of our presence, as well as the energy of the environment wherein it is being prepared. At the Tree of Life Café, our live-food creations vibrate with a deeply healing energy that affects all levels of creation.

The focus of this seven-day experiential course is to share with students the power of remaining present in the heart while preparing food. This is the true essence of conscious food preparation. This exciting intensive guides you through the basics of Phase 1.0 and 1.5 levels of conscious live-food preparation while immersing you in the Tree of Life experience. One is fully empowered to develop a Phase 1.0 and 1.5 delicious live-food cuisine after taking this course. Visit DrCousens .com for course content.

Spiritual Fasting Retreat

> I have done fasting, yoga, and meditation before, but never on the level of competence and integrity Dr. Cousens and his staff have designed to address medical, emotional, and spiritual concerns in one fully integrated, lovingly supportive program.
>
> **G. L. D., PhD, Tucson, Arizona**

My wife, Shanti Gold-Cousens, and I are longtime experienced juice fasters and host this retreat, applying spiritual juice fasting to unblock the divine source of youth, vitality, and transformation. On the Spiritual Fasting Retreat, we release our resistance to healing and open the body and mind to awaken to the Truth of who we are. Through the process of nonattachment to physical food, we open to spiritual nourishment and enjoy the spiritual feast of the four elements of air, earth (juices), water, and the sun (fire). Our spiritual fasting retreat is perhaps the most overall transformative workshop experience we offer. The Spiritual Fasting Retreat is the ultimate journey to the warrior within—inward and beyond to the One. During the retreat we offer the following:

- Seven days of fresh, organic juices
- Daily Shaktipat meditation
- Two days of live food to support reintroduction of food

- Authentic Native American Lakota sweat lodge (weather permitting)
- Daily Kali Ray TriYoga
- Nature walks
- Chanting from various traditions
- Spiritual discussions and seminars
- Mystical Shabbat and Havdalah
- Outdoor hot tubs
- Optional whole person healing evaluation (by appointment only)

The Spiritual Fasting Retreat, with two meditation sessions daily, supports you connecting to your Divine Truth, personal holy rhythm, and renewed life purpose. Spiritual fasting helps you not only detoxify and lose weight but also deeply experience all levels of your potential well-being. You do not know what feeling good is until you do a spiritual fast.

Through living in the Culture of Life, we become potentialists, seeing the true capabilities of everyone, individually and collectively, including ourselves. The transformed *you* that will arise through the Dr. Cousens's Diabetes Recovery Program—A Holistic Approach and living the Culture of Life will see with new, unique eyes. People often experience a physical, emotional, mental, and spiritual shift in themselves as they realize their true potential at each of these levels, living with a renewed mind, body, and spirit.

We eat and live in the Culture of Life as an act of love and consciousness, aware that we are each a person of great importance who can be vibrant and healthy and free of diabetes and inspire self-confidence, joy, and hope in others. We can do this just by the very simple act of living an authentic existence that acknowledges who we are. Therein, one is empowered to move beyond the processed diabetogenic realities of "modern" living to a Culture of Life in which few are ill, where we honor the inheritance of our ancestors, where we create a world that is safe for the health of future generations, and where all obtain the best possible food and quality of life.

Notes

1. *Am J Cardiol*, 2002, 90(suppl.): S551–S621.

2. Bronell and Puhl. "Bias, discrimination, and obesity." *Obesity Research*, 2001, 9: 788–805.[0]

3. Jensen, B. *Dr. Jensen's Guide to Better Bowel Care*. New York: Penguin-Putnam, 1999, p. 118.

CHAPTER 7

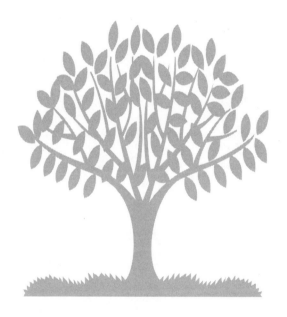

Culture of Life Cuisine

Introduction

We have now reached the tastiest part of this book, and we'll answer your questions about how to sustainably live and eat this moderate-low carbohydrate, live-food lifestyle. You've seen the research I've done with 120 people who ate approximately 25–45 percent complex carbohydrate intake of leafy greens, colored vegetables, and sprouts; 25–45 percent moderate fat; and 10–25 percent protein diet, all varied according to their constitution. As one reads about the profound antidiabetes and general health building power of this diet, it is useful to keep in mind that these findings are part of a cutting edge consensus shift away from a diet with a low-fat, high complex carbohydrate emphasis and toward a more healthy, green carbohydrate intake and a moderately higher fat intake. Surprisingly enough, according to my results, this live-food diet actually moves cholesterol to optimal levels and maintains omega-3s at safe, healthy zones, rather than pathological cholesterol levels below 159. It also dramatically decreases obesity, diabetes, and with high probability (based on its comparison results with research by Dr. Ornish and Dr. Esselstyn), decreases atherosclerotic cardiovascular disease (ASCVD) lesions.

What is interesting as we look at this, as I earlier pointed out in reference to the *Archives of Medicine* (2009), there is no correlation between a high cholesterol diet and an increase in heart disease. This is important because when I switched from a high carbohydrate to a moderate low carbohydrate diet for the diabetes healing program, I needed to increase one of the other macronutrients. Based on the totality of research and clinical experience, I choose to increase healthy, plant-based, raw fats. This dietary approach of a live-food, organic, moderate-low carbohydrate, moderate protein diet consists of organic, live, vegan cuisine, with high quality, plant-source carbohydrates, fats, and proteins. It should not be associated with the Atkins diet, which is not vegan and does not emphasize high-quality organic, live-food fats, proteins, and carbohydrates in any particular manner.

Another consideration is that on this diet there are no fat or protein restrictions or carbohydrate restrictions besides keeping to plant-source-only foods, green and colored vegetables, high-fiber foods, leafy greens, and sprouts. The caveat of this of course is that one can only eat so much. I have observed that the range of caloric intake for participants was approximately 2,000 calories daily. On this moderate and sustainable diet, people were able to eat 50 percent less, have increases sustained energy, and maintain a significant healing and maintenance energy for reversing diabetes, as well as weight and sustained weight loss. Weight loss is not the point of this diet. It is about healing and sustaining the reversal of diabetes. However as people reverse their conditions, they usually experience a return to their optimum weight. This is not just a diet for reversing diabetes; it is a diet for optimal health and weight.

It is useful to consider that we are unique individuals and have to find within this overall context the right balance for us. This is why I don't give single numbers, but a range: we are unique individuals and must find, within this context, the right balance for us.

For the treatment of diabetes and the maintenance of a diabetes free state, I recommend a range of 25–45 grams of carbohydrates during treatment and 35–50 grams in the maintenance stage. It is interesting to note that the idea of individualizing the diet according to constitution has been part of the Ayurvedic approach for about 3,000 years, but it has only been since the 1930s that Westerners have begun to approach it scientifically. Recent genetic research done at Stanford in 2012 on a phenomenon called the "phenotype diet" further validates the idea that we are unique individuals and do best if we individualize our diet to our unique metabolic constitutions.[1] This research identifies three of the key genes that determine how we can predict our dietary type. It is a new aid for clarifying our personal diet type. These Stanford research results suggest 25 percent of people need a low protein, high complex carbohydrate diet, which supports what have been my teachings since 1990. From my experience, approximately 35 percent of people do better on a lower fat moderate-high carbohydrate diet. The remaining 65 percent of people seem to do better with a moderately higher protein and higher fat, lower carb diet. In this context, people are advised to keep these individualizing principles in mind and thoughtfully apply them to our recipes in creating your most appropriate and effective daily dietary intake.

As I look at these delicious food recipes, I realize that this is not a restrictive diet. It is a delightful, delicious, enticing set of recipes that make living and eating the Phase 1.0 diet a culinary pleasure rather than an austerity. The purpose of this is to not only to enjoy yourself but to heal yourself and sustain yourself joyfully with this dietary way of life. I recommend that people stay on Phase 1.0, 100 percent live-food diet until their blood sugar is less than 100 and all blood tests are nondiabetic. After this, one is free to continue this or to move to a Phase 1.5 diet consisting of at least 80 percent live food. The recipes that have been selected and modified from the Tree of Life Café menu or created by Marcela Benson, MA (a graduate of my Spiritual Nutrition Masters Program) are for your culinary delight to support you in maintaining your diabetes-free lifestyle. They are arranged in a unique way for the flow of your day. There are breakfast, main meal, smaller meal, and snack recipes. These ideas may be played with and are meant to be starting points for your culinary creativity. This creative approach reflects the way we teach at the Tree of Life. In the Conscious Eating Course at the Tree of Life, food preparation is a creative, artful expression in appreciating that food is a love note from God.

To support people in Phase 1.0 healing diet, we have created an easy and original way to start thinking about planning individual menus. The flow and ease of the recipes were designed to empower people to begin the healing process right away. You can select from simple lists of choices for breakfast, main meals, smaller meals, snacks, and dessert menu options. This way you can more consciously and individually build your day-to-day menu according to your taste preference and lifestyle. When you are completely healed, you can expand your menu options with cooked recipes from the maintenance diet section, as you move to an expanded Phase 1.5 cuisine. If Phase 1.0 is too big of a leap for you, start by including into your life recipes and culinary techniques from the maintenance menu. Then build a lifestyle toward Phase 1.0.

Properly stocking your pantry and your refrigerator is key for success in this new endeavor. We have provided a comprehensive, beginning list to copy and take with you to an organic market. Some ingredients are hard to find in the organic markets but easy to get via the internet or at DrCousens.com. Becoming familiar with your ingredients will make the learning process much smoother. If you are sharing a kitchen space, you might want to make a special space for your products. If you are vulnerable to temptations or need time to adjust to this new lifestyle, creating a separate space in the pantry or the refrigerator will help you stay on track without distractions. If you are not sharing your kitchen with someone else (not doing Phase 1.0 or 1.5), it will best serve you to completely transform it! It takes some time until the old cellular memory is erased and replaced with the new, healthy one. Living with awareness and joy requires both spontaneity and preparation. Live food is for people who are interested in living fully and joyously. Once we start eating delicious live foods that nourish us, we are blessed with physical satisfaction and no longer crave what made us sick. As we shift toward our new lifestyle, it is difficult to return to our old, unhealthy habits because they no longer satisfy us or make us feel as good as our new cuisine. We wish you a smooth and easy transition toward radiant health!

May all enjoy the play of this cuisine as Marcela Benson, MA, (www .holisticnutritionstudio.com) leads us through this delightful experience of 159 recipes, tips, and ideas as seeds for you to reproduce your own delightful variations.

A Loving Piece of Advice: Throw Out Your Microwave!

A microwave oven decays and changes the molecular structure of the food by the process of radiation, making it a "radiation oven." The Soviet Union banned the use of microwave ovens in 1976. Yet more than 90 percent of American homes have microwave ovens. Because microwave ovens appear more convenient and energy efficient than conventional ovens, very few homes or restaurants are without them. The general perception, even among health professionals, is that whatever a microwave oven does to foods cooked in it doesn't have any negative effect on either the food or the consumer of the food. This is far from the truth. I actually cured two people from what was diagnosed as "chronic fatigue" by having them literally throw out their microwaves. The following five pieces of information, although not conclusive, are highly suggestive of the potential risks of using microwave ovens.

The first is a piece of news about a lawsuit in Oklahoma in 1991 concerning the hospital use of a microwave oven to warm blood needed in a transfusion. The case involved a hip surgery patient, Norma Levitt, who died from a simple blood transfusion. It seems the nurse had warmed the blood in a microwave oven. The implication is that microwaving the blood for the transfusion transformed the structure of the previously compatible blood, making it incompatible for transfusion.

The second is a report on microwaved baby formula, from *The Lancet* of December 9, 1989:

> Microwaving baby formulas converted certain trans-amino acids into their synthetic cis-isomers. Synthetic isomers, whether cis-amino acids or trans-fatty acids, are not biologically active. Further, one of the amino acids, L-proline, was converted to its d-isomer, which is known to be neurotoxic (poisonous to the nervous system) and nephrotoxic (poisonous to the kidneys). It's bad enough that many babies are not nursed, but now they are given fake milk (baby formula) made even more toxic via microwaving.

The third is a report on eating microwaved food, showing that eating microwaved food changes blood chemistry, titled "Comparative Study of Food Prepared Conventionally and in the Microwave Oven," published by Raum and Zelt in 1992:

> One short-term study found significant and disturbing changes in the blood of individuals consuming microwaved milk and vegetables. Eight volunteers ate various combinations of the same foods cooked different ways. All foods that were processed through the microwave ovens caused changes in the blood of the volunteers. Hemoglobin levels decreased and overall white cell levels and cholesterol levels increased. Lymphocytes decreased.

The fourth piece of information concerns the carcinogens created when the food is microwaved. In Dr. Lita Lee's book, *Health Effects of Microwave Radiation—Microwave Ovens*, and in the March and September 1991 issues of *Earthletter*, she stated that every microwave oven leaks electromagnetic radiation, harms food, and converts substances cooked in it to dangerous organ-toxic and carcinogenic products. Further research summarized in this article reveals that microwave ovens are far more harmful than previously imagined.

The fifth interesting piece of information is the Russian investigations published by the Atlantis Raising Educational Center in Portland, Oregon. Carcinogens were formed in virtually all foods tested. No test food was subjected to more microwaving than necessary. Here's a summary of some of the results:

- Microwaving prepared meats sufficiently to ensure sanitary ingestion caused formation of d-Nitrosodienthanolamines, well-known carcinogens.
- Microwaving milk and cereal grains converted some of their amino acids into carcinogens. Thawing frozen fruits converted their glucoside and galactoside containing fractions into carcinogenic substances.

- Extremely short exposure of raw, cooked, or frozen vegetables converted their plant alkaloids into carcinogens.
- Carcinogenic free radicals were formed in microwaved plants, especially root vegetables.

Russian researchers also reported a marked acceleration of structural degradation, leading to a decreased food value of 60 to 90 percent in all foods tested. Some of the changes were as follows:

- Deceased bioavailability of vitamin B complex, vitamin C, vitamin E, essential minerals, and lipotropics factors in all food tested
- Various kinds of damage to many plant substances, such as alkaloids, glucosides, galactosides, and nitrilosides
- The degradation of nucleoproteins in meats

Stocking Your Refrigerator and Pantry for Success

Superfoods and others

Spirulina
Blue and green algae
He shou wu
Reishi
Chaga
Noni
Tocotrienols
Whole psyllium husk

Sea vegetables

Raw nori Sheets
Kelp granules
Dulse granules
Sea palm
Alarea
Hijiki

Pacific arame

Pacific wakame
Sea lettuce
Irish moss

Dried and sun dried

Sun-dried tomatoes
Sun-dried olives

Fresh herbs

Basil
Parsley
Oregano
Thyme
Marjoram
Cilantro
Tarragon
Rosemary
Kaffir lime leaf
Ginger
Turmeric

Spices

Ground yellow mustard
Currie
Paprika
Garam masala
Cumin
Cinnamon
Turmeric
Cardamom
Nutmeg

Cayenne
Lavender
Chili powder
Hing (Asafoetida)
Italian Blend
Pizza seasoning
Pumpkin pie spice
Bay leaves
Carob

Oils and butters

Raw coconut oil
Hemp seed oil
Flax seed oil
Olive oil
Sesame seed oil
Coconut butter
Cashew butter
Almond butter
Tahini butter
Pecan butter
Walnut butter

Nuts and seeds

Sesame seeds
Black sesame seeds
Pumpkin seeds
Brown flax seeds
Golden flax seeds
Hemp seeds
Sunflower seeds
Chia seeds
Brazil nuts
Pine nuts

Walnuts
Pecans
Almonds
Cashews
Hazelnuts
Macadamias

Sweeteners

Xylitol
Stevia

Sprouts

Broccoli
Sunflower
Clover
Daikon
Wheat grass
Mug bean
Lentils
And many more!

Salts

Transformational Salts
Himalayan
Pink premier salt blend

Greens

Kale
Collards
Mustard
Tat soi
Spinach
Herbs
Sorrel

Lettuce
Sprouts
Purslane
Chard
Dandelion
Bok choy

Vegetables and nonsweet fruits

Tomato
Eggplant
Cabbage
Avocado
Green beans
Sunchokes
Cucumber
Radish
Fennel
Asparagus
Peas
Celery
Burdock
Red bell peppers
Broccoli
Lemon
Zucchini
Ginger
Hot pepper
Cauliflower
Lime

Remember there are over 20,000 edible plants in this planet (probably more). Explore and have fun on your culinary journey!

Know Your Ingredients

It is essential that before you venture into the supermarket, investing time and money for your new lifestyle, you become familiar with the ingredients and can recognize their quality. In this section, we focus on the quality of the ingredients because quality makes an important difference in your recipes' taste, satisfaction, and nutritional value. Most of the ingredients presented in this section can be found in the list "Stocking Your Refrigerator and Pantry for Success." We are providing a short explanation that will help you understand how to use and purchase these high quality ingredients. Many of these items are available in your local organic supermarkets or from the Culture of Life Store at DrCousens.com.

A Note about Nama Shoyu and Bragg's Amino Acids

These soy-based condiments are a popular flavoring agent for many raw-food chefs. They are not part of the phase 1.0 healing diet. The overall recent research has established many deleterious effects of soy, as previously discussed in this book. There is also a high likelihood that the "organic soy" is contaminated with GMO crops (soy being 92–96 percent GMO). It has also been shown that during the heat of processing (because all soy products are cooked), there is also a formation of naturally occurring MSG.

Green Leafy Vegetables

Among the most nutrient dense of all plant foods are the dark green, leafy vegetables, especially kale, dandelion, spinach, chard, collards, arugula, parsley, and green cabbage. These vegetables are high in alkaline minerals, protein, and chlorophyll. As such, they are regenerative, purifying, and highly potent foods.

Buying and Storing Nuts and Seeds

It is recommended that organic nuts and seeds be purchased directly by mail order from specialty suppliers. The nuts and seeds obtained from health food stores or conventional markets are susceptible to rancidity, as they may have been stored on the shelf for long periods of time. Ideally, nuts and seeds should be stored in the freezer or refrigerator to prevent the oils from going rancid. If this is not possible, store them in a cool, dark, dry place. Be especially careful with high-oil-content nuts and seeds, like Brazil nuts, macadamias, and pine/pignoli nuts. If they look yellow, it is likely that they are rancid.

Buying Oils

As suggested in Chapter 2, people with serious ASCVD would be prudent to minimize or eliminate olive oil and other saturated cooked or raw animal fats from their diet in their plant-source-only approach to healing atherosclerosis. In the same context, those people diagnosed with diabetes for more than a year have, with almost 100-percent certainty, a degeneration of the endothelium of the arteries, and are most prudent to avoid or minimize the use of olive oil until the diabetic physiology has been reversed completely for two years. I still recommend that one keep a 25–45 percent carbohydrate intake in Phase 1.0 and a 30–50 percent carbohydrate intake in Phase 1.5, a 10–25 percent protein intake, and approximately 25–45 percent of total calories from raw fats in the process of healing diabetes through a live-food diet. It is essential to avoid all trans and hydrogenated fats and all processed, junk food, especially white sugar and white flour.

The best oils to use in salad dressings are those high in omega-3; these include walnut, flax, chia, and hemp oils, as well as sesame oil, which is very high in antioxidants. Conventional cooking oils should be avoided, as they have been highly processed. Even "cold-pressed oils" could have been influenced by heat at some stage of processing.

Recommended oils include the following:

- Cold-pressed flax seed oil, which should be used within three weeks from date of pressing, as it is highly susceptible to rancidity

- Hemp seed oil, which should be used within six weeks from date of pressing, as it is highly susceptible to rancidity
- Chia seed oil
- Cold-pressed sesame, sunflower, and almond oils
- Coconut oil

Herbs and Spices

Where possible, we encourage you to use fresh herbs and whole spices. Their flavors are so much richer and delightful than their dried counterparts. Spices such as fennel, dill, cumin, clove, cinnamon, and cardamom can be bought in whole form and easily ground in a spice mill or coffee grinder. The quality of your spices will change the outcome of your recipes. Most people tend to overlook this, but for this reason it is important to buy only organic spices.

Stevia

Stevia is a sweet herb native to North and South America. Only one species, rebaudiana, tastes sweet enough to be called "sweet leaf" in Brazil and Paraguay, where it grows wild. Stevia is a great sweetener alternative. Recent research indicates that it does not raise the blood sugar level and may even lower it. Whole stevia leaf can be bought at health food stores or by mail order, or you can grow your own. Grind the whole leaf into a powder and add to food and teas for a sweet taste. You can also buy water-extracted stevia in liquid form from your local health food store in the supplements section. Avoid alcohol-extracted and refined forms of stevia. Unrefined stevia is dark green in color. At the Tree of Life online store, all varieties and flavors of stevia are available.

Xylitol

This is an alternative for sweetening your recipes and has a fresh, sweet taste. It can be used to transform any recipes that call for sweetness. Some people experience diarrhea when they use too much. It might be a good idea to try it in small quantities and see how you do with it.

Another option is to use a little xylitol in combination with stevia to get the best sweet taste without getting the runs. Most of our recipes called for ground xylitol (with a powdered, sugar-like texture). Not all xylitols are the same! Make sure you buy a non-GMO birch-tree xylitol. You can purchase xylitol at the Tree of Life store.

Flax Seed

Golden flax seed is packed with nutrition and is an essential daily addition to a healthy diet. Golden flax seed has greater nutritional value than the more common brown flax seed. It contains fiber, lignans, and short-chain omega-3 fatty acids, as well as both soluble and insoluble fiber, helping to clean your intestinal tract and promote regularity. Lignans provide a powerful support to the immune system and cellular health. Long-chain omega-3 fatty acids are essential for balanced brain chemistry. Flax seed is one of the main sources of omega-3 for a plant-source-only cuisine. I recommend 3 tablespoons for slow oxidizers and 3–6 tablespoons for fast oxidizers each day. Other long-chain omega-3 sources that contain the long-chain components DHA and EPA are blue-green algae (E3Live™) and the herb purslane. The conversion rate of short-chain omega-3 to long-chain is 1–3 percent. Adding 1 tablespoon of coconut oil to the flax seed more than doubles the conversion rate to 6–10 percent.

The seeds we are using can be ground in a spice mill or coffee grinder and used in many recipes, or they can simply be sprinkled on top of salads or granola or even fruit. When flax seed is soaked, the soaking water becomes thick and jelly-like, providing a versatile thickening and binding ingredient for many recipes.

Salt of the Earth

After much salt research, I have discovered a powerful salt called Transformational Salts™. It is a mixture of precious salts from all directions on the planet: the Andes Mountains, two areas in Hawaii, the Himalayas, and the Salt Lake area of Utah. These are harvested from beneath the earth and are thus protected from radioactive fallout. In the production of Transformational Salts, these earth salt elements are activated by scalar wave technology to bring the grounding and healing frequency of all four directions. They are strongly negatively charged and so help pull the positively charged toxins out of our systems. They are completely organic and raw. This is my highest recommendation for salt. After this, and still a great choice, is Himalayan salt, which comes from beneath the Himalayas. Because of the ongoing Fukushima catastrophe, I no longer recommend salt from the ocean.

Common table salt, which I do not recommend, lacks minerals and trace elements because it is purified and refined, leaving only sodium and chloride. After refining, common table salt is mixed with iodine, bleaching agents, and anticaking agents, which creates a pure white, free-flowing product. Even many salts labeled "sea salt" are washed or boiled, which removes minerals and trace elements, rendering them toxic to the human body. Any salt that has been heated in this manner is converted to a covalent form, which is difficult for the body to assimilate. Transformational Salts and Himalayan salt are very energizing and complete salts. Research indicates that sea salt is used by the body for mineralization, hydration, and to restore a healthy sodium-potassium balance for the lymph, blood, and extra cellular fluid.

Delicious, Creamy, and Alive Nut Butters

We recommend using high quality nut butters; not all butters are the same. The ones we have at our web store are stone ground and made from sprouted live nuts and seeds. Using sprouted live nuts and seeds with the stone grinding method results in the most delicious and beneficial nut butters.

High-quality almond butter is made from ground, raw, sprouted almonds. Likewise, tahini is the succulent butter ground from raw sesame seeds. Many commercial tahinis, almond butters, and other nut butters involve chemical pasteurization and exposure to intense heat in the grinding process. Thus their labels, which identify them as "raw," may be misleading.

Alive nut butters such as almond butter and sesame tahini are versatile ingredients for many types of recipes—particularly soups and salad dressings. Tahini is especially enhancing with its creamy, dairy-like texture and rich flavor. These butters make a great snack straight out of the jar, a dip for crudités, or a spread for raw bread or crackers. Research cited in this book shows, as an added benefit, that a regular intake of almonds is associated with up to a 21–23 percent decrease in LDL.

Hemp Seed

The tiny, shelled seed of the amazing hemp plant has a pleasant nutty flavor, similar to sunflower seeds. The seeds are packed with nutrients—they are an excellent source of the essential fatty acids (EFAs), delivering these EFAs in a balanced 3.75:1 ratio. Hemp seeds contain the rare fatty acid gamma-linolenic acid (GLA). Hemp seed is a source of complete protein, containing all the essential amino acids. It is equal to flax seed as a source of short-chain omega-3 fatty acids.

Unfortunately, most hemp seeds are irradiated upon import; however, our web store supplies truly live, organic hemp seeds, which we call hemp nuts. Hemp seed is great with granola, sprinkled on salads, and is especially tasty in tomato-based sauces. Hemp seed is a delicious substitute for other nuts and seeds in almost any recipe.

Olives

The healthiest olives are those that are water-cured or cured in Celtic sea salt. Olives are rich in monounsaturated fat, with high proportions of essential amino acids, vitamins E and A, beta-carotene, calcium, and magnesium.

Coconut Oil

Mature coconuts are used in the creation of health-enhancing coconut oil that is mostly solid at room temperature, so it is often referred to as *coconut butter*. Raw, unprocessed coconut oil smells fragrant like fresh coconuts, while most commercial coconut oils, including the brands commonly found in health food stores, are often deodorized and heat processed, and therefore they are not recommended. Cold-pressed coconut oil is available from Dr. Cousens's online store.

The saturated fats in coconut oil are medium-chain fats (triglycerides, or MCTs) and therefore unlike most other sources of saturated fats (long-chain triglycerides), which are stored in the body as fat reserves. The high MCTs found in coconut oil are easy to digest, even for people who typically have trouble digesting fats. In fact, MCTs actually assist the body in metabolizing fat efficiently. As such, coconut oil provides a readily available fuel source. Saturated fats are also an important building block for all the cells of the human body. As stated previously, coconut oil helps convert short-chain omega-3 fats to long-chain omega-3 fats.

Coconut oil has a high (50 percent or more) lauric fatty acid and caprylic acid content, from which it derives its antiparasitical, antiviral, and antifungal properties. Those with intestinal problems such as candida or other systemic infections can therefore benefit from the daily inclusion of coconut oil in their diet. Coconut oil can be added to nut mylks, dressings, desserts (acting as a thickener when chilled), and even soups. Coconut oil also makes an excellent skin lotion and massage oil.

Ready Made Ingredients in Your Organic Local Market

Non-soy miso is a great find. When purchasing any miso product, be sure to read the ingredient list. Many of these products do not include soy in the name but do contain it. Chickpea miso has a delicious savory flavor that can be used to enhance your soups, sauces, dressings, and any other preparation that you feel needs more flavor, including sweets.

Salad seasonings are useful to add to any salad or soup as a topping. This is a quick way to enhance both the nutrition and taste of your dish. At our web store, we carry Living Intentions Salad Booster.

Spirulina has 95 percent bioavailable protein. For some people, it may be an acquired taste. Others won't be able to stop eating it.

Fermented foods such as kim-chi and sauerkraut help to populate our intestines with beneficial microorganisms and aid us in a gentler transition to the Culture of Life.

Tocotrienols are rice bran solubles and a good source of vitamin E. They add a rich creamy texture to recipes. A tablespoon in a tea takes the place of milk, making it a good travel companion.

Food Preparation Equipment

High-quality equipment will make preparing live foods easier and faster. The purchase of quality equipment for the living-foods kitchen requires an investment, but the durability and the results are well worth the initial cost. Most of the items listed here are available from Dr. Cousens's online store.

Selecting a Chef's Knife

A good chef's knife is a necessity in the kitchen, but what is most important is that whatever knife you have is kept sharp. A sharp knife will make the job faster and easier. Purchase the best-quality knife and sharpener you can afford. A high-carbon steel blade is recommended, as it is the most durable material. Try it out in the store if possible, noticing how it feels in your hand. A good knife should have balance— like an extension of your arm.

Ceramic knives are an excellent alternative to steel because they do not lead to browning in fruits and vegetables due to oxidation caused by the metal, nor is there any subtle metallic taste imparted to the food. They will also last months, or even years, without sharpening. Ceramic is a very hard material, but brittle; these knives are susceptible to break-age if care is not taken in their use and handling.

For mincing fresh herbs, a cleaver with a slightly rounded blade is essential. Use a rocking motion, moving back and forth across the herbs, finely chopping them.

Blender

A high-speed blender is essential in the living-foods kitchen. House-hold blenders are unable to adequately process or achieve the desired smoothness when blending hard nuts and seeds—the motors will quickly burn out with this type of use. We recommend the Vita-Mix Super 5000 (the most versatile blender), the K-Tec HP3 blender, and the Tribest single-serving blender (great for traveling).

Juicer

The selection of a juicer for your living-foods kitchen should be carefully considered. Most home juicers are of the centrifugal type. The quality of the juice extracted from this type of juicer is less than ideal because as the centrifugal mechanism spins at high speed, it shreds the produce, which therefore oxidizes it more rapidly. Centrifugal juicers also tend to waste produce because they are unable to fully break down the cell wall and extract all the juices.

The very best is a juice press system, such as the Norwalk juicer, with a hydraulic pressing mechanism. At the Tree of Life Café, we use a commercial hydraulic press juicer. The juice from a hydraulic press keeps its energy for up to three days. The second best type of juicer is one that masticates the produce at low speeds and therefore preserves the health-giving qualities of the juice. Masticating juicers produce a very dry pulp, as the juices are completely extracted. The Super Angel juicer and Green Star juicer are perhaps the best masticating juicers currently available. They are capable of juicing all types of produce, including green leafy vegetables (even grasses), and can effectively homogenize nuts and seeds for pâtés. A less expensive option is the Omega single-gear masticating juicer. We recommend that you purchase the best juicer you can afford. Until you have your juicer, you can also make green vegetable juice with a high-speed blender by blending your produce with a little water and straining the juice through a nut mylk bag (a fine mesh bag) over a bowl or pitcher.

Food Processor

A high-quality food processor enables you to process vegetables in a variety of forms; it will also allow the processing of nuts and seeds to a variety of consistencies. Look for one with an 8- to 10-cup capacity. Cuisinart is a time-honored favorite brand, although there are many good food processors on the market today. In our recipes, we use the food processor with an S-blade option for many procedures.

Dehydrator

When looking for a dehydrator, it is important to choose one that is fan-operated, which provides even drying temperatures in the food. Many home round stackable models lack quality temperature controls.

We recommend Sedona and Excalibur dehydrators because of their efficient fan-operated systems, accurate temperature control, and ease of use and cleaning. The Excalibur has two different sizes: five trays or nine trays. The Sedona dehydrator has nine trays but is a bit smaller than the Excalibur. It has two fans, giving you the option to use half the dehydrator when needed. These tray systems, which slide in and out, allow you to adjust certain levels without disturbing other levels, as would be the case with the common circular stacking models.

Coffee Grinder, Spice Grinder, and Spice Mill

A coffee grinder can be used to grind whole spices, and it works perfectly for grinding your daily flax seed. A quality spice grinder may be more effective for grinding hard spices to a fine powder. You can also purchase a ceramic spice mill for each type of whole spice you use, such as black and white peppercorns, nutmeg, coriander, cardamom, cinnamon, cumin, caraway, and anise.

Spiral Slicer (Saladacco)

A spiral slicer, also called a *saladacco,* is necessary if you want to create pasta-like "noodles" from a variety of vegetables, such as zucchini and daikon. It is easy to make both flat ribbon "noodles" and super-thin angel hair "pasta" with this clever tool.

Mandoline

A most versatile kitchen tool, the mandoline is simple to use and will perfectly slice veggies and fruits thick or thin. With the switch of a blade, you can instantly julienne, grate, or shred. This is essential for making vegetable "pasta" for live-food lasagna and other "noodle" dishes.

Miscellaneous Tips

Dehydration

Low-temperature food dehydration is a technique that warms and dries food but will not destroy enzymes. It has been suggested by Edward Howell in his book *Food Enzymes for Health and Longevity* that food enzymes are destroyed when the food temperature reaches 115–120°. However, recent research by the Excalibur Dehydrator Company suggests that it is actually better to begin the dehydration process at 145° for the initial stage. The reasoning is that as the food is dehydrating, it literally "sweats out" the moisture it contains and thus creates cooling.

This information changes how I think about the entire process of food dehydration. It means that the safest way to dehydrate is to begin drying at 145° for a maximum of three hours for foods with a high water content. After this, the temperature is set in the "normal" range of 110–115° through the completion of the drying process. By doing this, we are limiting the potential of bacterial growth by reducing the time the food spends in the dehydrator. The longer that a food is in the dehydrator, the more potential exists for the enzymes to be destroyed, even at lower temperatures. Low-temperature dehydration for sustained time, as practiced for years by the live-food community, may not be safe because sustained low-temperature dehydration encourages bacterial growth and fermentation. At the Tree of Life, we feel that the new approach is both safer and more efficient. But note that this technique is only recommended for the Excalibur dehydrator because it is the one used in the research cited previously.

Salting and Massage

The technique of salting, as indicated in many recipes, helps to soften hard vegetables such as cabbage, kale, or broccoli. Salt causes the vegetables to release moisture as it breaks down the cell walls. Digestion is made easier when these fibers are broken down. Foods that are high in cellulose will wilt slightly, creating a texture similar to cooked food.

Green leafy vegetables can be "massaged" by using the hands to directly rub salt into the greens. This effect is further enhanced by adding a small amount of an acid, such as lemon juice or apple cider vinegar.

Soaking and Sprouting

Many nuts, seeds, and grains must be soaked and/or sprouted before they can be used in live-food cuisine. Soaking the seeds and nuts removes the enzyme inhibitors they contain, thereby activating a food's full nutritional potential. We recommend soaking most of your nuts and seeds for 20 minutes with 3 percent food grade hydrogen peroxide. For each cup of soaking water, use a tablespoon of hydrogen peroxide. This will remove any bacterial or fungal growth that may have occurred on the nuts and seeds. After 20 minutes, drain the nuts or seeds, rinse until the water is crystal clear, and cover with fresh water to soak for the remaining time.

Sprouting is a fun and easy way to grow your own organic high life force food. We encourage you to read *Sprouts: The Miracle Food*, a book by Steve Meyerowitz. Organic sprouts are available in health food stores and in some supermarkets. There may also be, in your local area, someone who is growing sprouts to sell privately, and sometimes these are of better quality because they are not commercially produced. When looking for a local source for sprouts, here are some questions to ask:

- Do they use spring or filtered water?
- Do they use food grade hydrogen peroxide?
- What kind of medium are they grown in and what additional supplements are used to enhance the nutritive value of the soil (e.g., ocean minerals and effective micro-organisms)?

The answers to these questions will help you to determine the quality of the sprouts and the level of knowledge of your local sprout grower.

Answers to Frequently Asked Questions

The following is a list of answers to frequently asked questions by people transitioning to the Culture of Life:

- If your food tastes bland, you may need a little more salt, herbs, or spices.
- If you are not sure how much salt, herbs, spice, or liquid to add to a recipe, begin with a small amount and keep adding it until you reach the desired effect. You can always add more, but if you add too much to start with, it can be difficult to redeem the recipe.
- If a dish comes out too spicy, you may be able to balance it with some fat (e.g., coconut butter, nut butter, or avocado).
- Don't be afraid to add new ingredients to any of your recipes. You might just be in for a great new culinary experience when you do.
- Sometimes simple foods are the most satisfying. For example, one of my favorite meals is avocado, hemp oil, and salt with a side of sauerkraut.
- Plan your meals and learn the ingredients. Ultimately it is the easiest way to eat.
- Chia porridge is the fast food breakfast of a healthy lifestyle.
- Once you get the hang of live food preparation, you will be able to make it in a flash.
- Plan your snacks to make sure you always have them available.
- Be open to trying new things several times. Some things are an acquired taste.
- If you are feeling a little light, nut butter, including coconut butter and avocado, will help to ground you.

- If you are still hungry after your meals, you may need to add more plant-based protein and fat to them.
- If you are having trouble digesting your foods, you may want to consider taking digestive enzymes and hydrochloric acid (HCl).
- The time it takes to adjust to this lifestyle is different for different people. Take the time to adjust at your own pace and enjoy the process.

Breakfast Menu Options for Phase 1.0 Healing Diet

Creamy vanilla porridge

Nut mylkshake with cinnamon and E3Live, and 2 raw crackers with nut cheeze, tomato, and basil

Green smoothie and raw biscotti

Chagachino (adaptogenic mushrooms supplement rishie, chaga, and/or he shou wu powder with warm nut mylk)

Granola

Biscotti with almond butter and nut mylkshake

Nogurt with flax seed crumbs

Chia seed porridge with cinnamon and coconut nut mylk

Chia smoothie

Cinnamon chia smoothie

Sesame seed mylk

Pumpkin seed mylk

Almond mylk

Walnut mylk

Cardamom bars with two icings

Star anise bars with lemon icing

Cinnamon bars

Lemon coriander bars with coriander icing

Muesli

Plate with tomatoes, avocados, cucumbers, and spirulina dressing

Nori cracker with sprouts and avocado

Main Meals Menu Options for Phase 1.0 Healing Diet

Simple kale salad

Spinach salad with avocado, bell pepper, celery, and dehydrated tomatoes

Stuffed tomatoes with pâté and mix salad with sprouts

2 raw crackers with chopped tomato, pepper, and basil

Nori sandwich with sun-dried tomato, hummus, alfalfa sprouts, and lettuce

Chopped salad

Baby greens salad with chopped vegetables with 2 raw crackers with nut cheeze, tomato slices, and dill

Caesar salad with a side of nut pâté

Yellow and green spaghetti zucchini with tomato sauce, mint pesto, or oriental dressing

Broccoli with bell pepper and nut cheeze

Flax wraps

Sushi nori or cucumber rolls

Taco shells

Guacamole with crackers

Tomato salsa

Pizza

Basil pesto

Indian-flavored shish kebabs

Coconut rice

Indian-style savory balls

Walnut savory balls

String bean dhal

Herb string beans

Kale salad with chipotle

Spinach salad with spirulina

Cabbage salad with caraway sesame tahini

Sea vegetable salad with sesame tahini

Wild greens salad with cactus pad dressing

Mock egg salad
Indian cabbage salad
Greek salad
Tabouli
Caesar salad
Asian noodle salad
Pad thai
Mediterranean falafels
Smaller Meals Menu Options for Phase 1.0 Healing Diet
Miso soup broth with chopped veggies
Cucumber coconut soup
Red pepper and miso soup
Spinach vegetable medley soup
Hemp spinach basil soup
Classic tomato soup
Gazpacho
Super green cactus chia soup
Aloe vera string bean soup
Aloe vera pad burdock cilantro soup
Green juice
Cracker with pâté
Dipping sauce with crudités
Side of hummus with zucchini chips
Live savory bell pepper bread with heirloom tomato almond cheeze
Green smoothie
½ avocado with sauerkraut and spirulina dressing

Snacks Menu Options for Phase 1.0 Healing Diet

Red minipeppers stuffed with nut pâté
Raw nut trail mix
Raw crackers with cultured cheeze and dill
Olives and pickles
Sauerkraut with nutbutter, spirulina, or any salad seasonings

Celery, red pepper, and cucumber sticks with hummus
Biscotti
Kale chips
Granola or muesli with nut mylk
2 tablespoons of hemp seeds
2 tablespoons spirulina with avocado, hemp seed oil, and salt
Sauerkraut with cashew butter and spirulina or any other salad
   seasonings
Zucchini chips

Diet Sweet Delights for Phase 1.0 Healing Diet

Creamy vanilla pudding
Halva
Bonbons
Chunky carob fudge
Ginger pudding
Key lime pie
Cinnamon mousse
Carob mousse

Maintenance Diet Options

Millet breakfast mix
Buckwheat meal (better than oatmeal)
Buckwheat tabouli
Simple lentil soup
Velvety red lentil soup
Quinoa salad
Sumptuous salad
Bean salad
Quinoa and black bean salad
Spiced kidney beans
Dhal

Amaranth
Millet, peas, and Indian spice
Quinoa and cabbage
Millet burgers
Lentil loaf
Chickpea stew

Breakfast Recipes for Phase 1.0 Healing Diet

Note: Xylitol comes in the form of granules; to obtain xylitol powder, grind with a coffee grinder or a high power blender.

Seed and Nut Mylks

Here are some tips, ideas, and uses for exquisite mylk:

- To clean, soak all your nuts and seeds for 20 minutes in water and add 1 or 2 tablespoons of hydrogen peroxide (3 percent or 10 percent food grade) to remove potential mold and bacteria. Rinse several times until clean. Soak your nuts/seeds overnight or for about 4–8 hours. If you do not need to use them right away, they can be refrigerated in clean water. Changing the water every day (while they are refrigerated) will keep them fresh and ready to use for several days.
- Add a pinch or two of Transformational Salts to bring out the flavor. It really works!
- Instead of water for your mylk base, you can use coconut water, herbal tea, or aromatic waters as your base. This technique will give a completely different palate to your regular mylk.
- You can also spice up your mylk with cinnamon, cardamom, nutmeg, ginger, vanilla, lemon, or coffee flavor.
- Save the pulp! When you make nut/seed mylk you will be left with the moist fiber/pulp. You can use this to make biscotti, challah, cookies and cinnamon rolls, and breads.

If you can't use it within two days, dehydrate it at 115° for a
few hours and grind (once completely dry and cool) to make
flour to use in those recipes at a later date. Store in airtight
containers in a cool, dry environment, and it will keep for
a couple of months. If you make the mylk with the flavors,
there is a greater chance that the pulp will ferment. The flour
or the pulp will smell stale or fermented if stored too long.

- Leave time for your mylk to chill for 1/2–1 hour in the
refrigerator before serving. Or you can blend with ice-cold
water for an instant chilled mylk.
- Nut/seed mylks are great on their own, over granola or
muesli, and as a base for smoothies, ice cream, various
soups, dressings, and raw entrees.

Here are directions for making seed and nut mylks:

Basic Mylk Recipe

2 cups nuts or seeds (cleansed and soaked overnight)
60-ounce liquid (depending on desired consistency)

Place nuts or seeds in the blender. Fill the blender with water. Blend
to a creamy consistency. Strain ingredients through a cheesecloth,
nylon mesh, or nut mylk bag into a bowl. Transfer to and store in
a glass container. Mylk will keep 3–4 days if stored in a glass jar or
pitcher. This basic recipe creates 1 full 64-ounce container of mylk.
Serves 4 16-ounce glasses. Mylk is delicious plain. As an option,
pour the mylk back into blender and add spices like cinnamon, nutmeg, star anise, cardamom, licorice root powder, and carob. You can
also add superfood and super herbs like green powders, spirulina,
chlorella, blue green algae, and/or maca chaga, reishi, and he shou
wu to boost the nutritional content. Serve as is, warmed or chilled.
To sweeten your mylk elixirs, use xylitol or stevia.

My Family's Favorite Mylk Combination

1 cup almond
½ cup sesame seeds

½ cup shredded coconut

60 ounces of water

Dash of Transformational Salts or Himalayan salt

Combine in a blender and blend until smooth.
Strain ingredients through a cheesecloth, nylon mesh, or nut mylk bag. Store in a glass pitcher, drink plain, or use for smoothies, cha-gachino, and other creations.

Sesame Mylk

2 cups sesame seed (soaked overnight)

60 ounces of water

For flavoring, add:

2–3 tablespoons cinnamon, powder

2 tablespoons maca

Pinch of Transformational Salts or Himalayan salt

Combine in a blender and blend until smooth. Strain ingredients through a cheesecloth, nylon mesh, or nut mylk bag.

Pumpkin Seed Mylk

2 cups pumpkin seed (soaked overnight)

60 ounces of water

Dash of Transformational Salts or Himalayan salt

Combine in a blender and blend until smooth. Strain ingredients through a cheesecloth, nylon mesh, or nut mylk bag.

For flavoring for a 16-ounce drink size, add:

1 teaspoon green superfood powder

1 teaspoon blue green algae

Pinch of Himalayan or sun-dried sea salt

2 tablespoons xylitol or stevia to taste

Almond Mylk

2 cups almond (soaked overnight)

60 ounces of water

Dash of Transformational Salts or Himalayan salt

Combine in a blender and blend until smooth, Strain ingredients through a cheesecloth, nylon mesh, or nut mylk bag,

For flavoring for a 16-ounce drink size, add:

¼ teaspoon cinnamon

Pinch of nutmeg

2 tablespoons of xylitol or stevia to taste

Walnut Mylk

2 cups walnuts (soaked overnight)

60 ounces of water

Dash of Transformational Salts or Himalayan salt

Combine in a blender and blend until smooth. Strain ingredients through a cheesecloth, nylon mesh, or nut mylk bag.

For flavoring for a 16-ounce drink size, add:

¼ teaspoon star anise, ground and sifted

Dash of licorice root powder

Pinch of salt

Coconut Mylk

2 cups shredded coconut or 1 or 2 cups of fresh mature coconut meat

60 ounces of water (If you are using fresh coconut, add the coconut water instead of water. If there isn't enough coconut water, just add more water.)

Dash of Transformational Salts or Himalayan salt

Combine in a blender and blend until smooth.

Creamy Vanilla Porridge

1 peeled zucchini or 1 cup zucchini, cut up

1 cup walnuts

1 tablespoon coconut butter or 1 avocado

4 drops of vanilla flavor or pinch of powder

1 tablespoon xylitol or stevia to taste

Water (approximately 3 ounces)

Pinch of Transformational Salts or Himalayan salt

Combine in a blender and blend, adding water a little at a time until very creamy. Serves 2 or 4.

Luscious Brazil Mylkshake

1 cup Brazil nuts

2 cups water

Combine in a blender and blend until smooth. Pour mixture into a nut mylk bag and squeeze until pulp is dry. (Reserve pulp for dehydration and later use as flour.)

Add:

1½ cups coconut meat

2 tablespoons vanilla extract or 2 vanilla beans (scraped or ground in a spice grinder)

2 tablespoons coconut oil

½ teaspoon salt

1 tablespoon orange zest

5 drops stevia or xylitol to taste

Blend again and enjoy!

Biscotti

1 cup nut pulp or nut flour

¼ cup flax, ground

½ cup pecans or walnuts, chopped

½ cup cashews, chopped

½ cup tocotrienols

¼ cup ground xylitol (grind to a powder, like powdered sugar)

¼ cup coconut butter

1 teaspoon Transformational Salts or Himalayan salt

Use the wet nut mylk pulp, or if you are using pulp flour, add ½ cup water or herbal tea until you reach dough-like consistency.

Mix all ingredients together and form into biscotti loaf, cut into 12 slices about ½-inch thick and 3-inches long. Dehydrate on 145 ° for 2 hours and 115° overnight.

Different flavor and variations ideas for biscotti:

5 drops of lemon essential oil and lemon rind

½ cup of carob and 1 tablespoon of pumpkin pie spice

5 drops vanilla flavor and 1 tablespoon ginger juice (see recipe in the juice section)

Cinnamon and vanilla to taste

Chagaccino

16 ounces nut mylk (it can be warmed to 115° before blending)

¼ teaspoon chaga

¼ teaspoon cinnamon

2 or 3 lavender flowers (optional)

3 or 5 drops of coffee flavor

1 drop orange or tangerine flavor (optional)

1 or 2 tablespoons xylitol or stevia to taste

Pinch of salt

After the mylk is warmed to 115°, put all the ingredients in the blender and blend. Serve in a cup with a little more cinnamon on top of the foam. Enjoy!

Granola or Muesli

1 cup walnuts (soaked overnight), chopped

1 cup sunflower seed (soaked overnight)

1 cup sesame seed (soaked overnight)

1 cup hemp seed

1 cup pumpkin seeds (soaked overnight)

¼ cup coconut oil

1 tablespoon pumpkin pie spice

¼ cup tocotrienol

¼ cup carob

1 teaspoon salt

Toss all whole nuts and seeds into bowl. Add oil, salt, and spices. Serve fresh as muesli or dehydrate on teflex/dehydrator trays on 115° overnight for a granola effect.

Nogurt with Flax Seed Crumbs

1 cup coconut water (for thinner nogurt)

4 coconut pulps

1 cup pecans or walnuts (soaked and rinsed well)

1 whole vanilla bean, scraped or ground, or vanilla essence to taste

2 tablespoons coconut oil

½ teaspoon salt

2 tablespoons ginger juice (see recipe in the juice section)

¼ cup lemon juice or 2 lemons, juiced

Stevia and/or xylitol to taste

Blend until creamy and completely smooth. Serves 4.

Flax Seed Crumbs

3 tablespoons golden flax seed

1 tablespoon tocotrienols

1 teaspoon xylitol powder or to taste

Pinch of salt

1 teaspoon cinnamon

Pinch nutmeg

1 tablespoon coconut oil

Put all the dry ingredients in a coffee grinder until flax seed is ground. Pour into a bowl and then add coconut oil. Mix with a fork to achieve a crumbly texture. You can use this mixture as a topping for nogurt, mylkshakes, muesli puddings, and so on. If you make this mixture salty without xylitol, cinnamon, or nutmeg, and instead use Italian spices, it is delicious for topping your salads, tomatoes, and soups!

Chia Seed Porridge with Cinnamon and Coconut Nut Mylk

1 cup coconut mylk or any other nut mylk

3 tablespoons chia seeds

1 tablespoon tocotrienols

1 tablespoon xylitol powder or stevia to taste

1 teaspoon cinnamon

Pinch of fresh-grounded nutmeg

Pinch of Transformational Salts or Himalayan salt

Put all the ingredients in a glass or a bowl, and stir with a fork until the chia has thickened. Refrigerate until next day for the perfect texture. Add more cinnamon on top and enjoy.

Cardamom Bars with Two Icings

Base:

1 cup hemp seeds, unsoaked, whole

1 cup brown sesame seeds, soaked, whole

1 cup sunflower seeds, soaked, whole

Keep the seeds whole. Toss into a bowl.

Cream:

1 cup coconut cream (dried mature coconut meat that has been blended into a cream)

¼ cup coconut oil blended with ½ cup hot water (120°)

¼ cup cardamom

¼ cup xylitol powder or stevia to taste

½ teaspoon Transformational Salts or Himalayan salt

Combine and blend until smooth.

Cardamom icing:

1 cup coconut cream butter

¼ cup hot water (120°)

2 tablespoons cardamom

½ teaspoon licorice root powder

¼ cup of xylitol powder or stevia to taste

Pinch Transformational Salts or Himalayan salt

Place all ingredients in blender and blend on high speed, to a smooth and spreadable consistency.

White licorice icing:

¾ cup coconut cream butter

3 tablespoons hot water

¾ teaspoon licorice root powder

¼ cup of xylitol powder or stevia to taste

Pinch Transformational Salts or Himalayan salt

Place all ingredients in blender and blend on high speed, to a smooth and pourable consistency.

Building the bars:

To the blended cream, add the whole seeds. Press mix into a flat rectangular glass container. Create cardamom icing and spread over the surface of the mix. Create white licorice icing and drizzle over the top of the cardamom icing. Chill until firm and cut into rectangles to serve. Serves 4–8, depending on size of bars. Bars will keep for up to 4 days, refrigerated.

Star Anise Bars with Lemon Icing

Base:

1 cup brown sesame seeds, soaked, whole

1 cup sunflower seeds, soaked, whole

1 cup chia seeds, unsoaked, mixed into the base

½–1 cup of water to rehydrate chia seeds

Toss all seeds into a bowl.

Cream:

1 cup coconut cream

¼ cup coconut oil, blended with ½ cup warm water

5 tablespoons star anise, ground and sifted

1 tablespoon xylitol powder

½ teaspoon Transformational Salts or Himalayan salt

Combine and blend until smooth.

Lemon icing:

½ cup coconut cream butter

2 tablespoons hot water

2 tablespoons lemon juice

1 teaspoon xylitol powder or stevia to taste

Optional: ¼ teaspoon lemon zest or a drop of lemon essential oil

Place all ingredients in blender and blend on high speed, to a smooth, spreadable consistency.

Building the bars:

Toss all seeds into a bowl and mix. Massage in the blended cream. Press into a flat rectangular glass container. Create lemon icing and spread over the mix. Chill, cut rectangles, and serve. Serves 4–8, depending on size of bars. Bars will keep up to 4 days, refrigerated.

Cinnamon Bars

Base:

1 cup walnuts, soaked, S-bladed

1 cup hemp, unsoaked

1 cup chia seed, unsoaked, mixed into the base

½–1 cup of water to rehydrate chia

Toss all seeds into a large mixing bowl.

Cream:

1 cup coconut butter

¼ cup coconut oil, blended with ½ cup hot water

¼ cup cinnamon

3 tablespoons xylitol or stevia herb, powdered to taste

½ teaspoon Transformational Salts or Himalayan salt

Combine and blend until smooth.

Building the bars:

Food process walnuts with S-blade to a finer consistency. Toss into bowl. Add hemp and chia whole. Blend and massage in cream. Pack into a large pan. Refrigerate and cut into squares and serve.

Lemon Coriander Bars with Coriander Icing

Base:

1 cup hemp seed, unsoaked, whole

1 cup brown sesame, soaked, whole

1 cup sunflower seed, soaked, whole

Toss all seeds into a bowl.

Cream:

1 cup coconut butter

¼ cup coconut oil, blended with ½ cup hot water

½ cup poppy seed

¼ cup coriander

¼ cup of powder xylitol or stevia herb, powdered to taste

½ teaspoon Transformational Salts or Himalayan salt

Combine and blend until smooth.

Coriander icing:

1 cup coconut butter

2 tablespoons hot water

2 tablespoons lemon juice

3 tablespoons coriander

1 teaspoon licorice root powder

2 tablespoons xylitol or stevia to taste

Pinch of Transformational Salts or Himalayan salt

Combine and blend to a spreadable consistency.

Building the bars:

Toss base seeds, whole, into the bowl. Massage in the blended cream. Pack into a flat rectangular glass container. Create icing in blender and spread over the mix. Decorate with ground and sifted coriander. Serves 4–8, depending on size of bars. Bars will keep for up to 4 days, refrigerated.

Main Meals Recipes for Phase 1.0 Healing Diet

The purpose of designing the main meal recipe section is for you to discover your unique optimal way of eating. Normally, we are taught to eat 3–4 square meals each day. While this may be true for some, we recognize that it is not true for all. Depending on your lifestyle, your body constitution (as described in *Conscious Eating*), and your oxidative profile, you may want to have one or two main meals daily. In the Phase 1.0 Healing Diet, we do not need to limit ourselves to "breakfast, lunch, and dinner" because with a live-food lifestyle you may eat your lunch for breakfast, or take your breakfast as a snack, or have a snack in place of dinner. It is important to relearn what you need in order to be truly satisfied. You should eat in a way that leaves you energetic and mentally alert. In this process, you will have ups and downs until you learn what works best for you without falling out of the Phase 1.0 Healing Diet. If you do not feel satisfied in daily eating, it usually means that you have not eaten particularly for your individual constitutional needs. For example, if you are a fast oxidizer, you may wish to add more spirulina or another vegan protein source to these recipes. Or if your Ayurvedic constitution type is more *vata* oriented, you may wish to add more coconut butter or avocado to these recipes. Learn your specific needs for the healing of your body and your transition to this new paradigm. Freely play in your live-food kitchen, and take time to organize your meals and mealtimes to best serve you. Take inspiration from these recipes and make them your own by altering the amounts of salt, oil, and other ingredients within the parameters of this healing diet. We encourage you to explore other recipes from online sources, books, or culinary magazines, substituting Phase 1.0 ingredients for ingredients that are not a part of this healing lifestyle.

Some of these recipes constitute an entire meal and others can be combined to make a meal. For example, use the guacamole and salsa in the tacos to create a main meal.

Tips and Ideas for Recipe Creation

Soup	Pâté	Dressing
Base: water, sun-dried tomato water, tomato, cucumber, tea, lemon/lime	Base: zucchini, nuts, seeds	Base: olive oil, avocado, water, tomato, cucumber, tea
Additions: vegetables of choice and spices/herbs	Additions: spices and herbs, minced or diced vegetables, olives	Additions: spices and herbs, vegetables
Thickeners: extra veggies, sun-dried tomatoes, tahini or other nut butters, avocado, oil, nuts, seeds	Liquid: lemon or lime juice, water, olive oil, olive brine, sun-dried tomato water	Thickeners: avocado, oil, nuts, seeds

Yellow and Green Spaghetti Zucchini

2 green zucchini

2 yellow zucchini

Cut the zucchinis with the spiral slicer (saladaco) and serve with tomato sauce or pesto. It can also be placed in the dehydrator with the solid sheet at 145° for 30 minutes to 1 hour for a warmer dish. Serves 2.

Broccoli with Bell Pepper and Cheeze

Veggies:

2 cups broccoli, sliced or chopped

1 cup red bell pepper, julienne cut

Seed cheeze in blender:

1 cup sunflower seeds

¼ cup olive oil (or other recommended oil to taste)

2 tablespoons lemon juice

½ teaspoon black pepper

¼ teaspoon Transformational Salts or Himalayan salt

½ bunch fresh cilantro

¼ teaspoon cayenne

¼ teaspoon hing (Hing is an Ayurvedic spice that tastes like onion.
   It has antiflatulence properties.)

2 teaspoons cumin

Kalamata olive water, to desired consistency (Note: This is the soak
   water that the olives are marinating in.)

Toss the bell pepper and broccoli and set aside. In food processor,
process the seeds to a butter or as much as possible. Add olive oil,
lemon juice, water, hing, black pepper, cayenne, and salt. Process to a
creamy consistency. Massage into broccoli and bell pepper and mix.
Eat as is or serve in a flax wrap, burrito style. Serves 1–2.

Flax Wraps

1 cup flax seed, ground, unsifted

1 cup seed flour, ground and sifted

2 tablespoons poppy seed, whole

½ teaspoon Transformational Salts or Himalayan salt

½ cup blessed water

Grind and sift dried seed pulp from cheeze into bowl (see the section on seed and nut cheeze) to create a "seed flour." Combine all
dry ingredients together. Add water a little at a time until you have
a dough-like texture that can be rolled out with a rolling pin. Roll
out dough and cookie cut 6-inch circles. Roll out each circle again to
achieve a very thin tortilla-style wrap. This is a basic flax wrap. Other
dried herbs can be added for a "savory wrap." Serves 1–2.

Sushi Nori or Cucumber Rolls

Sushi filling:

2 cups walnuts

Red and yellow bell pepper

2 tablespoons sesame oil

2 tablespoons lemon or lime juice

2 tablespoons ginger juice

½ teaspoon Transformational Salts or Himalayan salt

¼ teaspoon freshly ground black pepper

Dash cayenne

4–6 tablespoons fresh cilantro and/or basil, minced

Optional:

1 teaspoon lemongrass, ground in the spice mill

1 kaffir lime leaf, ground in the spice mill

For filling:

With an S-blade, process nuts in food processor. Add oil, lemon or lime juice, ginger juice, salt, pepper, and cayenne. If you are using any of the optional ingredients, add them at this time. Process to the consistency of pâté. Add the fresh herbs and process.

Julienne red bell pepper and yellow bell peppers and prepare other ingredients you may want to have in the roll, such as sunflower sprouts, red clover, alfalfa, and/or julienned greens.

For rolling:

Place filling on the bottom half of the nori sheet. Place bell peppers and sprouts over the top of filling. Begin rolling the filling in sheet to form a tube. Use a little water to seal the edges. Cut and serve.

For cucumber rolls:

Take both ends off of the cucumber. Use a vegetable peeler to peel all the skin off and discard. Use the vegetable peeler to peel the whole length of the vegetable. Keep peeling to get long thin strips of cucumber the same width of the vegetable peeler blade. Lay these strips overlapping each other approximately ¼ to ½ inch, achieving a 6- or 7-inch-width sheet. You can place nori over this and roll, or roll without nori, using the previously given directions for rolling.

Nori is a wonderful food. We often cut the sheets into quarters and fill them with a bit of salad, then fold over like a taco shape and enjoy. Serves 4.

Taco Shells

Use one of the basic cracker recipes. After 4 hours of drying, flip the crackers off the teflex onto a cutting board. Cookie cut the cracker with a 6-inch cookie cutter (or use a Rubbermaid 1-gallon circular jug top, for example). You may need to use a knife to cut through the dry parts. Shape the circle into a half-moon taco shell shape, using a washcloth folded into quarters as a spacer. With this method, you should be able to fold two shells over one cloth. Lay the shells on their side and dehydrate the remaining time. Fill shells with greens, guacamole, and salsa. Serves 4.

Guacamole

2 avocados
2 tablespoons lime juice
¼ cup minced cilantro
1 teaspoon cumin
¼–½ teaspoon Transformational Salts or Himalayan salt
Dice avocado and add remaining ingredients. Mash a bit to achieve a creamy texture. Serves 2–4.

Tomato Salsa

1½ cup ripe tomatoes, diced
1½ cup cucumbers, deseeded and diced
1 cup cilantro, finely chopped
1 tablespoon olive oil
1 tablespoon lime juice
Dash cayenne
Dash Transformational Salts or Himalayan salt

Combine tomatoes, cucumbers, and cilantro in a bowl. Stir in the lime juice, oil, spices, and salt. Serves 1–2.

Pizza

Pizza crust:

Use one of the bread recipes: Form dough into a ball and place in the center of a teflex sheet. Press the center of the ball into the sheet and form into a pizza crust shape. To avoid any cracks in the dough, use the palm of one hand to press and the other hand to guide the shape. If a crack begins to form, quickly attend to it by pressing it back together. Serves 4.

Pizza cheeze:

Use the basic seed cheeze recipe with the optional Italian seasoning and thyme. Or, as an alternative to the cheeze, use the basil pesto recipe.

Marinara:

1 red bell pepper

2 cups sun-dried tomato

½ cup sun-dried tomato water

¼ cup olive oil (or other recommended oil to taste)

1 clove garlic

2–4 tablespoons Italian seasoning

½ teaspoon black pepper

¼ teaspoon Transformational Salts or Himalayan salt

Place all ingredients in blender and process on high speed until combined. Serves 4.

Topping:

2 bell peppers, diced

1 zucchini, diced

1 clove garlic, minced

1 bunch of basil, shredded

¼ cup kalamata olives, pitted and minced

3 tablespoons Italian seasoning

2 tablespoons cold-pressed stone-ground olive oil

1 tablespoon kalamata olive water

½–1 teaspoon black pepper

¼ teaspoon Transformational Salts or Himalayan salt

Toss all ingredients into a bowl until vegetables are coated with the herbs, spices, and oil. Let marinate for a few minutes. Serves 4 when used as pizza topping.

Basil Pesto

2 cups walnuts

½ cup olive oil (or other recommended oil to taste)

½ teaspoon Transformational Salts or Himalayan salt

½ teaspoon black pepper

2 cups basil

1 or 2 garlic cloves (optional)

In food processor, process nuts with the S-blade until fine. Add remaining ingredients and process until very smooth. Serves 4 when used as pizza topping.

Indian-Flavored Shish Kebabs

Marinated vegetables:

1 zucchini, sliced on a diagonal

1 yellow bell pepper, cut into large panels

1 broccoli, separated into large florets

1 red bell pepper, cut into large panels

1 tomato, sliced

Marinate vegetables for 4 hours with Indian-style sauce (provided in the following list). Place marinated veggies on a shish kebab, alternating with Indian-style or walnut savory balls. Dehydrate on 145° for 2 hours. Serve over coconut rice. Serves 4.

Indian-style sauce:

1 cup olive oil (or other recommended oil to taste)

2 cups Brazil nuts

6 tablespoons lemon juice

2 tablespoons coriander seeds, ground

2 tablespoons ginger, minced

2 tablespoons cumin, ground

½ teaspoon turmeric powder

½–¾ teaspoon Transformational Salts or Himalayan salt

½ teaspoon hing

1 teaspoon freshly ground black pepper

½ teaspoon cayenne

½ cup ginger juice

½ bunch cilantro

½ bunch basil

Place all ingredients in blender and blend on high speed. Serves 4 when used as marinade for vegetables.

Optional Thai version:

Before blending, add 1 tablespoon lemongrass and 1 kaffir lime leaf.

Coconut Rice

1 mature coconut removed from shell and peeled, processed with
　S-blade in food processor to a fine consistency
½–1 teaspoon Transformational Salts or Himalayan salt
1 teaspoon black pepper
Dash cayenne

Toss the food-processed coconut and spices together. Serves 4 when
served with Indian-flavored shish kebabs.

Indian-Style Savory Balls

½ cup almonds, soaked
½ cup sunflower seeds, soaked
½ cup hemp seeds
½ cup celery, minced
¼ cup fresh lemon juice
1 tablespoon fresh ginger, grated
½ teaspoon Transformational Salts or Himalayan salt
2 teaspoons cumin
1 teaspoon coriander
Dash turmeric
Dash cayenne
Dash hing
Dash mustard seed
Dash fenugreek

Process all nuts and seeds in food processor and place into bowl.
Add remaining ingredients and mix to a texture that can be formed
into balls. Hint: Use an ice cream scooper that is 1½ inch in diam-
eter to form the balls. Dehydrate at 145° for 2 hours. Serves 4 when
served in combination with Indian-flavored shish kebabs.

Walnut Savory Balls

1 cup walnuts, soaked
1 cup sunflower seeds, soaked
¼ cup fresh basil or cilantro

1 tablespoon fresh ginger, grated

½ teaspoon Transformational Salts or Himalayan salt

Dash hing

Dash cayenne

Dash turmeric

Place nuts and seeds in food processor and process to a fine texture. Add remaining ingredients and process to a formable texture. Form into balls and dehydrate at 145° for 2 hours. Serves 4.

String Bean Dhal

1 cup string beans

1 cup avocado

¼ cup water

1 tomato

2 tablespoons olive oil (or other recommended oil to taste)

2 teaspoons Transformational Salts or Himalayan salt

1 teaspoon cumin

¼ teaspoon turmeric

⅛ teaspoon cayenne

⅛ teaspoon coriander

⅛ teaspoon mustard seeds

In the blender, combine 2 string beans with the remaining ingredients until smooth. Add additional water for consistency.

Cut remaining string beans in 2-inch lengths. In a mixing bowl, combine sauce and beans, and mix well. Serves 2.

Herb String Beans

¾ pound string beans

2 tablespoons olive oil (or other recommended oil to taste)

1½ tablespoons fresh parsley, chopped

1 tablespoon fresh mint, chopped

Ground pepper to taste

1 tablespoon lemon juice

2 teaspoon lemon zest

½ teaspoon Transformational Salts or Himalayan salt

Place beans in large bowl, add salt, and massage until beans are softened, around 5 minutes.

Whisk together remaining ingredients and toss with beans. Serve at room temperature. Serves 2.

Mediterranean Falafels

1½ cups walnuts, soaked

1½ cups unsoaked, sesame seeds, ground

½ bunch parsley

½ bunch cilantro

1 garlic clove

¼ bunch oregano

½ teaspoon black pepper

1 teaspoon salt

2 tablespoons olive oil

2 teaspoons cumin, ground

3 tablespoons lemon juice

Process herbs in food processor. Set aside. Process nuts as much as possible. Set aside. Grind seeds and mix with nuts and herbs. Add salt, lemon juice, and oil. Form into patties and dehydrate at 145° for 2 hours.

Pad Thai

Noodles:

4 zucchini

2 bell peppers, julienned

Sauce:

¾ cup water

1 cups almond butter

¼ cup sesame oil

2–3 tablespoons lime juice

Fresh ginger, peeled and sliced, to taste

Salt, to taste

Chili flakes, to taste

Black pepper, to taste

Toppings:

1 bunch cilantro, coarsely chopped

½ cup seasoned almonds, crushed

Make noodles from the zucchini using a spiralizer or spirooli (or V-slicer and then julienne). Set aside. To make the sauce, combine all the sauce ingredients in a blender and blend until smooth. Add the sauce to the zucchini noodles and bell peppers and mix well. Lay the seasoned noodles on a dehydrator sheet and set to 140° for half an hour to warm them up. To serve, put the seasoned noodles on a plate, add the toppings, garnish with a wedge of lime, and serve. Serves 2–4.

Stuffed Tomatoes with Pâté

2 or 4 tomatoes, medium size (core the tomatoes, taking
   everything out)

Pâté (see other recipes)

Prepare your favorite salad mix with sprouts. Stuff the tomatoes with the pâté. Add some delicious dressing of your choice and serve with 2 raw crackers with chopped tomato, pepper, and basil.

Nori Sandwich

Building your nori sandwich:

2 nori crackers (see other recipes)

Hummus (see other recipes)

Lettuce

Sun-dried tomato

Alfalfa sprouts or any other sprouts

Start with the nori cracker. Then lay all the ingredients on top. Finish with another nori cracker, and your sandwich is done!

Salads

Option 1:

1 bunch kale, chard, or collards, destemmed and chopped, or

Bok choy, napa, or other cabbages

½ teaspoon of Transformational Salts or Himalayan salt

Option 2:

1 bunch spinach or other favorite greens (arugula, lettuces, mustard greens, lamb's quarters, dandelion, or other wild greens), tossed with other ingredients listed as follows, and

¼–½ teaspoon Transformational Salts or Himalayan salt

Choose option 1 or 2, and add:

1 bell pepper (red, orange, or yellow), chopped or julienned

1 avocado, diced, and/or ¼ cup hemp seed

3–4 tablespoons lemon juice or 2 tablespoons apple cider vinegar

3 tablespoons hemp, olive, or sesame oil

Massage all ingredients adding the salt to taste. Serves 1.

Optional for any salad:

Sea vegetables, dulse (whole or flakes), nori (whole or torn sheets)

Superfoods, spirulina, or other green powders

Fresh herbs

Roots (burdock and/or radish)

Olives, whole or pitted

Spices (cumin, caraway, curry, coriander, turmeric) or other favorite spices

Dash of hing, cayenne, black pepper, and/or chipotle

Kale Salad with Chipotle

Base:

2 bunches of kale, destemmed and torn into bite size pieces

1 bunch parsley, minced and massaged with ½ teaspoon Transformational Salts or Himalayan salt

Add:

1 avocado, diced

1 bell pepper, julienne

Small handful of whole dulse cut with scissors

2–3 tablespoons of hemp or high-quality cold-pressed olive oil

3 tablespoons lemon or lime juice

½–1 tablespoon cumin

¼ teaspoon chipotle

Dash hing

Dash chlorella or other green powders

Toss and serve. Serves 1 or 2.

Spinach Salad with Spirulina

Base:

    1 bunch spinach, chopped and washed

    2 handfuls of baby lettuce

Add:

    1 avocado, diced

    1 bell pepper, julienned

    2–3 tablespoons hemp oil

    2–3 tablespoons lemon

    1 tablespoon spirulina or other green powders

    3–4 olives

    ¼ teaspoon turmeric

    ¼ teaspoon cayenne

    Dash hing

    ¼ teaspoon Transformational Salts or Himalayan salt

A little ground sesame or flax on top is also nice. Creates a small/ medium bowl of salad for 1 or 2.

Cabbage Salad with Caraway Sesame Tahini

Base:

    Half head cabbage, shredded or chopped, massaged with ½ teaspoon Transformational Salts or Himalayan salt

Add:

    1 bunch cilantro, chopped

    1 avocado, diced

    1 bell pepper, julienned

Dressing:

In blender, combine the following ingredients:

    ¼–½ cup ground sesame seed

    1 clove garlic, minced

2–3 tablespoons sesame oil

2–3 tablespoons lemon

2–3 tablespoons blessed water or olive brine, to desired consistency

1 tablespoon caraway

¼ teaspoon cayenne and/or black pepper

¼ teaspoon Transformational Salts or Himalayan salt

Blend until smooth.

Building the salad:

Massage dressing into salad ingredients and top with

Handful of red clover, alfalfa, or sunflower greens, or

1 tablespoon green powder superfood, or

Dulse flakes or kelp powder

Serves 1 or 2.

Sea Vegetable Salad with Sesame Tahini

Base:

1 bunch dinosaur kale, massaged with

¼ teaspoon Transformational Salts or Himalayan salt

Add:

1 cup whole dulse, cut into strips with scissors

1 tablespoon kelp powder

1 bunch cilantro or parsley

½ cup chopped spinach

1 avocado, diced, or hemp seed

1 bell pepper, julienned

1 tablespoon spirulina

Dressing:

In blender, combine the following ingredients:

¼–½ cup sesame seed, ground

1 clove garlic, minced

2–3 tablespoons sesame oil

2–3 tablespoons lemon juice

2–3 tablespoons blessed water or olive brine, to desired consistency

¼ teaspoon turmeric

¼ teaspoon cayenne and/or black pepper

¼ teaspoon Transformational Salts or Himalayan salt

¼ cup unchopped fresh herb basil or cilantro (optional)

Blend until smooth.

Building the salad:

Massage dressing into salad ingredients and top with a handful of red clover, alfalfa, or sunflower greens. Serves 1 or 2.

Wild Greens Salad with Cactus Pad Dressing

Base:

1 bowl full of baby greens

1 or 2 handfuls of wild greens (lamb's quarters, dandelion, or wild mustard)

Add:

1 avocado, diced

1 bell pepper, julienned

¼ cup young raw nopal cactus pad, diced or julienned (Note: Remove thorns by scraping surface of pad and rinsing.)

Dressing:

In blender, combine the following ingredients:

1 young raw nopal cactus pad (Note: Very young cactus pads without thorns may be blended without the scraping technique.)

¼ cup hemp seed

¼ cup cilantro, fresh, unchopped

2–3 tablespoons hemp, sesame, or cold-pressed olive oil

2 tablespoons lemon

3 tablespoons blessed water

¼ teaspoon Transformational Salts or Himalayan salt

Blend until smooth.

Building the salad:

Massage dressing into salad ingredients. Serves 1 or 2.

Mock Egg Salad

Sauce:

¾ cup cashew

½ cup hemp oil

¼ cup lemon juice

¾ cup water

½ teaspoon turmeric

1 teaspoon Transformational Salts or Himalayan salt

Blend all ingredients in the blender until creamy and set aside.

Salad:

½ head cauliflower

1 celery stick, finely chopped

¼ cup red pepper, finely chopped

½ cup pickles, finely chopped, or wild capers

¼ cup green onion or chives, finely chopped

1 teaspoon fresh ground pepper

Process the cauliflower with an S-blade until finely chopped (smaller than rice). Put the cauliflower with the rest of the ingredient including the sauce and mix. Serve a scoop on top of any salad, and garnish with fresh ground pepper and parsley. Serves 4.

Indian Cabbage Salad

1 cup fresh parsley, chopped fine

1 cup walnuts, soaked and chopped

½ head green cabbage, shredded

½ head purple cabbage, shredded

Mix vegetables in large bowl.

Dressing:

1 cup almonds, soaked

1 cup water

4 tablespoons lemon juice

1 tablespoon olive oil

1 teaspoon each of curry powder, salt, and ground cumin

1 teaspoon fresh ginger, grated

Blend until smooth. Stir into vegetables. Serves 4

Greek Salad

4 tomatoes, diced

2 cucumbers, diced

1 bell pepper, diced

2 tablespoons olive oil

8 olives, chopped

Salt and pepper to taste

Mix together in large bowl. Serves 4.

Live Tabouli

2 heads cauliflower, finely ground in food processor

½ cup lemon juice

1 cup olive oil

4 teaspoon black pepper

¾ teaspoon sea salt

2 bunches fresh parsley, chopped

1 bunch fresh mint, chopped

2 bunches fresh cilantro, chopped

1 bunch fresh tarragon

1 cup olives, pitted and chopped

5–6 tomatoes, sliced

In a large bowl, combine all ingredients and mix thoroughly. Serves 6–8.

Caesar Salad

1 cup soaked sesame seeds

2 nori sheets

2 tablespoons lemon juice

2 teaspoon salt

1 garlic clove
1 cup water
1 teaspoon fresh ground pepper
½ cup olive oil
Brine (juice from olive jar)

Put aside the Nori sheets and blend all ingredients until creamy. Add the nori to the blender and blend a little more until you can see little speckles of nori spread evenly trough the dressing. Pour over chopped romaine. Choose any of the pâté recipes and serve on top. Serves 4.

Asian Noodle Salad

2 cucumbers, cut into noodles
½ red bell pepper, cut into matchsticks
¼ head red or green cabbage, shredded
Handful cilantro, chopped
Handful basil, chopped

Combine all ingredients in a large bowl. Toss with dressing. Serves 4.

Simple Kale Salad

Base:
2 bunches of kale, destemmed and massaged with ½ teaspoon
   Transformational Salts or Himalayan salt
Add:
1 avocado
4 tablespoons hemp seed
2–3 tablespoons of hemp or high-quality cold-pressed olive oil
3 tablespoons lemon or lime juice

Mix with the kale and enjoy. Serves 1 or 2.

Spinach Salad with Avocado and Olives

Base:
1 bunch spinach, chopped and washed

Add:

1 avocado, diced

10 grape tomatoes

2–3 tablespoons hemp oil

2–3 tablespoons lemon

3–4 olives

¼ teaspoon Transformational Salts or Himalayan salt

A little ground sesame or flax on top is also nice. Creates a small/medium bowl of salad for 1 or 2.

Chopped Salad

Chopped vegetables:

¼ cup cucumber, finely cubed

¼ cup red bell pepper, finely chopped

¼ cup tomatoes, finely cubed and without the seeds

½ cup avocado, cubed

¼ cup green onion

¼ cup red radish, finely cubed

¼ cup black olives, finely chopped

3 tablespoons cilantro

1 tablespoon mint, finely chopped

3 tablespoons sesame oil

3 tablespoons soaked almonds, finely chopped

1 tablespoon fresh lemon juice

½ tablespoon apple cider vinegar

1 teaspoon Transformational Salts or Himalayan salt

Mix all ingredients together and put on top off a bed of your favorite sprouts or salad. This recipe is also nice if you add spirulina dressing on top for garnish. Serves 2.

Baby Greens Salad with Chopped Vegetables

Set a bed of mixed baby greens on a plate and put aside.

Chopped vegetables:

¼ cup cucumber, finely cubed

¼ cup red bell pepper, finely chopped

¼ cup tomatoes, finely cubed and without the seeds

¼ cup green onion

3 tablespoons of cilantro

1 tablespoon mint, finely chopped

¼ tablespoon hemp seeds

3 tablespoons hemp oil

1½ tablespoons fresh lemon juice

1 teaspoon Transformational Salts or Himalayan salt

Pepper to taste (optional)

Mix all the ingredients and toss. Serve on top off the baby green salad. You can also add (on the side) 2 raw crackers, spread with nut cheeze, topped with a tomato slice and dill.

Pâté

Pâtés can be used as is; with a salad; wrapped in nori sheets, lettuce, or cabbage leaves; spread on crackers; or used in main-course dishes, such as stuffed vegetables. They will keep in your refrigerator for a few days. After that, it is a good idea to recycle them into a dehydrated snack. Dehydrating takes the water content out of the pâté, preserves it for a longer time, and transforms into a whole new taste and experience.

Here are some tips, ideas, and uses for pâté:

- Spread a thin layer over a nori sheet and dehydrate overnight. This is a great way to make nori crackers that can be eaten alone or used as a bread to make sandwiches.
- Spread a ½-inch thick line of pâté along the edge of the nori cracker. Paint the rest of the nori sheet with lemon juice and roll into a thin nori cigar. Dehydrate overnight. This makes a great snack.
- Scoop the pâté with small ice cream scooper to a dehydrator tray (using a mesh sheet). Dehydrate overnight. This makes crispy half round balls that you can add to your salads or zucchini pasta dishes.

- Cut nori sheets in half or in three equal strips. Put on about 2 or 3 tablespoons of pâté. Roll into a thick short roll (like a big, thick Cuban cigar). Cut into 2-inch pieces. Dehydrate overnight and enjoy beside your salad or as a great snack.
- Put the pâté back in the blender and add more lemon, water, oil, salt, and some more spices to make a salad dressing. Depending on how much liquid you use, it can also be transformed into a dip.
- Spread the pâté on a solid dehydrator sheet about ¼-inch thick and cut into 2-inch by 2-inch squares. Dehydrate for 2 hours at 145° and turn it over onto an open mesh sheet and dehydrate overnight. This makes great crackers, too.
- Use the same technique as given previously but cut into ½-inch squares and use as croutons for salads or soups.

Here are directions for making pâté:

Basic Pâté Recipe

3 cup sunflower seeds (soaked 12 hours, rinsed, drained) or nut of choice

¼ cup lemon juice, or more to desired taste

¼ cup raw organic tahini, or favorite oil

4 tablespoons parsley, chopped

1 teaspoon salt

Optional:

1 cup vegetable of choice: celery, red bell pepper, fennel

Blend in a food processor, stopping occasionally to scrape down seeds from the side. Add water as necessary to create a smooth consistency. Serves 6.

Pranic Pâté

2 cups hazelnuts

1 cup sunflower seeds, soaked

First process the hazelnuts in a food processor with an S-blade. Then process again with seeds.

Add:

1 cup sun-dried tomatoes, soaked

¼ cup lime juice

1 teaspoon salt

1 teaspoon hing

½ teaspoon black pepper

Process again until the tomatoes are well combined and the pâté is smooth.

Then mix in:

¼ cup parsley, freshly minced and destemmed

1 teaspoon rosemary, freshly minced

1 teaspoon thyme, freshly minced

1 teaspoon oregano, freshly minced

¼ cup basil, freshly minced

¼ cup olives, pitted and chopped

¼ cup celery, minced

¼ cup bell pepper, minced

Serve on nori sheets, flax crackers, or with a fresh salad. Serves 6–8.

Lemon Almond Herb Pâté

2 cups almonds, soaked

⅓ cup olive oil

½ cup lemon juice

½ cup water

1.5 teaspoon salt

1 teaspoon fresh chives, minced

1 teaspoon fresh thyme, minced

1 teaspoon fresh oregano, minced

Process almonds in food processor until finely ground. Gradually add liquid (oil and lemon) until smooth. Add water as needed to achieve a pâté consistency. Process herbs at the end. Serve on crackers, nori sheets, cucumber slices, or other desired veggie. Serves 4.

Herb Pâté

1½ cups almonds (soaked 12 hours, rinsed, drained)
¾ cup pine nuts
¼ cup of favorite herb (tarragon, sage, marjoram, rosemary)
2 tablespoons lemon juice
2 tablespoons olive oil
1 teaspoon garlic, minced, or a pinch of hing
2–3 tablespoons water, for consistency
1 teaspoon salt

First process pine nuts and almonds until ground. Add in the remaining ingredients. Drizzle in enough olive or flax oil while processing for a smooth consistency and a rich flavor. Serves 4.

Indian Bliss

1 cup sunflower seeds (soaked 12 hours, rinsed, drained)
1 cup almond pulp (fresh and moist from mylk making)
2 tablespoons raw, organic tahini
1 clove of garlic or ¼ teaspoon hing
½ tablespoon dill weed (or other favorite herb)
½ tablespoon cumin
½ tablespoon curry
Pinch cayenne
1 teaspoon fresh ginger, minced
½ teaspoon fresh turmeric, minced
2 teaspoon salt or more to taste

First process sunflower seeds and almonds until ground. Add in the remaining ingredients. Drizzle in enough olive or flax oil while processing for smooth consistency. Serves 4.

Under the Sea Pâté

2 cups almonds (soaked overnight)
½ cup celery, diced
¼ cup red pepper, diced
¼ cup green onions, chopped

3 tablespoons lemon

3 tablespoons olive oil

1 teaspoon salt

¼ cup dulse flakes

1 tablespoon kelp

Fresh ground pepper to taste

Process the almonds in a food processor with an S-blade. Add lemon, oil, and spices. Mix the celery, green onion, and bell pepper by hand. Serves 4.

Pink Pâté

2 cups almonds or sunflowers seeds (soaked overnight) or cashews

2 red peppers, seeded and chopped

3 tablespoons lemon

3 tablespoons olive oil

1 teaspoon salt

½ cup celery, diced

¼ cup green onions, chopped

½ cup wild capers or chopped green olives

Fresh ground pepper to taste

Process the nuts in a food processor with an S-blade. Add red peppers, lemon, oil, and salt. Process to combine. Mix the celery, green onion, and wild capers by hand. Serves 4.

Smaller Meals Recipes for Phase 1.0 Healing Diet

Includes soups, crackers, breads, seed cheeze, dips, dressings, juices, smoothies, and aromatic waters.

Soups

Miso Soup Broth with Chopped Veggies

2 cups water, warmed to 115°

4 tablespoons miso (nonsoy)

Blend all ingredients until smooth. Garnish with vegetables as desired: chopped avocado, parsley, bell pepper, nori, cilantro, celery. Serves 1 or 2.

Cucumber Tahini Soup

1–2 cucumbers
3 tablespoons tahini
1 teaspoon dried dill
½ teaspoon salt
½ teaspoon ginger, minced
3 tablespoons lime juice
Pinch cayenne
1½ cucumbers, diced
Olive oil, for garnish

Place all ingredients, except diced cucumber and olive oil, into blender. Blend until smooth. Pour into serving bowls and garnish with oil and diced cucumbers. Serves 2–3.

Red Pepper and Miso Soup

½ red pepper
4 tablespoons chickpea miso (nonsoy miso)
4 cups water (115° warmed)
2 tablespoons of tocotrienols
¼ inch ginger
Salt and pepper to taste

Blend all ingredients until smooth. Serves 2.

Spinach Vegetable Medley Soup

In bowl:
1 bell pepper (red or yellow), diced
2 ribs of celery, diced
½ bunch or 2 cups spinach, minced with S-blade in food processor
1 avocado, diced
½ bunch of cilantro or basil, S-bladed to mince
¼ cup sun-dried tomato, blended to a creamy texture in blender

2 tablespoons pumpkin seed, whole

1 tablespoon Italian seasoning

1 tablespoon cumin

1 tablespoon hemp, coconut, sesame, or cold-pressed olive oil

1 tablespoon lemon or ½ tablespoon apple cider vinegar

1 tablespoon sun-dried tomato water

½ tablespoon kalamata olive brine or apple cider vinegar

¼–½ teaspoon Transformational Salts or Himalayan salt

Dash cayenne

Dash hing

1 cup rooibos, nettle, or dandelion tea (recipe follows)

2–4 tablespoons nonsoy adzuki or chickpea miso (optional)

For superfood option, add 1 tablespoon spirulina, green powder, and/or 1 tablespoon of maca root powder

Toss all prepared ingredients into a pot. Warm to 100˚ and serve. Serves 1–2.

Note: This soup can be made in many different varieties by substituting various greens, herbs, and spices.

To make tea:

½ cup dry tea

3 cups hot water

Steep for 20 minutes and strain.

Hemp Spinach Basil Soup

1 small zucchini

1 rib of celery

1 bell pepper

½ bunch spinach or kale

¼ bunch of basil

¼ cup hemp seeds

½ cup olive brine, or 1 tablespoon of apple cider vinegar
    and ½ cup water

2 tablespoons hemp, sesame, or stone-ground cold-pressed olive oil

2 tablespoons lemon juice

2 tablespoons ginger juice

Dash cayenne

Pinch of chipotle

¼ teaspoon Transformational Salts or Himalayan salt

Chop the zucchini, celery, and bell pepper into similar size pieces. Tear the spinach or kale into pieces. Place all ingredients, except basil, in blender and blend on high speed. Chop the basil leaves and blend in lightly. Serves 1–2.

Classic Tomato Soup

1–2 cups sun-dried tomato

2 medium tomatoes

¼ cup sun-dried tomato water

¼–½ cup hemp seeds or sunflower seeds

2 tablespoons hemp oil or stone-ground cold-pressed olive oil

2 tablespoons lemon juice

2 tablespoons ginger juice

Dash Transformational Salts or Himalayan salt

Dash hing

Dash black pepper

Blessed water to desired consistency

Toss all ingredients into blender and blend on high speed. Serves 1–2.

Gazpacho

2 medium tomatoes

1 bell pepper

1 young raw nopal cactus pad, spines removed, or ½ cucumber

¼ cup hemp oil or stone-ground cold-pressed olive oil

Dash Transformational Salts or Himalayan salt

Dash black pepper

Dash hing

Dash cayenne

Toss all ingredients into blender and blend on high speed. Serve 1–2.

Super Green Cactus Chia Soup

1 young raw nopal cactus pad, spines removed

4 cups greens (kale, spinach, lamb's quarters, baby lettuces, or other favorite greens)

¼ cup hemp oil or stone-ground cold-pressed olive oil

¼ cup chia seeds or hemp seeds

2–4 tablespoons lemon juice

2–4 tablespoons ginger juice

1–3 teaspoons kelp powder

1–3 teaspoons maca root powder

Dash black pepper, cayenne, turmeric, and hing

Dash Transformational Salts or Himalayan salt

1 cup blessed water or more to desired consistency

Toss all ingredients into blender and blend on high speed. Serves 1–2.

Aloe Vera String Bean Soup

1 cup aloe vera, outside skin removed

1 cup string beans

2 cups greens (collards, kale, baby lettuces, spinach, or chard)

1 cup cilantro, chopped, loosely packed

¼ cup hemp oil or stone-ground cold-pressed olive oil

2–4 tablespoons lemon juice

2–4 tablespoons ginger juice

1–3 teaspoon kelp powder or other green superfood powders

Dash black pepper, cayenne, and hing

Dash to ¼ teaspoon Transformational Salts or Himalayan salt

1 cup blessed water to desired consistency

Toss all ingredients into blender and blend on high speed. Serves 1–2.

Aloe Vera Pad Burdock Cilantro Soup

1 cup aloe vera, diced, without the skin

1 cup cactus pad, diced

1 cup celery, roughly

1 cup cilantro, chopped, loosely packed

¼ cup burdock

2 teaspoons lemon juice

3 tablespoons stone-ground cold-pressed olive oil

1 tablespoon pumpkin seed oil

Dash to 1¼ teaspoon Transformational Salts or Himalayan salt

Dash cayenne

Dash black pepper

Dash hing

Toss all ingredients into blender and blend on high speed. Serves 1.

Crackers and Breads

Tools needed: Blender for grinding, large mixing bowl, food processor, S-blade, knife, cutting board, spice grinder or coffee grinder, dehydrator, dehydrator trays, teflex dehydrator sheets, and off-set spatula for spreading crackers.

Here are some tips, uses, and ideas for crackers and breads:

- For crackers and high moisture content breads, start the dehydration process on a teflex sheet. When the cracker or bread is semidry, place a tray with a mesh sheet on top face down. Flip both trays upside down so the cracker or bread ends up on the tray with the mesh.

- Use any leftover pâté to make crackers. You can thin the pâté slightly in order to spread it on the dehydrator tray, or you can process it with celery and flax seed.

- Use any leftover soak water from sun-dried tomatoes instead of water to add extra flavor.

- Lightly pat down sesame seeds or poppy seeds or any other seasonings on top of the crackers before dehydrating.

- To make breads airier and springier, add 1 cup of psyllium husk to any recipe that uses 2 cups of flour. Recipes that use more than 2 cups will need more psyllium. Use a 2:1 flour to psyllium ratio.

- Add 1 cup of blended young coconut meat to any recipe that uses 2 cups of flour for a heavenly light and creamy texture.
- You can always add both the psyllium and the coconut to your recipe, but if you do, you will also need to increase the herbs, spices, and salt to reach the desired flavor.

Here are directions for making crackers and breads:

Herby Chili Pepper Flax Crackers

4 cups golden flax, ground, soaked in sun-dried tomato water
    or blessed water
4 cups nuts or seeds, soaked, ground with S-blade or added whole
    if seed is small
4 cups sun-dried tomato, ground to a puree
½ cup poppy seed, whole
½ cup Italian seasoning
2 bunches cilantro or basil or other fresh herbs
3 tablespoons cumin seed, ground in spice or coffee grinder
1 tablespoon kelp, powdered
1 teaspoon chipotle
¼ teaspoon cayenne
1 teaspoon black pepper
3½ teaspoons Transformational Salts or Himalayan salt

Grind and soak flax in blessed water or sun-dried tomato water for 10 minutes in a large bowl. Roughly chop the herbs and mince with the S-blade in a food processor. Toss into the bowl. Grind soaked nuts or seeds with S-blade to a fine consistency, toss into the bowl, or if using whole seed, toss into the bowl whole. Grind sun-dried tomato to a puree, and toss into the bowl. Add salt, kelp, and spices. Stir. Spread on teflex dehydrator trays. Dehydrate for 4 hours. Flip the crackers onto a mesh sheet, removing the teflex sheet, and dehydrate for 12 more hours. Crackers will keep up to 3 weeks if stored in a cool, dry environment. Creates 9 trays of crackers.

Seedy Tomato Herb Crackers

2 cups flax seed, whole, soaked

2 cups nuts or seeds, soaked, ground with S-blade or added whole
    if seed is small

¼ cup ground flax seed

¼ cup poppy seed

¼ cup thyme

¼ cup Italian seasoning

1 bunch fresh herbs (marjoram, oregano, or basil)

1½ teaspoon Transformational Salts or Himalayan salt

¼ teaspoon hing

Pinch cayenne and/or chipotle

1 cup sun-dried tomato, soaked and blended

Mix all ingredients in a bowl. Spread on Teflex dehydrator sheets,
and dehydrate for 4 hours. Flip and dehydrate for 12 more hours.

Sun-Dried Tomato Bread

Base:

2 cups fresh nut/seed pulp or flour

2 cups sun-dried tomato, soaked and S-bladed to a puree

1 bunch basil

1 bunch of oregano or marjoram

½ cup poppy seed

½ cup Italian seasoning

¼ cup thyme

1 tablespoon olive oil

½ teaspoon Transformational Salts or Himalayan salt

Dash to ¼ teaspoon hing

Combine all ingredients.

Add:

2 cups golden flax, ground

Mix the flax into the base to achieve a dough-like texture. If using
dried nut or seed flour, you may need to add more liquid elements:

½–1 cup kalamata olive brine and/or sun-dried tomato water, added a little at a time to reach a cookie-dough consistency.

Mold dough into a loaf. Slice ⅜ to ½ inches thick. Lay on mesh trays and dehydrate for 2 hours.

Savory Bell Pepper Bread

Base:

2 cups fresh nut/seed pulp or flour

2 bell peppers, minced (red or yellow, or mixed)

1 to 2 bunches cilantro or basil, chopped with S-blade in a food processor

1 bunch fresh oregano or marjoram

½ cup poppy seeds

1 cup dried Italian seasoning

½ teaspoon Transformational Salts or Himalayan salt

½ teaspoon hing

Dash to ¼ teaspoon cayenne or chipotle

1 tablespoon olive oil

Combine all ingredients.

Add:

2 cups golden flax, ground

Mix the flax into the base to achieve a dough-like texture. If using dried nut or seed flour, you may need to add more liquid elements: ½–1 cup kalamata olive brine and/or sun-dried tomato water, added a little at a time to reach a cookie-dough consistency.

Mold dough into a loaf. Slice ⅛ to ½ inches thick. Lay on mesh trays and dehydrate for 2 hours.

Cumin Herb Bread

Base:

6 cups seed pulp or flour

3 bell peppers, minced with S-blade

1½ teaspoon salt

1 cup cumin, ground

1–2 bunch cilantro, chopped with S-blade in a food processor

½–1 cup poppy seeds

½–1 teaspoon hing

¼ teaspoon cayenne

2 tablespoons olive oil

Combine all ingredients.

Add:

6 cups golden flax, ground (optional if using dried nut or seed flour)

Additional liquid elements:

2–3 cups kalamata olive brine and or sun-dried tomato water (added a little at time to cookie-dough consistency). Note: The additional liquid elements may be necessary when you are using nut or seed flours.

Mold dough into a loaf. Slice ⅜ to ½ inches thick. Lay on mesh trays and dehydrate for 2 hours. Serve.

Dill Herb Bread

Base:

6 cups seed pulp or flour

2 bell peppers, minced with S-blade in a food processor

1½ teaspoon salt

½ cup dried dill

2–3 bunch dill, S-bladed

½–1 cup poppy seeds

¼ teaspoon cayenne

2 tablespoons olive oil

Combine all ingredients.

Add:

6 cups golden flax, ground (optional if using dried nut or seed flour)

Additional liquid elements:

2–3 cups kalamata olive brine and or sun-dried tomato water (added a little at time for a cookie-dough consistency). Note: The additional liquid elements may be necessary when you are using nut or seed flours.

Mold dough into a loaf. Slice 3/8 to ½ inches thick. Lay on mesh trays and dehydrate for 2 hours. Serve.

Oregano Cilantro Herb Bread

Base:

6 cups sesame seeds, seed pulp or flour

1½ teaspoon salt

1 cup dried Italian seasonings

2–3 bunch cilantro

2 bunch fresh oregano

½–1 cup poppy seeds

1 teaspoon hing

1 teaspoon cayenne

2 tablespoons olive oil

Combine all ingredients.

Add:

6 cups golden flax, ground (optional if using dried nut or seed flour)

Additional liquid elements:

2–3 cups kalamata olive brine and or sun-dried tomato water (adding a little at time for a cookie-dough consistency). Note: The additional liquid elements may be necessary when you are using nut or seed flours.

Mold dough into a loaf. Slice 3/8 to ½ inches thick. Lay on mesh trays and dehydrate for 2 hours. Serve.

Seed and Nut Cheezes

Almond Fermented Cheeze

4 cups almonds, soaked and peeled

4 cups water

¼ teaspoon ultra probiotic powder

Put the peeled almonds and 4 cups of water in a high-speed blender and blend until creamy. Add the probiotic by hand. Scoop the almond cream into a nut mylk bag. Close the bag tight with the string. Place the bag on a strainer with a heavy weight on top to press the water out of the almond cream. Let it ferment overnight for about 14 to 18 hours. Take out of the bag and season with salt, apple cider vinegar, and lemon to taste. The amount of lemon and vinegar will depend and how your fermented cheeze comes out. Taste the cheeze after you add the salt and see if it is tangy enough for you. Otherwise, add a little more lemon and vinegar to accentuate the tanginess of the cheeze. Form into balls the size of your hands (like a tennis ball), then roll on top of fresh ground pepper and flatten to 2- to 3-inch wheels. This will make about 6 wheels and it will last for about 2 months refrigerated. You can season with many other spices like turmeric and paprika. If you are going to roll your cheeze with fresh herb like chives, dill, or mint, make sure you use within 7 days.

Feta

1 cup nut/seed pulp (wet or dry)
3 tablespoons lemon juice
3 tablespoons olive oil
2 tablespoons thyme (optional)
Salt and pepper to taste

Put all the ingredients in a bowl and mix with a fork until it starts to stick together and forms crumbs. Eat as is or on top of salads. Serves 2–4.

Seed Cheeze

Base:
  1 bunch fresh herb, cilantro, or basil, S-bladed in food processor
  2 cups sunflower seeds or soaked walnuts, ground with an S-blade
Add:
  4–6 tablespoons stone-ground cold-pressed olive oil or hemp oil
  2 tablespoons lemon juice
  2 tablespoons kalamata olive brine
  2 tablespoons sun-dried tomato water
  ¼–½ teaspoon Transformational Salts or Himalayan salt

Dash cayenne or chipotle

Dash hing or 1 clove of garlic

Optional:

¼ cup Italian seasoning

2 tablespoons thyme

Process herbs in food processor with S-blade and set aside. Grind sunflower seeds in a food processor to a fine texture. Add remaining ingredients and herbs to the food processor container, and process to a creamy texture. Serves 4.

Brazil Nut, Olive, and Herb Cheeze

1 cup sunflower seeds

1 cup Brazil nuts

¼ cup olive oil (or other recommended oil to taste)

2–4 tablespoons lemon juice

Dash hing

½ tablespoon black pepper

¼–½ teaspoon Transformational Salts or Himalayan salt

2 tablespoons thyme or Italian seasoning, dried

1 cup kalamata olives, minced

¼ cup oregano or dill, fresh, chopped

Kalamata olive brine water or blessed water, to desired texture

Process nuts and seeds to a butter or as much as possible. Add olive oil, lemon, hing, black pepper, salt, and dried herbs. Process with enough kalamata olive brine to reach a creamy consistency. Pour or scoop into a bowl, then mix in olives and fresh herbs by hand. Serves 4.

Dips

Hummus

8 ounces sprouted chickpeas (garbanzo beans)

¼ cup lemon juice

¼ cup olive oil

2 tablespoons tahini

1 clove garlic

3 ounces water

Hot water (145°) for soaking

Soak chickpeas in the hot water for 10 to 15 minutes. Put all the ingredients in the blender and blend until creamy. Serve in a plate and decorate with paprika. Drizzle olive oil on top. Serves 4 to 6 as a side dish.

Red Pepper Dipping Sauce

1 bunch cilantro

4 cups bell pepper

1 cup tomato

2 cups almond (prepared according to instructions in "Soaking and Sprouting" section)

¼ cup hemp or olive oil

½ cup lemon juice

½ teaspoon Himalayan Salt

1 clove garlic

Chop cilantro and set aside. Blend bell pepper with all the ingredients until creamy. Add the chopped cilantro and serve. If you desire as a dressing, put back into the blender and add water to the dip until it reaches salad dressing consistency.

Mayonnaise

½ cup hemp seeds

1 cup macadamia nuts

¼ cup lemon juice

½ cup olive oil

1 teaspoon mustard seed (ground)

1 teaspoon salt

Blend all ingredients until smooth.

Red wasabi variation:

Set aside ½ of the mayo and add:

½ cup red bell pepper, roughly chopped

4 tablespoons ginger juice

2 tablespoons dulse flakes

2 tablespoons wasabi powder

Blend until smooth.

Green wasabi variation:

With the other ½ of the mayo, add:

3 kale leaves, destemmed

4 tablespoons ginger juice

2 tablespoons wasabi powder

Blend until smooth.

These two variations are a great accompaniment to sushi!

Sour Cream

Base:

2 cups sunflower seeds, soaked or use young coconut pulp

½ cup sesame seeds, soaked

½ cup lemon juice

½ cup olive oil

3 teaspoons salt

Water

Blend until very creamy, adding water to reach sour cream consistency.

Dill Sunflower Dip

2 cups sunflower

¼ cup olive oil

¼ cup lemon juice

1 teaspoon salt

¼ cup dill, chopped

⅕ cup green onions (optional)

Blend all the ingredients except dill and the green onions until creamy. Blend the dill and the green onions by hand and serve.

Variation for tzatziki:

1 teaspoon cumin

½ cup fresh herbs, cilantro, and/or parsley, finely chopped

2 cups cucumbers, cubed or sliced

Add cumin to the mix and blend again. Mix the fresh herbs by hand. In a bowl, add the cubed cucumber and pour the sauce on top. Decorate with green onions. Serves 8 as a side dish.

Spinach Cream

3 cups spinach

1 cup cashews

2 tablespoons lemon juice

1 tablespoon ginger juice,

1 teaspoon coriander

½ cup water

½ teaspoon salt

½ teaspoon white pepper or to taste

Blend all together in the blender and serve in a bowl. Use celery sticks or red pepper sticks to dip or any bread cracker recipe. If you have any leftovers, you can always use to coat your nori sheet and make a delicious new nori cracker.

Tomato Dipping Sauce

6 sun-dried tomatoes, soaked

1½ cups tomatoes, cubed

2 tablespoons lemon juice

2 tablespoons, ginger juice, or a small piece of ginger about 1 inch

¼ teaspoon salt

¼ teaspoon white pepper

¼ teaspoon paprika

¼ teaspoon curry

¼ teaspoon turmeric

¼ cup cilantro, finely chopped

½ cup green onion, finely chopped

Put the cilantro and the green onion aside. Mix all the ingredients in the blender and blend to make the sauce. Pour into a bowl and add the cilantro and the green onions. Use with vegetables sticks, crackers, or on top of zucchini pasta.

Dressings

Here are some tips, ideas, and uses for dressings:
- Any salad dressing can be used to make nori crackers. Just spread on top of the nori sheet and dehydrate.
- Use any leftover salad dressing to marinate zucchini chips and dehydrate.
- Massage any dressing into kale or any other greens and dehydrate to make chips.
- Use any salad dressing and drizzle on top of your quinoa, millet, amaranth, or buckwheat.
- If you are not sure how much salt you like, just start with a little and increase until you arrive to the right taste.
- When you use ginger in your recipes, the taste and the intensity varies according to the type of ginger and how long the ginger has been at the store. Start adding a little and then more until you arrive at the right taste.
- Use herbal teas instead of water in your salad dressings to add a different twist.

Here are directions for making dressings:

Café House Dressing

1 inch fresh ginger
¼ cup lemon juice
5 tablespoons miso
¼ cup sesame oil
¾ cup water
Salt to taste

Blend all ingredients until smooth. Makes about 1½ cups of dressing.

Tomato Dressing

½ cup sun-dried tomato, rehydrated
½ cup sunflower seeds
½ cup blessed water
¼ cup sun-dried tomato water
2 tablespoons olive oil or sesame oil
1 tablespoon lemon juice
½ tablespoon ginger
Dash Transformational Salts or Himalayan salt
Dash cayenne
Dash hing

Blend all ingredients until smooth. Makes about 2 cups of dressing.

Tahini Dressing

1 cup sesame seeds
½ cup kalamata olive brine or ½ cup blessed water with a dash
   of salt
3 tablespoons lemon juice
2–3 tablespoons tomato soak water
2 tablespoons ginger juice
3 tablespoons olive oil (or other recommended oil to taste)
1 tablespoon sesame oil
1 tablespoon cumin
¼ teaspoon black pepper
Dash Transformational Salts or Himalayan salt
Dash cayenne
Dash hing

Blend all ingredients until smooth. Makes about 2 cups of dressing.

Avocado Caraway Dressing

1 avocado
3 tablespoons lemon juice
3 tablespoons ginger juice

2 teaspoons caraway

¼ teaspoon black pepper

Dash cayenne

Dash hing

1 cup kalamata olive water or blessed water with a dash to ¼
teaspoon of Transformational Salts or Himalayan salt

Blend all ingredients until smooth. Makes about 1½ cups of dressing.

Dulse Dressing

1 avocado

3 tablespoons lemon juice

3 tablespoons dulse flakes

2 tablespoons ginger juice

¼ teaspoon black pepper

1 cup blessed water

Dash to ¼ teaspoon Transformational Salts or Himalayan salt

Pinch cayenne

Blend all ingredients until smooth. Makes about 1½ cups of
dressing.

Cumin Caesar Dressing

1 avocado

3 tablespoons lemon juice

3 tablespoons ginger juice

2 tablespoons olive oil (or other recommended oil to taste)

1 tablespoon cumin

¼ teaspoon black pepper

1 cup kalamata olive water or blessed water with a dash to
¼ teaspoon of Transformational Salts or Himalayan salt

Dash cayenne

Dash hing

Blend all ingredients until smooth. Makes about 1½ cups of
dressing.

Creamy Italian Dressing

1 cup tomato
1 avocado
¼ cup olive oil
1 teaspoon Italian seasoning
2 tablespoons lemon juice
¼ teaspoon black pepper
Dash hing
Dash Transformational Salts or Himalayan salt
½ bunch fresh oregano

Blend tomato with olive oil, lemon juice, avocado, hing, spice, salt, and pepper. Chop oregano. Mix into dressing and blend lightly. Makes about 2 cups of dressing.

Thai-Style Caesar Dressing

1 avocado
3 tablespoons lime juice
½ kaffir lime leaf and/or few sprigs of cilantro for variation
1 teaspoon minced lemon grass or a sprig of basil, for variation
2 tablespoons sesame oil or hemp seed oil
2 tablespoons ginger juice
¼ teaspoon black pepper
1 cup blessed water
Dash to ¼ teaspoon Transformational Salts or Himalayan salt
Pinch cayenne

Blend all ingredients until smooth. Makes about 2 cups of dressing.

Hemp Seed Dressing

½ cucumber
¼ cup hemp oil
2 tablespoons ginger juice
2 tablespoons lemon juice
½ cup hemp seed
¼ cup basil

2 tablespoons oregano, fresh

Dash Transformational Salts or Himalayan salt

Blend cucumber with hemp oil, ginger juice, and lemon juice. Add hemp seed and blend. Chop basil and oregano. Mix into dressing. Makes about 1½ cups of dressing.

Creamy Italian Dressing with Brazil Nuts

½ cucumber

2 tablespoons lemon juice

2 tablespoons ginger juice

¼ cup olive oil

½ cup Brazil nuts

¼ cup fresh basil, chopped

2 tablespoons fresh oregano, chopped

Dash Transformational Salts or Himalayan salt

Blend cucumber with lemon juice, ginger juice, and olive oil. Add Brazil nuts and blend. Mix chopped basil and oregano into dressing. Makes about 1½ cups of dressing.

Hemp Seed Ranch Dressing

1 cup hemp seeds, unsoaked

½ cup sunflower seeds, soaked

¾ cup olive oil

¼ cup lemon juice

¼ cup water

1 tablespoon jalapeno, chopped

¾ teaspoon salt

¼ teaspoon black pepper

1 tablespoon dried dill

Blend all ingredients until smooth.

Then add:

½ cup fresh parsley

½ cup fresh cilantro

Blend just until herbs are mixed and the dressing is speckled green. Add more water if needed. Makes about 3 cups of dressing.

Spirulina Dressing

1 avocado
½ cup lemon juice
3 tablespoons hemp
1 tablespoon spirulina
¼ teaspoon salt
¼ cup water, as needed to thin consistency
Pinch cayenne pepper

Blend ingredients in a blender. Add water as needed to reach desired consistency. Makes about 1½ cups of dressing.

Sea Goddess Dressing

½ ounce dried wakame, soaked 5 minutes until soft
½ cup almonds, soaked
½ cup water
1 tablespoon tahini
1 tablespoon miso
Dash nutmeg
Dash cayenne
Salt and pepper, to taste

Blend all ingredients until smooth. Makes about 1½ cups of dressing.

Spinach Tahini Dressing

3 cups spinach
1 cup fresh basil
½ cup celery
½ cup tahini
¼ cup fresh oregano
1 tablespoon Italian seasonings

1 cup celery juice or 2 stalks celery with ¾ cup of water or tea

1 teaspoon lemon juice

1 teaspoon salt

Blend all ingredients until smooth. Makes about 2 cups of dressing.

Quick Tahini Dressing

2 cups sesame seeds, unsoaked

¼ cup lemon juice

1 cup water

2 tablespoons miso

Black pepper to taste

Blend until creamy. Add more water for desired consistency. Makes about 3 cups of dressing.

Juices

Green Juice

80 percent celery and cucumber

20 percent leafy greens (kale, spinach, collards, chard, parsley, cilantro, etc.)

Additions:

Bell pepper

Burdock root

Fresh ginger root

Fennel

Fresh turmeric

Radish

Base for one juice:

2 cucumbers

¼ head of celery

4 kale leaves or the equivalent of any other leafy greens

Run vegetables through a juicer along with selections from the additions to suit your taste and enjoy!

V-6 Juice

3 cups tomatoes
1 celery stalk
1 cucumber
Dash salt
Dash pepper
Cayenne to taste
Lemon/lime to taste

Blend all ingredients until smooth.

Ginger Juice

2–4 inches of ginger, peeled and chopped
1 cup water

Blend in a high-speed blender and strain through a nylon mesh seed or nut mylk bag, cheesecloth, or a natural-fiber seed or nut mylk bag. You can also make pure ginger juice by juicing the ginger in a masticating juice. However, you will have to adjust the quantities you use in the recipes because the juice will be much stronger tasting.

Smoothies

Basic Green Blender Full

3 bell peppers (red, orange, yellow, or mixed)
½–1 avocado
3 cups greens (spinach, kale, collards, cilantro)
2 tablespoons lemon juice
2 tablespoons ginger juice (see recipe in the juice section)
2 cups blessed water

Blend all ingredients until smooth. Creates 1 full Vitamix blender. Serves 1–2.

Green Smoothie

1 young coconut, pulp and water
½ or 1 bunch of lettuce, collards, kale, or spinach

3 tablespoons green superfoods powder

1 tablespoon maca

Blend all ingredients until smooth. Serves 1.

Chia Smoothie

3 tablespoons chia

16 ounces any nut mylk

1 teaspoon Chaga

3 dry lavender flowers

1 tablespoon xylitol or stevia to taste

Pinch of salt

Ground the chia seeds in the coffee grinder and then blend all ingredients until smooth. Serves 1.

Chia Chai Smoothie

3 tablespoons chia

1 teaspoon cinnamon

Pinch of nutmeg, microplaned

Pinch cardamom

Ginger juice, to taste

Pinch of Transformational Salts or Himalayan salt

2 tablespoons xylitol or stevia, whole leaf, powder to taste

16 ounces of any nut mylk (if you want you can add ice to it too)

Blend all ingredients until smooth. Serves 1.

Aloe Vera and Lemon Smoothie

2 cups aloe vera

1 tablespoon lemon juice

1 teaspoon blessed water

Blend all ingredients until smooth. Serves 1.

Cinnamon Chia Smoothie

1 cup chia seeds

2–3 tablespoons cinnamon

1 tablespoon carob

½ nutmeg, microplaned

1 teaspoon cardamom

½ teaspoon Transformational Salts or Himalayan salt

¼ teaspoon stevia, whole leaf, powder, or ½–1 dropper of liquid

8 cups blessed water, or 7 cups blessed water plus 1 cup ice

Toss all dry ingredients into the blender with half of the water (and ice, if using), and blend. Add remaining water and blend until smooth. Serves 1–2.

Aromatic Waters

Our health is affected by the quality and the quantity of water we drink. Water produces hydroelectricity when it rushes through the cell membrane, producing a molecular exchange and making the whole body work properly.

With the lack of proper fluid flow, nothing communicates well, leaving us vulnerable to disease. At the Tree of Life all our water (even the bathing water) is purified through reverse osmosis, and filters are tested regularly. I also use distilled drinking water. I distill our water with a home water distiller. I recommend adding minerals back to the water using ionic minerals or a pinch of Transformational Salts or Himalayan salt, structuring the water using Crystal Energy. All of these items are available at Dr. Cousens's online store.

A good measure to know that you are well hydrated is urinating every 90 to 120 minutes. A hydrated body produces clear, colorless urine. In this section, we show you ideas on how to flavor your water to awaken the consciousness to drink sufficient water. It is a great idea to have water with you at all times. Most of the time we are not really hungry—we are thirsty! Having plenty of water throughout the day will help you stay on track, making your transition to better eating habits much easier. The most important thing you can do for your water is restructuring its vibration by blessing it!

Water with Mint Leaves and Fennel

1 bunch of fresh mint
½ fennel
About 60 oz of water
Pinch of Transformational Salts or Himalayan salt

Put all the ingredients in a pitcher with water, stir, and let it rest for 1 hour. Serve throughout the day.

Water with Peppermint Oil and Lemon Slices

5 drops food-grade peppermint oil
1 lemon sliced very thin
Pinch of Transformational Salts or Himalayan salt

Put all the ingredients in a pitcher with about 60 ounces of water, stir, and let it rest for 1 hour. Serve throughout the day.

Herbal Iced Tea

Herbal tea of your choice

Make a big pitcher and refrigerate. Keep in mind that what you do not use you can substitute for water in all your recipes.

Ginger Lemonade with Stevia and/or Xylitol

½ inch of ginger
2 lemons peeled and cut in four
Pinch of Transformational Salts or Himalayan salt
Xylitol or stevia to taste
32 ounces cold water

Put all the ingredients in the blender and blend. Strain and serve.

Lemonade

1¼ cup lemon juice
16 ounces water
Pinch of Transformational Salts or Himalayan salt
Xylitol powder or stevia to taste

Put all the ingredients in a 16-ounce glass and enjoy.

Jamaica Flower Sun Tea

1½ ounces dried Jamaica flowers (hibiscus flowers)
64 ounces spring water
Pinch of Transformational Salts or Himalayan salt

Put the Jamaica flower and the water in a glass container with a lid over it. Place in a very sunny window or outside where the sun will shine on it. Let it sit until the water takes a deep pomegranate color. It will take about 4 to 6 hours, depending on the warmth of the day. Strain the tea into a pitcher and enjoy warm, room temperature, or cold. You can add stevia or xylitol if you wish to enjoy a sweet drink.

Snacks Recipes for Phase 1.0 Healing Diet

This section will give you an overall idea of what you can eat between meals or take with you during the day. Being prepared with some easy snacks will help you to avoid eating foods that are not part of the Phase 1.0 Healing Diet. If you are a person that needs to snack, be prepared. Also, nowadays it is possible to find a raw section at your local organic market where you can find ready made snacks that you can buy. Just read the ingredient list and make sure they fit into the Phase 1.0 Healing Diet. We will provide a list of snacks that we have already prescreened and can be purchased at Dr. Cousens's online store. The easiest thing to do is to carry nuts, seeds, and dehydrated food.

List of snacks:

It's Alive: Crackers and Seeds
Gone Nuts: Marinara, Chipotle, Cilantro/Lime
Fragmints: Assorted Flavors: Lemon, Berry, Peppermint, Wintergreen, Cinnamon, and so on
Kale Krunchies: Mega Green, Herbs de Provence, Sassy Spice
Nuts and nut butters
Noni Land: Coconut Crisps
Rejuvenate Foods: Kim Chi and Sauerkraut
Aimee's Living Magic: Crackers and Cereals
Sea Vegetables: Nori, Kombu, Wakame, Hijiki, Laver, Alaria, Sea Lettuce, Dulse

Red Minipeppers Stuffed with Nut Pâté

1 or 2 red mini peppers cut in half

2 to 3 tablespoons nut pâté

Cut the mini peppers in half and stuff with any nut pâté. Eat as is or dehydrate for 2 hours and then eat.

Raw Nut Trail Mix

½ cup walnut

½ cup almonds

½ cup pumpkin seeds

½ cup sunflower seeds

½ cup pecans

Soak with 3 or 10 percent hydrogen peroxide (food grade) for 20 minutes and then rinse well. Soak with clean water for six more hours. Drain the water and season. For a simple delicious seasoning, just sprinkle with Transformational Salts and dehydrate at 115° for 24 hours or until crispy. They will be nice and crunchy, ready to eat, and better than roasted nuts! Seal in an airtight container and use as needed. They will be good for about 1 month.

Variation in flavors:

Savory: 1 tablespoon of turmeric, salt to taste, 1 teaspoon cinnamon, 1 teaspoon cardamom

Sweet: 1 tablespoon cinnamon, pinch of salt, 2 teaspoons xylitol, 1 tablespoon maca

Italian: ½ tablespoon olive oil; Italian seasoning; fresh tomatoes, cubed; garlic powder or fresh, crushed red pepper (for a spicy flavor).

Mix all with trail mix and dehydrate in mesh tray until all is crispy.

Pickles

¾ cup unpasteurized apple cider vinegar

1 cup filtered or spring water

1 teaspoon Transformational Salts or Himalayan salt

2 teaspoons ground pickling spice (which you can buy already blended) or just use 2 or 3 whole garlic cloves cut in half or

quarters, 1 tablespoon of chopped fresh or dry dill, and ½ table
spoon peppercorns

1 cucumber cut into ¼-inch thick rounds or into long segments

1 small daikon radish peeled ¼-inch thick pieces, round

¼ fennel, cut in quarters

Put vinegar, water, salt, and pickling spice or the fresh spices into a
1-quart mason jar with lid. Tighten the lid and shake to combine the
ingredients. Add the vegetables to the jar, close tightly, and shake
well to distribute pickling spice. Let sit for at least 5 hours or overnight, and then refrigerate. Use only cucumbers or a combination of
other vegetables like red radish, ginger, and so on. Pickles are great
on their own or combined into salads or on top of crackers. For a
pickle relish, put your pickle mix in the food processor with little bit
of stevia or xylitol and grind. Use this pickle relish on top of avocados, salads, breads, and all your other wonderful creations.

Kale Chips

4 bunches of lacinato kale, washed and without the stem

1 cup hemp seeds

Sauce:

1 cup hemp seed

¼ cup hemp seed oil

¾ cup of water

½ cup of lemon

Salt and pepper to taste

Blend until creamy. Put all the lacinato kale in a bowl and then put
all the sauce on top, with 1 cup of hemp seeds. Massage to evenly
coat the kale. Place the whole preparation on 2 or 3 mesh trays, all
bunched up, and dehydrate at 115° overnight until crispy. It's a delicious snack you can eat any time!

Sauce Variations:

For a simple preparation you can use olive oil, lemon, salt and
pepper.

Use any dressing you might have left over.

Use other leaves like curly kale, rapini leaves, beats, or daikon
leaves.

Use any leftover pâté and add more lemon, oil, or water to make a sauce.

Sauerkraut

Tools needed:

Mandolin

Glass jar, quart size, with an air lock setup

Ingredients:

1 cabbage, large

1–3 teaspoons salt

⅛ teaspoon ultra probiotic

Shred the cabbage with a mandolin very thin or to the desired consistency of the final product. It can also be done in a food processor with a slicing attachment. Sprinkle with salt and massage the cabbage with your hands until it becomes soft and gives off water. Mix in the probiotics and pack in the 1-quart glass jar (with an air lock setup). Make sure water is covering the cabbage completely. If the cabbage did not give off enough water, add spring water to cover 1–2 inches above the cabbage line. Allow the cabbage to culture for about 3 to 10 days at room temperature. Once the sauerkraut is finished, move to a new glass jar and store in the refrigerator. Aging the sauerkraut in the refrigerator for 4–6 weeks improves the flavor.

Variation:

For a more complex flavor, add caraway seeds or combine with sea vegetables like dulse or alaria.

Zucchini Chips

6 zucchinis

Slice the zucchinis with a mandolin; place the zucchini vertically to get ⅛-inch thick round chips. Season with salt, pepper, vinegar, and olive oil and dehydrate on mesh trays until crispy. You can use any salad dressing for seasoning, too. When you place zucchini chips on the trays, make sure they are not on top of each other because they will stick together as they dehydrate.

Phase 1.0 Healing Diet Sweet Delights Recipes

Although all the sweet delights recipes are Phase 1.0, we recommend only eating them occasionally or as a party food. For some people, sweet taste can trigger old cellular memories and might encourage unintentional deviation from the healing path. It is best to keep away from sweet tastes until you are completely healed.

Creamy Vanilla Pudding

1 zucchini (about ½–¾ cup, chopped)

1 cup cashews

2 tablespoons xylitol

5 drops of liquid stevia

2 tablespoons psyllium husk

¾ cup water

Pinch of salt

Pinch of vanilla powder

9 drops of vanilla flavor

Put all ingredients in a blender and blend. The psyllium husk takes a few minutes to thicken into a pudding texture. Let it rest for 3 minutes in the blender and blend again. Chill and serve. Serves 2–3.

Halva

2 cups whole sesame seeds (light brown color)

6 tablespoons coconut butter

1 cup cashew

½ cup xylitol powder

2 droppers full of vanilla flavor

1 teaspoon Transformational Salts or Himalayan salt

Wash in hydrogen peroxide (food grade) and then soak the sesame for 4 hours. Dehydrate for about 12 hours at 115° until the seeds are dry again. The washing and soaking takes the bitter flavor out of the sesame seeds. Grind the sesame seeds and the cashews in a spice grinder or a high power blender. Put all the ingredients in a food processor with an S-blade and process until they form a dough. Take out and shape into a loaf. Refrigerate until it becomes hard. Cut with a sharp knife into ¼-inch slices and enjoy with your friends!

Bonbons

½ cup shredded coconut

¼ cup xylitol powder

2 cups cashew

¼ teaspoon Transformational Salts or Himalayan salt

6 tablespoons coconut butter

Put the shredded coconut on top of a cutting board and set aside. Powder the ¼ cup of xylitol by putting it in a coffee or spice grinder. Put all the ingredients except the shredded coconut in the food processor with S-blade and process until they form a dough-like consistency. Make balls about 1-inch round. To decorate, roll the balls with the shredded coconut. Makes 30 delicious bonbons.

Variations:

Add different spices for diverse flavors. Use this recipe as a base and then add cinnamon, vanilla, ginger, camu camu, or carob.

Ginger Pudding

Pulp of 4 young coconuts

5 drops of vanilla flavor

2 tablespoons ginger juice (see recipe in Juice section) or 1-inch piece of fresh root

2 tablespoons xylitol or stevia to taste

Blend until very smooth. Serve in a cup and drizzle with cinnamon.

Cinnamon Mousse

1 cup cashew

½ cup nut mylk or water

1 yellow zucchini

2 tablespoons coconut butter

½ cup xylitol

¼ teaspoon salt

¼ teaspoon nutmeg

5 drops of vanilla essential oil

½ tablespoon cinnamon

Process all ingredients in a food processor until very smooth. Chill and enjoy! Serves 4.

Key Lime Pie

Crust ingredients:

½ cup whole flax seed (ground)

½ cup tocotrienols

¼ cup almond flour

¼ cup coconut oil

3 tablespoons xylitol powder

¼ teaspoon salt

Cream filling ingredients:

1 cup hydrated Irish moss

3 cups cashew/coconut mylk (1 cup cashews and 1 cup shredded coconut with 3 cups of water, blended and strained)

¾ cup lime juice

½ tsp lemon essence

½ cup xylitol

Pinch salt

1 cup coconut oil

To make the crust:

Combine all ingredients in a bowl. Press into a spring form pan.

To make the filling:

Blend the Irish moss with the mylk, lime juice, lemon essence, xylitol, and salt until completely smooth. Add coconut oil and blend for about 30 seconds only, to avoid saponization of coconut oil. Pour the filling on top of the base and chill until firm. Serves 8–10.

Angel Wings Sabayon Cake

Crust:

2¼ cups almond flour

6 tablespoons xylitol powder

¾ cup tocotrienols

⅓ cup coconut butter

½ cup coconut oil

⅛ tsp salt

42 drops vanilla essence (nonalcoholic)

Angel wings cream:

1 scant cup coconut butter

⅓ cup xylitol

22 drops vanilla essence

1¼ cup water

Pinch of salt

Sabayon ingredients:

1 cup cashews

1 cup shredded coconut

4 cups water

Pinch of salt

½ cup sabayon tea (recipe follows)

1 sachet cho-wa (chinese supplement, optional)

½ tablespoon chaga

5 dropperfuls Earth Drops: Wild Ginseng

⅞ cup xylitol

1 cups hydrated Irish moss packed

½ cup coconut oil

1 teaspoon ceylon cinnamon

To make crust:

Mix all ingredients in a bowl with a fork until the mixture is crumbly. Press ¾ of mixture into the bottom of a 10-inch spring form pan. Set aside.

To make sabayon:

Blend the cashews, shredded coconut, water, and salt to and strain to smooth mylk. Put back in the blender and add tea, chaga, ginseng, xylitol, Irish moss, and cho-wa (if using). Blend until smooth. When the mixture is smooth, with the blender still running, add the coconut oil and cinnamon. Pour mixture on top of the base in the spring form pan.

To make angel wings cream:

Blend coconut butter, xylitol, vanilla essence, water, and salt. Pour into the cake to create a swirling effect. Sprinkle the reserved ½ cup of crumb mixture on top. Freeze for 1 to 2 hours until firm, then refrigerate. Serves 10–12.

Note: This recipe makes a large cake that makes 16 servings. To make a smaller cake, half the ingredients and use a 7- or 8-inch spring form pan.

Sabayon tea:

3 tablespoons chicory root

2 tablespoons roasted dandelion

1 tablespoon rhodiola

2 cups spring water

Put all herbs into a bowl. Heat the water to a simmer and pour over the herbs. Allow the herbs to steep for 20 minutes.

This recipe makes 2 cups. The tea can be diluted further and used as a tea with nut mylk or on its own.

Maintenance Diet Recipes: 20 Percent Cooked Meal Options

We recommend expanding to the maintenance diet once you are completely healed. When you prepare the recipes in this section, you will be able to observe a variety of techniques, such us adding salt at the end of the cooking process, adding raw veggies to a small portion of cooked seeds, using a lead-free clay pot for cooking, and so on. These recipes are designed to help you become aware of the healthiest ways to cook and also what to eat if you are going to be cooking. For some people, it might be a big leap to go from an American junk food diet to a completely organic live-food Phase 1.0 healing diet. Those who want to do it but feel it will be a big stretch may want to consider starting from this section and gradually moving to a Phase 1.0 diet.

Millet, amaranth, buckwheat, and quinoa are usually described as grains, but while they are indeed granular, they are in fact seeds. Seeds are lower in carbohydrates and often higher in protein and other nutrients. They also have a lower glycemic index than grains (wheat, rice, oats, etc.). Quinoa, millet, buckwheat, and amaranth contain no gluten. These seeds are delicious, nutritious, and very easy to cook and sprout.

To cook these seeds, it is best to use clay pots or a rice cooker, although it is not necessary.

Cooking Measurements for Clay Pot Cooking or a Rice Cooker

Millet	Quinoa	Amaranth	Buckwheat
Soak for 20 minutes in hydrogen peroxide (food grade)	Soak for 20 minutes in hydrogen peroxide (food grade)	No need to soak	Soak for 20 minutes in hydrogen peroxide (food grade)
1 cup millet	1 cup quinoa	1 cup amaranth	1 cup buck wheat
1 cup water	¾ cup water	¾ cup water	¾ cup water
Yields 3 cups when cooked	Yields 2¾ cups when cooked	Yields 2 cups when cooked	Yields 3 cups when cooked

Basic Cooking and Cleaning Directions for Your Seeds

Cover your seeds (except amaranth) generously with water and soak for 20 minutes, adding 2 tablespoons of 3 or 10 percent food-grade hydrogen peroxide. After 20 minutes, rinse several times until the water comes out clean and clear.

Put the desired amount of seeds with the recommended amount of water in a clay pot or rice cooker. Bring to a boil and then simmer (30 minutes for millet, 25 minutes for quinoa, 20 minutes for buckwheat, and 25 minutes for amaranth). Once it is cooked, fluff with a fork and drizzle with coconut or hempseed oil and add salt to taste.

Notes:

- Buckwheat groats are an exception to these directions because they are porous and absorb the water quickly. They do best if water is boiling before they are added. Cover and return to a boil once groats are in pot. Turn heat to low and steam for the specified time.

- Buckwheat, millet, and quinoa are always best prepared by cleaning with hydrogen peroxide and then rinsing in a fine strainer for 2 minutes or until the water comes out clean. Quinoa has what is called the saponins, a natural protective coating, that will give a bitter flavor if not rinsed off before cooking.
- There is no need to clean amaranth with hydrogen peroxide. Just measure, give a quick rinse, add water, and cook.
- Don't cook your Transformational Salts or Himalayan salt. Always add at the end to conserve most of the minerals intact.

Buckwheat Breakfast Meal (Better than Oatmeal)

1 cup buckwheat grouts, raw
¾ cup water
1 teaspoon cinnamon
1 tablespoon shredded coconut
1 cup nut mylk
2 teaspoon tocotrienols (optional)
Dash of salt

Cook the buckwheat only with water, bring to a boil, and simmer for 20 minutes. Put the buckwheat in a bowl and add the rest of the ingredient and enjoy! Serves 2 or 3.

Millet Breakfast Mix

½ cup cooked millet (see chart)
2 tablespoons chopped walnuts, almonds, or pecans
Nut mylk to cover

Millet is an alkaline grain. Flavor with your favorite spices, such as cinnamon, cardamom, vanilla, coconut flakes, and coconut oil. Add a pinch of salt and sweeten with licorice root powder, xylitol, or stevia. Serves 1.

Buckwheat Tabouli

1 cup buckwheat
½ cup red pepper, finely chopped

¼ cup celery, finely chopped
¼ cup cilantro, finely chopped
1 cup parsley, finely chopped
½ cup cucumber, finely chopped
½ avocado, small cubed
2 tablespoons lemon juice
2 tablespoons olive oil
¼ teaspoon salt

Cook the buckwheat and set aside to cool down. Add the rest of the ingredients, mix, and serve. Serves 2 or 4.

Simple Lentil Soup

4 cups lentils, washed and picked through for any pebbles
1–2 bay leaves
4 tomatoes, chopped
1 big onion, chopped (optional)
3 stalks celery, chopped
1 or more cloves garlic, minced (optional)
Salt and pepper to taste

In a pot, cover lentils (plus a couple inches above) with water. Add all other ingredients. Bring to a boil until lentils are tender (30–60 minutes). Toss in chopped parsley and shallots if desired before serving. Drizzle on top with coconut oil. To make the soup thicker or have a more intense flavor, add a tomato paste:
½ cup dry sun-dried tomatoes, blended to a paste in a blender or clean coffee grinder

Velvety Red Lentil Soup

2 yellow onions, diced (optional)
2 cups red lentil (or any lentil desired)
6 cups water
2 cups chopped vegetables of choice (celery, red bell pepper, spinach, kale)
1 teaspoon ground pepper
Salt to taste

Put the lentils and onions in a pot and cover with 2 cups of water. Cover and simmer for 25 minutes. Meanwhile, heat the remaining 4 cups of water. Remove lentils from heat and ladle into a blender. Add 2 cups of chopped vegetables and blend with 4 cups of hot water. The blending is what makes this soup velvety smooth. Serves 4.

2 tablespoons of chickpea miso or 1 teaspoon of Herbamare (organic herb seasoning) will add a different twist to this velvety soup.

Quinoa Salad

1 cup cooked quinoa

1 tablespoon coconut oil (or other recommended oil to taste)

¼ teaspoon Transformational Salts or Himalayan salt

In a medium bowl, combine:

2 celery stalks, diced

¼ red onion, diced (optional)

2 tomatoes, diced

1 bunch cilantro, chopped

½ bunch parsley, chopped

1 tablespoon coconut oil

1 clove of garlic (optional)

1½ tablespoons lemon juice

Toss all the ingredients in the cooked quinoa and serve. Season with salt and pepper to taste. Serve warm or chilled. Serves 2.

Sumptuous Salad

3 cups amaranth cooked (cooled)

1 cup cooked beans of choice (cooled)

2 cups diced vegetables of choice (colored bell peppers, celery, spinach, cucumber, tomato)

1 cup nuts or seeds, chopped

¼ red onion (optional)

½ bunch minced herb of choice (cilantro, basil, oregano, thyme, parsley)

2 tablespoons olive oil (or other recommended oil to taste)

1 teaspoon Transformational Salts or Himalayan salt

1 clove garlic, minced

1 teaspoon lemon or lime juice

This is a great quick and easy salad and the beans are a great source of protein! This fast and healthy complete meal serves 4.

Bean Salad

4 cups green beans (cooked or raw)

2 cups black beans (cooked)

2 cups kidney beans (cooked)

2 cups chickpeas (cooked)

2 cups celery, diced

2 cups red bell pepper, diced

1 red onion, thinly sliced (optional)

⅔ cup lemon juice (option: apple cider vinegar)

⅓ cup olive oil (or other recommended oil to taste)

25 drops stevia (optional)

Salt and pepper to taste

Warm together in a large pot for 5 minutes while stirring. Remove from heat and let sit for 30 minutes to 1 hour. Serve warm or chilled. This dish will last a few days in the fridge. Serves 6 generously.

Quinoa and Black Bean Salad

1 cup cooked quinoa (see chart)

2 scallions, sliced thin

½ cup tomatoes, chopped

½ cup celery, chopped

½ cup red bell pepper, chopped

1 cup cooked black beans (see chart)

Toss in a large mixing bowl.

Dressing:

4 tablespoons olive oil

2 tablespoons lemon juice

1 small clove garlic, minced (optional)

Salt and pepper to taste

½ bunch cilantro, minced

Whisk together ingredients. Toss with quinoa and bean mixture.
Serves 4.

Spiced Kidney Beans

4 cups cooked kidney beans

2 tablespoons olive or coconut oil (or other recommended oil
to taste)

1½ onions, chopped (optional)

2 inches ginger root, peeled and minced

4 cloves fresh garlic, peeled and minced

6 large tomatoes, chopped

1–2 teaspoons Transformational Salts or Himalayan salt

½ tablespoon curry powder

½ teaspoon turmeric powder

¼ teaspoon paprika

¼ teaspoon cumin seeds, ground

½ cup sun-dried tomatoes, dry, ground in a coffee grinder or
blender (to thicken)

½ bunch fresh cilantro or parsley, chopped

½ lemon or 1 lime, juiced (optional)

Toss all ingredients in a large mixing bowl. To enhance flavor, let sit
before serving (as long as you can, up to overnight in the fridge).
Serves 2.

Dhal

2 cups water

1 cup red lentils

1 cup chopped cabbage

2 tomatoes, chopped

1 hot green chili pepper, chopped or whole (optional)

1 tablespoon olive or coconut oil

1 teaspoon cumin seeds, ground

¼ teaspoon turmeric powder

Salt and lime to taste

¼ bunch cilantro, chopped

Wash lentils and cook in the water on medium-low heat for 20 minutes.

In separate pot, heat the oil on medium heat. Then add cumin, stirring for 30 seconds. Add chili and cabbage, and sauté until softened. Set aside.

When lentils are soft, mash them and add into the cabbage pot. If the mixture is too thick, add water to reach the desired consistency. Add turmeric and salt. Remove from heat. Toss in cilantro, tomatoes, and lime juice. Serves 2.

Amaranth

1 cup amaranth

¾ cup water

1 small garlic clove, minced (optional)

1 medium onion, diced (optional)

1 tablespoon coconut or olive oil

Salt and pepper to taste

Dried chili flakes or cayenne powder to taste

In a pot, combine first four ingredients. Bring to a boil, and reduce to a simmer. Cover and steam amaranth for 25 minutes. Remove lid and stir in remaining ingredients. Serves 2.

Millet, Peas, and Indian Spice

2 cups green split peas

4 cups water

2 stalks celery, chopped

½ onion, chopped (optional)

1 teaspoon coconut oil

2 tablespoons curry powder

2 teaspoons cumin, ground

1 garlic clove, pressed (optional)

1½ teaspoon Transformational Salts or Himalayan salt

Dash of cayenne (optional)

1¼ cup millet, hulled

Bring the water, with the peas, ¼ cup onion (optional), spices, and oil to a boil and simmer 35 minutes. Stir in the millet. Cover and steam for 20 minutes. Remove from heat. Stir in ¼ cup onion (optional) and the celery. Let sit 10 minutes, covered. Toss with 2 tablespoons coconut oil and serve. Serves 4.

Quinoa and Cabbage

1 cup quinoa

¾ cup water

2 tomatoes

⅓ head coarsely chopped cabbage

Ground pepper, salt, cilantro, and dill, for seasoning to taste

Simmer quinoa and water for about 15 minutes, then add remaining ingredients and continue simmering until cabbage is soft, 5–10 minutes. Serves 2.

Millet Burgers

1 cup raw millet (1 cup raw millet yields about 3 cups cooked)

2 cups cooked lentils or any other beans

¼ cup celery, finely chopped

½ cup red pepper, finely chopped

1 cup green onions, finely chopped

1 cup parsley, finely chopped

2 garlic cloves (optional)

½ teaspoon cumin

½ teaspoon Transformational Salts or Himalayan salt

Cook 1 cup of millet and then put in the food processor with an S-blade. Process the cooked millet with the rest of the ingredients until it is well blended and sticking together. Form into 12 round balls and flatten into burgers. Place the burgers you plan to eat on a baking pan lightly coated with coconut oil. Bake at 400° for 20 minutes, turn the burgers, and bake for 10 minutes more. Freeze the remaining burgers for a later date. Top the burgers with slices of avocado and heirloom tomato. Drizzle with salt and olive oil and serve with your favorite salad.

Lentil Loaf

2 cups lentils, cooked

1 cup amaranth

1 cup red pepper, finely chopped

1 cup parsley

½ cup zucchini, shredded

½ teaspoon all spice

½ teaspoon salt

½ cup flax seed, grounded

2 garlic cloves, crushed

Cook 1 cup of amaranth and set aside to cool. Once the amaranth has cooled down, place all the ingredients in the food processor with an S-blade and processes until all is evenly mixed. In a 9-inch by 5-inch loaf pan, bake the mixture for 1 hour at 400°. Let it cool, cut, and serve with your favorite salad.

Chickpea Stew

1 cup raw chickpeas (yields 2 cups cooked)

¼ cup red pepper, chopped

¼ cup celery, chopped

¼ cup green onion, chopped

¼ cup water

½ teaspoon curry powder

½ teaspoon salt

1 garlic clove

Cook the chickpeas for the indicated amount of time. In a blender, add 1 cup of cooked chickpeas with the rest of the ingredients, including the ¼ cup of water. Blend until it becomes a cream; then pour over the remainder of the chickpeas. Heat once more and serve on top of quinoa and decorate with fresh parsley. Serves 2 or 3.

Bean and Legume Cooking

Bean (1 cup dry)	Cups water	Cook time	Cups yield
Adzuki (Aduki)	4	45–55 minutes	3
Anasazi	2½–3	45–55 minutes	2¼
Black beans	4	1 hour–1½ hours	2¼
Black-eyed peas	4	1 hour	2
Cannellini (white kidney beans)	3	45 minutes	2½
Cranberry bean	3	40–45 minutes	3
Fava beans, skins removed	4	40–50 minutes	1
Garbanzo beans (chickpeas)	3½	1–3 hours	2
Great northern beans	4	1½ hours	2⅔
Green split peas	4	45 minutes	2
Yellow split peas	6	1–1½ hours	2
Green peas, whole	3	1–2 hours	2
Kidney beans	2¼	1 hour	2¼
Lentils, brown	2	45 minutes–1 hour	2¼
Lentils, green	3	30–45 minutes	2
Lentils, red	4	20–30 minutes	2–2½
Lima beans, large	4	45 minutes–1 hour	2
Lima beans, small	4	50–60 minutes	3
Lima beans, Christmas	2½	1 hour	2
Mung beans	3	1 hour	2
Navy beans	3	45–60 minutes	2⅔
Pink beans	3	50–60 minutes	2¾
Pinto beans	4	1½ hours	2⅔

Basic Cooking Directions

Begin by washing beans and discarding any discolored or deformed ones. Check for small rocks and twigs and remove.

Beans cook quicker if soaked overnight for 8 hours, covered a couple inches over with water. Strain the soak water off before cooking.

Sometimes beans will take longer to cook. This may be due to the use of hard water, or the beans may have been dried for a longer period of time. If this is the case, soaking them for 24 hours and changing the water 2 or 3 times during the soaking period speeds up the cooking.

Soaking also aids in breaking down the complex sugars (oligosaccharides), which challenge the digestive system and cause gas.

Some herbs that help in the digestion of beans can be added during cooking. For example, use bay leaves, cumin, winter or summer savory, or fresh epazote (available in Hispanic markets). Many people from India maintain the tradition of chewing on dried fennel seeds or drinking a cup of fennel tea at the end of a legume meal to aid the digestion.

As a general rule of thumb, 1 cup of dried beans will yield about 2½ to 3 cups of cooked beans.

Quick-Soak Method for Dried Beans

When time is limited, you can wash and pick beans and put them in a stock pot with water, covering by 3 inches. Bring to a boil and boil for 10 minutes. Then cover and allow to soak for 1 hour. Discard the soak water, add fresh water, and cook until tender.

Cooking Fresh Beans

Two methods are used: boiling and steaming. To boil the beans, drop the shelled beans into boiling water. Cover and boil gently for 5–10 minutes. Flavor while cooking, with onion, garlic, herbs of your choice, and a dash of salt added to the water.

To steam the beans, put around an inch of water in the bottom of a pot, and put beans into a steamer basket that fits in the pot. Cover the pot, and steam the beans over boiling water for 5–10 minutes.

Fava Beans

These beans require a bit of different handling before cooking. They are usually peeled after cooking, as leaving the skins on will give the beans a bitter flavor. To peel, use a paring knife and peel one end, then squeeze the opposite end and the bean will slip out easily.

These are general guidelines. Some varieties of grains and beans will require different cooking times than those specified in the chart. This will depend on the variety of the bean. The variation will only be a matter of a few minutes. If you are cooking packaged beans with directions, always follow the recommendations on the package for the variety you have.

Those new to natural foods can choose to discover how easy it is to prepare good, wholesome meals that rely on whole grains and legumes as the center of their meals. Here is a useful website to begin your discovery: www.vegparadise.com/charts.html.

Summarizing Thoughts

People suffer from preventable evils, and the people perish for lack of knowledge.

    "The Golden Verses" in *Fragmenta Philosophorum Groecorum*

It is important to appreciate this program as a logical extension of past research that extends back to the 1920s, when Dr. Max Gerson healed Dr. Albert Schweitzer from Type-2 diabetes with a live-food diet. Over a period of 40 years, I have seen a variety of people heal diabetes naturally with live foods and fasting. All I have done differently with the Dr. Cousens's Diabetes Recovery Program—A Holistic Approach is to take the next logical and common-sense step. As Ralph Waldo Emerson said, "Society is always taken by surprise by any new example of common sense." The common sense, in this case, is that I have utilized the power of 100 percent live foods and green juice fasting to create a rapid genetic and epigenetic upgrade. I have found that by taking the next evolutionary step, supported by clinical experience and employing a diet that is based on those principles, clients move away from a phenotypic expression of diabetes to a phenotypic expression of health and well-being. I have done the obvious and made a common-sense move by making the green juice fast and 25–45 percent carbohydrate, live-food plant-source diet the most powerful approach to healing diabetes naturally. Consistently with this approach, within one to four days, many clients are off all medications. In one week the fasting blood sugar (FBS) number for many Type-2 diabetics comes into normal range, and in three weeks, the FBS is normal for 24–61 percent of the Type-2 diabetics.

Depending on the degree of complications, 70 percent of the Type-2 diabetics' FBS may take longer to come into a nondiabetic range, but the end result is often a normal fasting blood glucose level. As with all human issues of healing, one is not able to issue a 100 percent guarantee, but my clinical experience at this point has been that this is the case for the majority of our Type-2 non-insulin-dependent diabetes mellitus (NIDDM) clients within three weeks, if they are fully attentive to the program. In this context, most people also see their blood chemistry, cholesterol, and C-reactive protein return to normal during this time.

Notes

1. Nelson, M D, Prabhakar, P, Kondragunta, V, Kornman, K S, Gardner, C. "Genetic phenotypes predict weight loss success: The right diet does matter." Presented at the American Heart Association's Joint Conference—50th Cardiovascular Disease Epidemiology and Prevention and Nutrition, Physical Activity and Metabolism—2010, San Francisco, CA (March 25, 2010). Nelson and Gardner represent Stanford University; all others represent Interleukin Genetics, Inc.

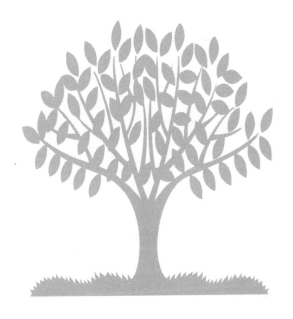

More Information on
Dr. Cousens's Programs

Dr. Cousens's Diabetes Recovery Program—A Holistic Approach is renowned throughout the world for its high success rate and impeccable design. Participants often find themselves completely off their insulin and other medications by the end of the 3-week program and, if not, have nearly always significantly reduced their doses. Blood sugar rates become lower and much steadier as guests immerse themselves in the life-promoting foods and lifestyle advocated at our center. Based on 40 years of experience of treating diabetes naturally, this program is masterfully designed for the comprehensive healing of chronic diabetes degenerative syndrome (CDDS), in which high blood sugar is just a symptom. Presently 61 percent of Type-2 non-insulin-dependent diabetes mellitus (NIDDM) participants and 24 percent of Type-2 insulin-dependent diabetes mellitus (IDDM) participants are healed within 21 days. In Type-1 diabetes, insulin levels are reduced by an average of 70 percent, with 21 percent cured.

Other Tree of Life programs include the following:

- Holistic Vegan Vacations
- Whole Person Health Assessments
- 21-Day Transformation Programs
- Spiritual Fasting Retreats
- 10-, 17-, and 24-Day Juice Fast Detoxification Programs
- Zero Point Programs
- Conscious Eating Courses
- Expanding Culinary Joy Courses
- Dr. Cousens's Spiritual Nutrition Masters Degree Program
- Sustainable Veganic Farming Masters Degree Program

For more information on Dr. Cousens's Diabetes Recovery Program—A Holistic Approach and other Tree of Life transformative programs, please visit DrCousens.com.

It is also a program that, on a metacommunication level, ultimately makes the point that one has to love oneself enough to want to heal oneself. When one follows this diet and way of life, it is easier to love oneself and want to maintain one's self-healing.

GLOSSARY

ACE inhibitor—Type of drug used to lower blood pressure. It may also help prevent or slow the progression of kidney disease in people with diabetes.

acute—Happening for a limited period of time and/or coming on abruptly.

adrenal glands—Two organs sitting on top of the kidneys that make and release hormones such as adrenaline (epinephrine).

albuminuria—Having an excess amount of protein called albumin in the urine. Albuminuria may indicate kidney disease.

aldose reductase inhibitor—A class of drugs under investigation as a way to prevent eye and nerve damage in people with diabetes.

alpha cell—A type of cell in the pancreas that makes and releases the hormone glucagon.

angiopathy—A disease of the blood vessels (arteries, veins, and capillaries) that occurs when someone has diabetes for a long time.

antigens—Substances that cause an immune response in the body. The body perceives the antigens to be harmful and thus produces antibodies to attack and destroy the antigens.

arteriosclerosis—A group of diseases in which the artery walls get thick and hard, slowing blood flow.

artery—A large blood vessel that carries blood from the heart to other parts of the body.

atherosclerosis—One of many arteriosclerosis diseases in which fat builds up in the large and medium-size arteries.

autoimmune process—A process by which the body's immune system attacks and destroys body tissue that it mistakes for foreign matter.

beta cells—Cells that make the hormone insulin, which controls blood glucose levels. Beta cells are found in areas of the pancreas called the Islets of Langerhans.

bladder—A hollow organ that urine drains into from the kidneys. From the bladder, urine leaves the body.

blood glucose—The main sugar that the body makes from the food we eat. Glucose is carried through the bloodstream to provide energy to all the body's living cells.

blood glucose monitor—A machine that helps measure the amount of glucose in the blood.

blood pressure—The force of the blood against the artery walls. Two levels of blood pressure are measured: the highest, or systolic, occurs when the heart pumps blood into the blood vessels, and the lowest, or diastolic, occurs when the heart rests.

blood sugar—See blood glucose.

blood urea nitrogen (BUN)—Waste product produced by the kidneys. Raised BUN levels in the blood may indicate early kidney damage.

callus—Thick, hardened area of the skin, generally on the foot, caused by friction or pressure. Calluses can lead to other problems, including serious infection and even gangrene.

capillary—The smallest blood vessel in the body.

capsaicin—A colorless irritant that gives hot peppers their hotness. Used for an ointment made from chili peppers to relieve the pain of peripheral neuropathy.

carbohydrate—One of three main groups of foods in the diet that provide calories and energy. (Protein and fat are the others.) Carbohydrates are mainly sugars (simple carbohydrates) and starches (complex carbohydrates, found in whole grains and beans) that the body breaks down into glucose.

cataract—Clouding of the lens of the eye.

CDDS—Chronic diabetes degenerative syndrome. A causative theory of diabetes that includes FBS patterns and postprandial spike pathologies.

cholesterol—A substance similar to fat that is found in the blood, muscles, liver, brain, and other body tissues. The body produces and needs some cholesterol for hormone synthesis.

chronic—Lasting a long time. Diabetes is an example of a chronic disease.

corn—A thickening of the skin of the feet or hands, usually caused by pressure against the skin.

creatinine—A chemical in the blood that is eliminated through urine. A test of the amount of creatinine in the blood and/or urine indicates if the kidneys are working properly.

diabetes mellitus—A chronic degenerative aging disease secondary to a toxic genetic and epigenetic downgrade, which may involve a disruption in leptin and insulin signaling, leptin and insulin resistance, and chronic parainflammation.

diabetes pills—Pills or capsules that are taken by mouth to help lower the blood glucose level. These pills may work for people whose bodies are still making insulin. Some are associated with up to 250 percent more heart disease and death.

diabetic eye disease—A disease of the small blood vessels of the retina of the eye in people with diabetes. In this disease, the vessels swell and leak liquid into the retina, blurring the vision and sometimes leading to blindness.

diabetic ketoacidosis—High blood glucose with the presence of acidity ketones in the urine and bloodstream, often caused by taking too little insulin or during illness. It can be life threatening.

diabetic kidney disease—Damage to the cells or blood vessels of the kidney. Often fatal five years after beginning dialysis.

diabetic nerve damage—Damage and pain to the nerves of a person with diabetes. Nerve damage may affect the feet and hands, as well as major organs.

dialysis—A method for removing waste such as urea from the blood when the kidneys can no longer do the job. There are two types of dialysis: hemodialysis and peritoneal.

diphtheria—An acute, contagious disease that causes fever and problems for the heart and nervous system.

diuretic—A drug that increases the flow of urine to help eliminate extra fluid from the body.

EKG—A test that measures the heart's action. Also called an electrocardiogram.

endocrine glands—Glands that release hormones into the bloodstream and affect metabolism.

end-stage renal disease (ESRD)—The final phase of kidney disease.

epinephrine—A hormone, also called adrenaline, secreted by the adrenal glands and helping the liver release glucose. The principal blood-pressure-raising hormone. Used medicinally as a heart stimulant and muscle relaxant in bronchial asthma.

fasting blood sugar (FBS)—The blood sugar level taken first thing in the morning before eating or drinking.

fats—One of the three main classes of foods and a source of energy in the body. (Protein and carbohydrates are the other two.)

fiber—Substance in food plants that helps the digestive process, lowers cholesterol, and helps control blood glucose levels.

flu—An infection caused by the influenza virus. A contagious viral illness that strikes quickly and severely. Signs include high fever, chills, body aches, runny nose, sore throat, and headache.

gangrene—Death or pervasive decay of body tissue, usually caused by loss of blood flow.

gastroparesis—A form of nerve damage that affects the stomach.

gestational diabetes—A type of diabetes that can occur in pregnant women who have not been known to have diabetes before. Although gestational diabetes usually subsides after pregnancy, many women who have had gestational diabetes develop Type-2 diabetes later in life.

gingivitis—A swelling and soreness of the gums that, without treatment, can cause serious gum problems and disease.

glaucoma—An eye disease characterized by increased pressure in the eye.

glomeruli—Tiny blood vessels in the kidneys where the blood is filtered and waste products are eliminated.

glucagon—A hormone that raises the blood glucose level. When someone with diabetes has a very low blood glucose level, a glucagon injection can help raise the blood glucose quickly.

glucose—A sugar in our blood and a source of energy for our bodies.

glucose tolerance test—A test that shows how well the body deals with glucose in the blood over time; used to see if a person has diabetes. A first blood sample is taken in the morning before the person has eaten; then the person drinks a liquid that has glucose in it. After one hour, a second blood sample is taken and then, one hour later, a third.

glycogen—A substance composed of sugars that is stored in the liver and muscles and releases glucose into the blood when needed by cells.

glycosylated hemoglobin test—A blood test that measures a person's average glycosylated hemoglobin in the red blood cell in the three-month period before the test.

glycosylation—The process in which glucose binds to, chemically alters, and damages proteins. These altered proteins are called advanced glycation end products (AGEs). Over time, AGE proteins may accumulate in the cells and interfere with normal cell functioning. Glycosylation is accelerated in people with diabetes, and complications with eyes, kidneys, and the circulatory system are associated with AGE proteins.

HDL (high-density lipoprotein)—A combined protein and fatlike substance that lowers cholesterol and usually passes freely through the arteries. Sometimes called "good cholesterol."

heart attack—Damage to the heart muscle caused when the blood vessels supplying the muscle are blocked, such as when the blood vessels are clogged with fats (a condition sometimes called hardening of the arteries).

hemodialysis—A mechanical way to remove waste products from the blood. See also dialysis.

hemoglobin (Hgb)—The substance in red blood cells that carries oxygen to the body's cells.

HgbA1C—A test that sums up how much glucose is nonenzymatically bound to the hemoglobin during the past three months.

high blood glucose—A condition that occurs in people with insulin and/or leptin resistance, prediabetes, and diabetes when their blood glucose levels are too high. Symptoms include having to urinate often, being very thirsty, losing weight, and a general accelerated aging process.

high blood pressure—A condition where the blood circulates through the arteries with too much force on the artery walls. High blood pressure tires the heart, harms the arteries, and increases the risk of heart attack, stroke, and kidney problems.

hormone—A chemical that special cells in the body release to help other cells work. For example, insulin is a hormone made in the pancreas to help the body use glucose as energy.

human insulin—Laboratory-made insulins that are similar to insulin produced by the human body.

hyperesthesia—One of different changes in nerve function in extremities, expressed with numbness and tingling.

hyperglycemia—See high blood glucose.

hypertension—See high blood pressure.

hypoglycemia—Also called low blood glucose. A condition that may be independent of diabetes in which there is an imbalance in the endocrine system in which the blood sugar drops rapidly or too low. The problem is usually with pancreatic, adrenal, thyroid, pituitary/pineal, or ovarian/testicular imbalances.

immunization—Sometimes called vaccination; a shot or injection that theoretically protects a person from getting an illness by making the person "immune" to it. Evidence does not necessarily support the theory.

impaired glucose tolerance (IGT)—Blood glucose levels that are higher than normal but not so high as to be considered diabetes.

implantable insulin pump—A small pump placed inside the body to deliver insulin on demand from a handheld programmer.

impotence—A condition where the penis does not become or stay hard enough for sex. Some men who have had diabetes a long time become impotent if their nerves or blood vessels have become damaged.

influenza—See flu.

inject—To force a liquid into the body with a needle and syringe.

insulin—A hormone that helps the body use blood glucose for energy. The beta cells of the pancreas make insulin. When people with diabetes can't make enough insulin, they may have to inject it from another source.

insulin-dependent diabetes mellitus (IDDM)—See Type-1 diabetes.

insulin pump—A beeper-sized device that delivers a continuous supply of insulin into the body.

insulin reaction—A response to a too-low level of glucose in the blood; also called hypoglycemia.

insulin receptors—Sites on the outer part of a cell that allow the cell to join with insulin.

insulin resistance—Occurs when the different functions of the insulin hormone are blocked. It may force the pancreas to overproduce up to four times the amount of insulin to compensate. May result in inflammation, scarring, and destruction of the beta cells of the pancreas from exhaustion and burn-out.

intensive therapy—A method of treatment for Type-1 diabetes in which the goal is to keep the blood glucose levels as close to normal as possible. Also recommended for Type-2 diabetes.

ketoacidosis—See diabetic ketoacidosis.

ketones—Fat breakdown products that the brain, heart, and some other tissues of the body may use for energy.

ketosis—A condition when ketone bodies build up in body tissues and fluids. Ketosis can lead to ketoacidosis.

kidney—One of the twin organs found in the lower part of the back. The kidneys purify the blood of all waste and harmful material. They also control the level of some helpful chemical substances in the blood.

kidney disease—Also called nephropathy, kidney disease can be any one of several chronic conditions that are caused by damage to the cells of the kidney.

LDL (low-density lipoprotein)—A combined protein and fatlike substance. Rich in cholesterol, it tends to stick to the walls in the arteries. Sometimes called "bad cholesterol."

lente insulin—An intermediate-acting insulin.

low blood glucose—A condition that occurs in people with diabetes when their blood glucose levels are too low from excess insulin or oral hypoglycemics and in nondiabetics. Symptoms include feeling anxious or confused, feeling numb in the arms and hands, and shaking or feeling dizzy.

meal plan—A guide to help people get the proper amount of calories, carbohydrates, proteins, and fats in their diet.

microalbumin—A protein found in blood plasma and urine. The presence of microalbumin in the urine can be a sign of kidney disease.

nephropathy—See diabetic kidney disease.

neuropathy—See diabetic nerve damage.

Neutral protamine hagedorn (NPH) insulin—An intermediate-acting insulin

non-insulin-dependent diabetes mellitus (NIDDM)—See Type-2 diabetes.

obesity—Excessive accumulation and storage of fat in the body. The degree of overweight when people have 20 percent or more extra body fat for their age, height, sex, and bone structure.

oral glucose tolerance test (OGTT)—A test to see if a person has diabetes. See also glucose tolerance test.

pancreas—Organ in the body that makes insulin so that the body can use glucose for energy. The pancreas also makes enzymes that help the body digest food.

paresthesia—One of different changes in nerve function in extremities, expressed with numbness and tingling.

periodontitis—Gum disease in which the gums shrink away from the teeth. Without treatment, it can lead to tooth loss.

peripheral neuropathy—Nerve damage associated with diabetes that usually affects the feet and legs.

peritoneal dialysis—A mechanical way to clean the blood of people with kidney disease.

plaque—A film of mucus that traps bacteria on the surface of the teeth. Plaque can be removed with daily brushing and flossing of teeth.

polydipsia—Great thirst that lasts for long periods of time.

polyphagia—Great hunger.

polyunsaturated fats—Fat that comes from vegetables.

polyuria—Excessive, frequent urination.

protein—One of the three main classes of food. (Fats and carbohydrates are the other two.) Proteins are found in many foods, including greens, legumes, and algae. Leafy greens are 30 percent protein.

proteinuria—Presence of too much protein in the urine; may signal kidney disease.

pumice stone—A special foot care tool used to gently file calluses as instructed by one's health care team.

regular insulin—A fast-acting insulin.

retina—Center part of the back lining of the eye that senses light.

retinopathy—See diabetic eye disease.

risk factors—Traits that make it more likely that a person will get an illness. For example, a risk factor for developing Type-2 diabetes is having a family history of diabetes.

saturated fat—Fat that comes from animals.

secondary diabetes—Diabetes that develops because of another disease or because of taking certain drugs of chemicals.

self-monitoring blood glucose—A way for people with diabetes to find out how much glucose is in their blood. A drop of blood from the fingertip is placed on a special coated strip of paper that "reads" (often through an electronic meter) the amount of glucose in the blood.

sorbitol—A sugar alcohol produced by the body, which, if levels get too high, may cause damage to the eyes and nerves.

stroke—Damage to a part of the brain that happens when the blood vessels supplying that part are blocked, such as when the blood vessels are clogged with fats (a condition sometimes called hardening of the arteries).

sucrose—Table sugar; a form of sugar the body must break down into a simpler form before the blood can use it.

support group—A group of people who share a similar problem or concern. The people in the group help one another by sharing experiences, knowledge, and information.

syringe—Device used to inject medications or other liquids into the body tissues. An insulin syringe has a hollow plastic or glass tube with a plunger inside. The plunger forces the insulin through the needle into the body.

transcutaneous electric nerve stimulation (TENS)—A treatment for painful neuropathy.

triglyceride—A type of blood fat.

Type-1 diabetes—An auto-immune condition in which the pancreas makes so little insulin that the body can't use blood glucose as energy. Type-1 diabetes most often occurs in people younger than age 30 and must be controlled with daily insulin injections.

Type-2 diabetes—A condition in which the body either makes too little insulin or can't use the insulin it makes to use blood glucose as energy. Type-2 diabetes has typically occurred in people older than age 40, but increasingly appears in children today and can often be controlled through meal plans and physical activity plans. Some people with Type-2 diabetes have to take diabetes pills or insulin.

U-100—A unit of insulin, meaning 100 units of insulin per milliliter or cubic centimeter of solution.

ulcer—A break or deep sore in the skin. Germs can enter an ulcer so that it may be hard to heal.

ultralente insulin—A long-acting insulin.

urea—One of the chief waste products of the body. When the body breaks down food, it uses what it needs and throws the rest away as waste. The kidneys flush the waste from the body in the form of urea, which is in the urine.

urine testing—A test of urine to see if it contains glucose and ketones.

vaccination—A shot given to theoretically protect against a disease. Vaccinations have been associated with a 147 percent increase in Type-1 diabetes.

vitrectomy—An operation to remove the blood that sometimes collects at the back of the eyes when a person has eye disease.

yeast infection—A vaginal, blood, sinus, or colon infection that is usually caused by a fungus. Women who have this infection may feel itching, burning when urinating, and pain, and some women have a vaginal discharge. Yeast infections occur more frequently in women and men with diabetes because of the high blood glucose.

INDEX

Other Books by Gabriel Cousens, MD

Conscious Eating

Depression-Free for Life

Tachyon Energy (with David Wagner)

Rainbow Green Live-Food Cuisine

Spiritual Nutrition: Six Foundations
for Spiritual Life and the Awakening of Kundalini

Creating Peace by Being Peace

There Is a Cure for Diabetes

Torah as a Guide to Enlightenment

ABOUT THE AUTHOR

Gabriel Cousens, MD, MD (Homeopathy), DD, Diplomate American
Board of Holistic Medicine, Diplomate in Ayurveda, a holistic medical doctor with 40 years of success
in healing diabetes naturally, is the
founder and director of the Tree
of Life Foundation and Tree of
Life Rejuvenation Center U.S. in
Patagonia, Arizona. He is also an
acknowledged spiritual teacher,
the leading Essene teacher in the
United States and the world, as well
as an ordained rabbi. He is a gradu-
ate of Amherst College, where he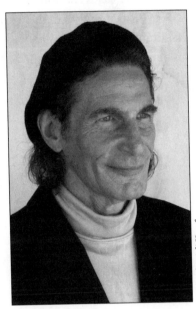

Photo by Adi Yosef

published his first scientific paper in the *Journal of Biochemical and
Physics Acta* and was captain of an undefeated football team. He was
inducted into the National Football Hall of Fame as a scholar-athlete.
Cousens received his MD from Columbia Medical School in 1969 and
completed his psychiatric residency in 1973.

He is a best-selling author and the creator of Dr. Cousens's Diabetes
Recovery Program—A Holistic Approach. Dr. Cousens uses the modal-
ities of diet, nutrition, naturopathy, Ayurveda, Chinese medicine, and
homeopathy blended with spiritual awareness in the healing of body,
mind, and spirit. He facilitates spiritual, nutritional, and lifestyle support seminars and has given seminars on nutrition through the United
States, Canada, Mexico, Nicaragua, Costa Rico, Panama, Peru, Argentina, Uruguay, Ecuador, Ethiopia, Cameroon, New Guinea, Turkey,
Greece, Morocco, Lebanon, Egypt, Israel, Ghana, Nigeria, South Africa,
Australia, New Zealand, England, Italy, Spain, France, Amsterdam,

Denmark, Sweden, Switzerland, Czech Republic, Germany, Poland, Croatia, India, Singapore, Bali, Thailand, and Hong Kong. Through his books, media, and body-mind-spirit transformative programs at the Tree of Life Rejuvenation Center, Dr. Cousens is recognized as a leading medical authority in the world on live-food nutrition, diabetes, and healing diabetes naturally. His Tree of Life Rejuvenation Center U.S. in Patagonia, Arizona, is the only location where he facilitates the full Dr. Cousens's Diabetes Recovery Program—A Holistic Approach. He is happily married, a father of two, and a grandfather of three.

AUTHOR'S NOTE

Please note: Nothing in this book is intended to constitute medical advice or treatment. For development of an individualized diet or the use of fasting cycles, it is advised that any person first consult his or her holistic physician. It is important that he or she remain under the doctor's supervision throughout any major shift in diet or while fasting. I consider it dangerous and do not recommend doing this on your own if you are on insulin or have Type-1 diabetes. I strongly recommend using these teachings under medical supervision or attending our 21-Day Dr. Cousens's Diabetes Recovery Program—A Holistic Approach at Dr. Cousens's Tree of Life Rejuvenation Center U.S. in Patagonia, Arizona.

We have referred to a variety of studies, a few of which have involved animals. In no way does this mean that we endorse the use of animal studies for scientific purposes, and when data were available to illustrate points without using these studies, we have done so. Animal studies, particularly studies in which the animals have been sacrificed, interfere with the peace between the animal world and the human world.